Mental Health in Historical Perspective

Covering all historical periods and geographical contexts, the series explores how mental illness has been understood, experienced, diagnosed, treated and contested. It will publish works that engage actively with contemporary debates related to mental health and, as such, will be of interest not only to historians, but also mental health professionals, patients and policy makers. With its focus on mental health, rather than just psychiatry, the series will endeavour to provide more patient-centred histories. Although this has long been an aim of health historians, it has not been realised, and this series aims to change that.

The scope of the series is kept as broad as possible to attract good quality proposals about all aspects of the history of mental health from all periods. The series emphasises interdisciplinary approaches to the field of study, and encourages short titles, longer works, collections, and titles which stretch the boundaries of academic publishing in new ways.

More information about this series at
https://link.springer.com/bookseries/14806

Ana Antić

Non-Aligned Psychiatry in the Cold War

Revolution, Emancipation and Re-Imagining the Human Psyche

palgrave
macmillan

Ana Antić
Department of History
University of Copenhagen
Copenhagen, Denmark

ISSN 2634-6036 ISSN 2634-6044 (electronic)
Mental Health in Historical Perspective
ISBN 978-3-030-89448-1 ISBN 978-3-030-89449-8 (eBook)
https://doi.org/10.1007/978-3-030-89449-8

Cover image: courtesy of the Yugoslav Cinematheque

This Palgrave Macmillan imprint is published by the registered company Springer Nature Switzerland AG
The registered company address is: Gewerbestrasse 11, 6330 Cham, Switzerland

Acknowledgments

The idea for this book started many years ago, when I was a postdoctoral fellow in the history department at Birkbeck, University of London, where I met a wonderful group of colleagues and friends. Dora Vargha, Johanna Conterio, David Brydan, Marcie Holmes, Louise Hyde, Joanna Bourke have been a wonderful support network and provided kind and constructive criticism, brainstorming sessions and much more as I was trying to make sense of my new archival material. Special thanks go to Daniel Pick, whose unwavering support and friendship have been exceptionally important. My understanding of the field has benefited enormously from our many conversations about psychoanalysis, the Cold War and European history, and from his and Jacqueline Rose's delightful and challenging History and Psychoanalysis reading group.

At the University of Exeter, a lot of colleagues were extremely patient and generous, offering to read my drafts and discuss my semi-developed arguments and ideas. Martin Thomas, James Mark, Stacey Hynd, Nandini Chatterjee and many others in the Centre for Global and Imperial History worked hard to ensure a dynamic research culture, organising a series of seminars and informal discussions which shaped my thinking, and challenged me to reframe my own contributions to the field of global history. This was also a great place to work in medical humanities, and I'm very grateful to Rebecca Williams, Kate Fisher and the Centre for Medical history for their kindness and support.

In the course of researching the book, I was very lucky to get to know Mr. Tomislav Krsmanovic, whose commitment to documenting psychiatric abuses and state breaches of human rights has been admirable, and who generously shared with me his comprehensive personal archive. Without it, and without our insightful and moving conversations, this book would not be the same, and he has my deepest gratitude.

In the recent years, I moved away from East European history into the field of the history of global and transcultural psychiatry, and this book partly reflects that transition. As I was formulating my own research path in the historiography of global psychiatry and decolonisation, and trying to understand Eastern Europe's place in it, the exceptional research and support of many colleagues in this growing field have been incredibly valuable. Thanks are due to Liz Lunbeck, Jonathan Sadowsky, Nancy Hunt, Katie Kilroy-Marac, Dagmar Herzog, Ursula Read, Matthew Heaton, Marco Ramos, Omnia El Shakry, Romain Tiquet, to name just a few, whose thoughtful and nuanced contributions enriched my own analysis and interpretations in immeasurable ways.

My new colleagues at the University of Copenhagen deserve a special mention. I am particularly grateful to Morten Heiberg and Tina for their incredible generosity and faith in my research, and for welcoming me so warmly. Sacra Rosello, Alex Knopf, Kristoff Kerl, Sofie Steinberger and Maria Damkjær became an instant workplace family, who continue to inspire me with their brave and rigorous research, and with whom I'm planning many future projects. It has been delightful to work with Lamia Moghnieh, a superb medical anthropologist and friend, on our new project 'Decolonising Madness', and to get her kind and insightful feedback on my work.

As always, my greatest gratitude goes to my family—to my mother, Marica Antic, without whose unconditional support and faith in me nothing would ever be possible, and to my husband, Carl Bjerstrom, who remains my kindest, most generous and affectionate brainstorming partner. Their love has been vital to this (and every other) project in more ways than I could describe, and this book is dedicated to them.

Contents

CHAPTER 1

Introduction

This book tells an intricate story of socialist Yugoslavia's 'psy' disciplines—a complex, dynamic and internally contradictory professional field, whose participation in multiple transnational and global networks shaped its development, clinical character and political-ideological orientation in a genuinely unique manner. Yugoslavia's 'psy' professions certainly availed themselves of the country's peculiar geopolitical position, and the relative liberalism of its socialist path, and grew into an exceptionally influential and socially and politically engaged clinical and intellectual field. Because of that, this book offers more than a mere narrative of the disciplines' historical development. In the first instance, it argues that psychiatry, psychoanalysis and psychotherapy serve as a perfect lens through which Yugoslavia's multiple globalisations as well as resultant internal political contradictions can be understood and re-evaluated, as they combined punitive and repressive practices with a serious and focused interest in personal emancipation and struggle against social and political authoritarianism. But histories of psychiatry in this small but vital socialist country also opens up broader European and global perspectives, offering a unique insight into the nature of professional, cultural and political relations across the Iron Curtain. The coming chapters thus explore an important case study in transnational cooperation in order re-assess the history of exchange and collaboration across ideological boundaries in

A. Antić, *Non-Aligned Psychiatry in the Cold War*, Mental Health in Historical Perspective, https://doi.org/10.1007/978-3-030-89449-8_1

Cold War Europe, describing how the human mind and its potentials and pathologies were re-imagined and debated in this complex and tense political context. Furthermore, the book contributes to the growing literature on socialist globalisation and exchanges between the Second and Third Worlds, emphasising the role and participation of Eastern Europe and its 'psy' experts in debates about decolonisation, political and psychiatric universalism, and the 'global psyche'. Finally, it demonstrates that Yugoslav socialist 'psy' sciences were not 'hostages of the state' nor producing knowledge and expertise on the communist state's demand. They were themselves constitutive of the socialist experience and ideology, took an active part in broader discussions of socialism's shortcomings and achievements, and provided patients, artists and social scientists with the language and conceptual equipment for working out what the Yugoslav version of Marxism might mean in different social and cultural spheres.

In the recent years, the field of the history and sociology of communist psychiatry has seen significant growth, and scholars have successfully begun to revise the image of communist psychiatry as static, monolithic and entirely subordinated to the whims of dictatorial political regimes.[1] Indeed, in the Eastern bloc the 'psy' disciplines eventually developed in a variety of different directions. While socialist governments did consider certain schools of thought or therapeutic frameworks politically less appropriate, following the 1950s Eastern Europe's—including Soviet—'psy' sciences were characterised by a notable diversity of clinical approaches and practices.[2] Moreover, communist psychiatric professionals

[1] Sarah Marks and Mattjew Savelli, eds, *Psychiatry in Communist Europe*, London: Palgrave Macmillan, 2015; Greg Eghigian, 'Was There a Communist Psychiatry? Politics and East German Psychiatric Care, 1945–1989', *Harvard Review of Psychiatry*, 2002, 10:6, 364–368; Benjamin Zajicek, *Scientific Psychiatry in Stalin's Soviet Union: The Politics of Modern Medicine and the Struggle to Define 'Pavlovian' Psychiatry, 1939–1953*, PhD dissertation, University of Chicago, 2009; Christine Leuenberger, 'Socialist Psychotherapy and Its Dissidents', *Journal of the History of the Behavioural Sciences*, 2001, 37:3; Hannah Proctor, *Psychologies in Revolution: Alexander Luria's 'Romantic Science' and Soviet Social History*, Basingstoke: Palgrave Macmillan, 2021.

[2] R. J. Decarvalho and Ivo Cermak, 'History of Humanistic Psychology in Czechoslovakia', *Journal of Humanistic Psychology*, 1997, 37:1, 110–130; S. Hoskovcová, J. Hoskovec, A. Plháková, M. Sebek, J. Svancara, and D. Voboril, 'Historiography of Czech Psychology', *History of Psychology*, 2010, 13:3, 309–334; B. Buda, T. Tomcsanyi, J. Harmatta, R. Csaky-Pallavicini and G. Paneth, 'Psychotherapy in Hungary During the Socialist Era and the Socialist Dictatorship', *European Journal of Mental Health*, 2009, 4:1, 67–99; Alberto Angelini, 'History of the Unconscious in Soviet Russia: From Its

and practitioners were not isolated from the rest of the world: they remained relatively open to Western influences, and maintained relationships with colleagues from outside the socialist bloc.[3]

In their edited volume on psychiatry in socialist Eastern Europe, Sarah Marks and Matthew Savelli draw attention to this complex and dynamic nature of the 'psy' disciplines across the region, and to their multifaceted political outlook and purposes.[4] This book proceeds in a similar vein, and presents Yugoslav psychiatry, psychotherapy and psychoanalysis as vigorous, thoroughly internationalised and often professionally progressive.[5] In her ground-breaking book on Czechoslovak socialist sexology, Liskova argues that sexology experts were far from enslaved by the authoritarian state, and that their profession was robust and influential enough to directly affect the state's politics and management of sexuality and family life, while their concepts and ideas were reflected in social and individual behaviour more generally. In the Yugoslav case, from the 1950s on psychiatric, psychotherapeutic and psychoanalytic concepts and language spread beyond the consulting room, and informed a variety of political and cultural discourses. Just like in the case of Czechoslovak sexologists, Yugoslav 'psy' experts' relationship to power was complex and varied—it was, at different times, tactical, loyal, critical, subordinated—but this was by no means a marginalised, irrelevant or politically subjugated profession. Until the devastating wars of Yugoslav succession, Yugoslav 'psy' disciplines were not only exceptionally quick to adopt Western theories and therapeutic techniques; they were genuinely experimental and innovative in a broader European and global context, and pioneered both clinical practices and interpretive frameworks.

However, recent scholarship on communist psychiatry has also tended to emphasise its similarity with Western mental health sciences, rightly

Origins to the Fall of the Soviet Union', *International Journal of Psychoanalysis*, 2008, 89:2, 369–388.

[3] Greg Eghigian, 'Care and Control in a Communist State: The Place of Politics in East German Psychiatry', in Marijke Gijswijt-Hofstra et al., ed., *Psychiatric Cultures Compared: Psychiatry and Mental Health Care in the Twen-tieth Century*, Amsterdam: Amsterdam University Press, 2005, 183–199.

[4] Savelli and Marks, *Psychiatry in Communist Europe*.

[5] Here, the argument is not dissimilar from Katerina Liskova's analysis of sexologists in socialist Czechoslovakia: Katerina Liskova, *Sexual Liberation, Socialist Style*, Cambridge: Cambridge University Press, 2018.

arguing against the othering and exoticisation of East European psychiatric professionals and their activities. But in their efforts to demonstrate that there were no fundamental clinical or intellectual differences between East and West European psychiatry—that the former was not merely an extended repressive arm of the East European authoritarian regimes but a legitimate medical field—some scholars have effectively negated that socialist 'psy' disciplines had anything particularly socialist about them.[6] In this regard, my argument in this book differs significantly. Yugoslav psychiatry, even though Westernised and internationalised to an exceptionally large extent, was fundamentally shaped by its direct engagement with the broader Marxist ideological context. Its political involvement was consistent and extremely important throughout the period but it could not be reduced to manipulation or subordination by the government and its repressive apparatus. The 'psy' disciplines in Yugoslavia earnestly contributed to some of the core political and social debates of the time, and many practitioners reflected very carefully on their own profession's role within the broader framework of socialist revolution and humanist Marxism.

Communist psychiatry, therefore, should be viewed as a distinct intellectual field, marked by unique professional characteristics and developments which went beyond both coercion and simple Westernisation. In that sense, the history of psychiatry and psychoanalysis in socialist Yugoslavia encapsulates very well the regime's political and intellectual complexities. While psychoanalysis became an important site for formulating social and political critique, and for interrogating shortcomings in Yugoslavia's efforts to implement the theory of workers' self-management, both psychoanalysis and psychiatric institutions could be mobilised for devising extremely repressive and violent policies towards political dissidents. Neither a mere political tool nor a replica of Western psychiatric and psychotherapeutic practices, Yugoslav 'psy' disciplines developed into a unique and truly original professional, clinical and intellectual field in Cold War Europe.

Recent historical and anthropological research has demonstrated the broader social, political and intellectual significance of psychoanalysis in the second half of the twentieth century. Dagmar Herzog, Marco Ramos,

[6] Matthew Savelli, 'Beyond Ideological Platitudes: Socialism and Psychiatry in Eastern Europe', *Palgrave Communications*, 2018, 4:45. https://doi.org/10.1057/s41599-018-0100-1.

Jennifer Lambe and others have explored the exceptionally close relationship that developed between psychoanalysis and politics in the aftermath of the Second World War, arguing that, in the 1960s, 1970s and 1980s, the discipline became much more than a clinical or therapeutic technique. Leading psychoanalysts from Germany, Western Europe, United States, Latin America engaged with a variety of broader social, religious and political issues, so that psychoanalysis evolved into a conceptual instrument for cultural and political criticism, and provided inspiration for radical and progressive interventions in a series of non-medical and non-psychiatric fields.[7] Moreover, in different parts of the world, psychoanalysis and psychoanalysts often styled themselves as natural allies of revolutionary political activism, developing conceptual tools and analytic frameworks for discussing and practicing radical politics.

Eastern Europe has so far remained cut off from these historiographical discussions, perhaps because of the longstanding assumption that the discipline of psychoanalysis was politically suppressed and marginalised in this region. But socialist psychoanalysis and psychotherapy in Yugoslavia played an exceptionally important role in both medical and political discussions about the nature of Marxist praxis and workers' self-management. This book explores the fascinating and complex relationship between Yugoslav psychoanalysis (and other 'psy' disciplines) and broader socio-political, cultural and intellectual fields. The coming chapters will demonstrate that it was in a small socialist East European country that some of the most radical ideas regarding an activist psychoanalysis developed as early as the late 1950s, well before comparable developments ensued in Western Europe, for instance. Moreover, Yugoslav psychoanalysts styled themselves not only as perceptive social critics and politically subversive intellectuals, but also as direct revolutionaries in their everyday clinical practice. Even though they participated in broader social and political discussions, their primary field of political action and involvement was the consulting room, in which they proposed to directly transform archaic social relations and promote self-management by undoing traditional Yugoslav patriarchal and authoritarian families.

[7] Dagmar Herzog, *Cold War Freud: Psychoanalysis in an Age of Catastrophes*, Cambridge: Cambridge University Press, 2016; Anne-Emanuelle Birn and Raul Necochea Lopez, eds, *Peripheral Nerve: Health and Medicine in Cold War Latin America*, Durham: Duke University Press, 2020.

Yugoslav psychoanalysis, psychiatry and psychotherapy were certainly unique—uniquely liberal and Westernised—in the East European context. Recent research has convincingly demonstrated that psychoanalysis was not banned or extinguished in the rest of socialist Eastern Europe either, but in most countries it was confined to various degrees of underground existence, and integrated in therapies and approaches labelled as 'dynamic' or 'psychotherapeutic'.[8] On the other hand, Yugoslav 'psy' disciplines openly discussed their intellectual, theoretical and clinical indebtedness to leading psychoanalytic figures, as well as their ongoing collaborations with and reliance on contemporary British, French and American schools of psychoanalysis. Moreover, several leading Yugoslav psychiatrists explicitly endeavoured to reinforce what they perceived as a close link between Marxism and psychoanalysis, and spent their careers demonstrating that the two theories were eminently combinable and complementary in a revolutionary political context: for instance, Yugoslavia's leading psychoanalyst and military psychiatrist Vladislav Klajn famously declared in public that one side of his heart was Freudian and the other Marxist.[9] This was despite the fact that East European socialist governments tended to see psychoanalysis as 'politically subversive' and incompatible with materialist notions in psychology.[10]

However, this book argues that the status and mission of Yugoslav psychoanalysis remained unmatched outside the socialist camp too,

[8] See Eghigian, 'Was There a Communist Psychiatry?'; Leuenberger, 'Socialist Psychotherapy and Its Dissidents'; Ana Antic, 'The Pedagogy of Workers' Self-management: Terror, Therapy and Reform Communism in Yugoslavia After the Tito-Stalin Split', *Journal of Social History*, 2016, 50:1, 179–203.

[9] Klajn was a veteran partisan fighter with the rank of colonel of the Yugoslav army and a high-ranking Communist Party functionary as well as a practising psychoanalyst. Following his medical studies and specialization in psychiatry, Klajn underwent two years of training analysis with Nikola Sugar between 1938 and 1940, and was a permanent member of Sugar's psychoanalytic circle in interwar Yugoslavia. In turn, Nikola Sugar, the first Yugoslav psychoanalyst who supervised the first generation of postwar analysts in the country, was a member of the Viennese and Budapest psychoanalytic societies, completed his own training analysis with Felix Boehm, and also worked closely with Paul Schilder (Petar Klajn, *Razvoj psihoanalize u Srbiji*, MA thesis, Unviersity of Belgrade, 1980, 107).

[10] Alexander Etkind, *Eros of the Impossible: The History of Psychoanalysis in Russia*, Routledge, 1997; Martin A. Miller, *Freud and the Bolsheviks: Psychoanalysis in Imperial Russia and the Soviet Union*, New Haven: Yale University Press, 1998; Leuenberger 'The End of Socialism and the Reinvention of the Self: A Study of the East German Psychotherapeutic Community in Transition', *Theory and Society*, 2002, 31:2.

because it was only in Yugoslavia that progressive psychoanalytic clinical practice and theoretical ambitions dovetailed so closely with the government's revolutionary agenda and increasing reliance on humanist Marxism. While Western radical and politically engaged psychoanalysis generally existed on the social and political margins, Yugoslav psychoanalysts and psychotherapists were given an opportunity to become directly involved in the process of revolutionising individual psyches as well as familial and social relationships in order to build a socialist alternative to Marxism-Leninism. In many ways, despite the persistence and co-existence of a variety of psychiatric and psychotherapeutic schools of thought on the Yugoslav soil, this particular version of revolutionary psychoanalysis and psychotherapy came to dominate mental health discussions as well as the work of outpatient psychiatric clinics throughout the socialist period. Furthermore, once Yugoslavia dissolved in a violent conflict in the 1990s, it was psychoanalytic concepts and frameworks that primarily informed not only discussions about PTSD or war trauma, but also broader political interpretations of the war, its causes and social and cultural effects.

Yet another aspect contributed significantly to the exceptional nature of Yugoslav socialist psychiatry—its unique involvement with the global South, and its participation in discussions about global transcultural psychiatry and decolonisation. Yugoslav psychiatrists and psychotherapists were arguably the only socialist East European representatives in this debate and in the broader field of global psychiatry. Their theoretical and clinical involvement was, again, fundamentally shaped by their Marxist background, by the geopolitical peripherality of their own country of origin, as well as by Yugoslavia's position as the founding member and one of the leaders of the Non-Aligned Movement. At the same time, their contributions to global and transcultural psychiatry were tightly linked with their experiences and concerns in the Yugoslav context, so that this engagement with the global South shaped the way psychiatry was conceived of and practiced in Yugoslavia itself. In that sense, Yugoslav psychiatry in the Cold War was not only Marxist but also 'non-aligned': its revolutionary and activist ethos was informed by its practitioners' transcultural clinical and anthropological research into revolutionary conditions and personalities in the decolonising world, and into alternative, non-Western frameworks of mental illness and healing.

By tracing Yugoslav psychiatrists' efforts to establish links and communication models between Western, Eastern and (global) Southern epistemological systems and networks, I aim to inscribe the region of Eastern Europe in the broader history of global medical and psychiatric knowledge production. The recent years have witnessed growing scholarly interest in the emergence and development of transcultural psychiatry in the aftermath of the Second World War. In particular, historians and anthropologists have looked at the decolonisation of psychiatry on a global scale, and at attempts by a variety of mental health professionals to re-define some of the core principles of international and global psychiatry in order to move away from the racist colonial psychiatric framework.[11] This is still a highly under-researched field, however, and in the existing literature the emergence of post-colonial transcultural psychiatry has been represented as mainly driven by Western psychiatrists and anthropologists, with important participation of some African and Asian professionals.[12] The role of socialist Eastern Europe has been entirely omitted, even though Eastern Bloc countries took part in these global discussions. This book zooms in on Yugoslav contributions to the field, and explores for the first time the role of socialist psychiatry in the creation of post-colonial global psychiatric frameworks. Yugoslavia was the only socialist state which sent psychiatrists and other mental health workers to the Global South as part of technical assistance and exploratory clinical missions, and these professionals intervened in the theory and practice of global post-colonial psychiatry in important and original ways. Their interventions were unique precisely because they were shaped by both Western education and socialist ideological background of anti-colonialism and non-alignment.

The literature on Cold War encounters between the socialist bloc and the 'Third World' is growing, and it largely focuses on networks of political activists and technological experts, and on university student

[11] Matthew Heaton, *Black Skin, White Coats: Nigerian Psychiatrists, Decolonization, and the Globalization of Psychiatry*, Athens: Ohio University Press, 2013; Yolana Pringle, *Psychiatry and Decolonisation in Uganda*, Basingstoke: Palgrave Macmillan, 2019; Jonathan Sadowsky, *Imperial Bedlam: Institutions of Madness in Colonial South West Nigeria*, University of California Press, 1999.

[12] Alice Bullard, 'Imperial Networks and Postcolonial Independence: The Transition from Colonial to Transcultural Psychiatry', in S. Malone and M. Vaughan, eds, *Psychiatry and Empire*, Basingstoke: Palgrave Macmillan, 2007.

exchanges,[13] while historical accounts of medical collaboration remains rather limited.[14] This book engages with the dynamic field of the history of socialist internationalism and globalisation, exploring how an atypical East European state participated in East–South exchanges, and how those connections and networks were affected by Yugoslavia's multifaceted professional and political collaborations with the West. I explore how socialist globalisation shaped the legacies of colonialism in the Global South, and address the role of East European actors (and states) in global discussions and processes related to decolonisation. The existing scholarship on Eastern Europe and on the history of psychiatry tells us virtually nothing about the role of psychiatrists and mental health experts in such exchanges. Through a study of how such experts from Eastern Europe redefined the relationship between individual psyche, race and culture, this account aims to shed much needed light on socialist states' understandings not only of anti-colonialism and racism but also of 'human nature'. In the context of Yugoslav historiography, the book makes an argument that it is important to look beyond diplomacy and foreign relations—to broader social and cultural phenomena and discussions—when analysing the history of the Non-Aligned Movement.[15]

The story of Yugoslav psychiatry, moreover, is important because it opens an unexpected window onto the broader history of cultural and

[13] See James Mark, Artemy Kalinovsky, and Steffanie Marung, eds, *Alternative Globalizations. Eastern Europe and the Postcolonial World*, Bloomington: Indiana University Press, 2020; Maxim Matusevich, *No Easy Row for a Russian Hoe: Ideology and Pragmatism in Nigerian-Soviet Relations*, 1960–1991, Trenton, NJ: Africa World Press, 2003; Matusevich, 'Probing the Limits of Internationalism: African Students Confront Soviet Ritual', *Anthropology of East Europe Review*, 2009, 27:2, 19–39; Quinn Slobodian, ed., *Comrades of Color: East Germany in the Cold War World*, New York: Berghahn Books, 2015; Benjamin Tromly, 'Brother or Other? East European Students in Soviet Higher Education Establishments', 1948–1956, *European History Quarterly*, 2014, 44:1, 80–102; Lukasz Stanek, 'Architects from Socialist Countries in Ghana (1957–1967): Modern Architecture and Mondialisation', *Society of Architectural Historians' Journal*, 2015, 74:4, 416–442; James Mark and Peter Apor, 'Socialism Goes Global: Decolonization and the Making of a New Culture of Internationalism in Socialist Hungary 1956–1989', *Journal of Modern History*, 2015, 87, 852–891.

[14] See, for instance, Dora Vargha, 'Technical Assistance and Socialist International Health: Hungary, the WHO and the Korean War', *History and Technology*, 2020, 36:3–4.

[15] Nataša Mišković, Harald Fischer-Tiné and Nada Boškovska Leimgruber, eds, *The Non Aligned Movement and the Cold War: Delhi, Bandung, Belgrade*, Routledge, 2014; Tvrtko Jakovina, *Treća strana hladnog rata [The Third Side of the Cold War]*, Zagreb: Fraktura, 2011.

professional contacts and exchanges across the Iron Curtain. Seeking to undermine traditional narratives of Cold War divides, this book explores the dynamic relationship between Eastern and Western Europe, and traces the political and broader social impact of these lively professional and cultural exchanges.[16] As we will see in the coming chapters, despite being a socialist and non-aligned country, Yugoslavia was deeply involved in West European and North American professional networks and its political and cultural life was decisively shaped by such engagements across the ideological boundaries.[17]

The role of the 'psy' disciplines in the creation of such transnational networks between socialist Eastern Europe and the Western world has so far been completely neglected, even though it is particularly important as it demonstrates how socialist understandings of some of the core concepts relating to human psyche, 'human nature' and social relationships were developed in a complex conversation which traversed political, ideological and cultural boundaries. These concepts were central to a range of political discussions in socialist Yugoslavia, and such transnational psychiatric collaborations had a transformative impact on the country's political debates. At the same time, while scholars have traditionally tended to emphasise the 'Westernisation' of socialist Eastern Europe which resulted from such exchanges, I propose to view Yugoslavia as a true testing ground and a site for genuine transnational interpenetration of different cultural, professional and political models. Rather than merely Westernising the country or minimising its differences from the Western world, this rich cooperation produced unique solutions, theories and forms of practice which combined Western insights with socialist concerns and innovative Marxist agendas. Moreover, these crossings of the Iron Curtain will be placed in a broader transnational context, showing that the East–West connections both informed and were informed by Yugoslavia's relationships with the Global South.

[16] Yale Richmond, *Cultural Exchange and the Cold War: Raising the Iron Curtain*, Philadelphia: Pennsylvania State Unviersity Press, 2003; Sune Bechmann Pedersen and Christian Noack, eds, *Tourism and Travel during the Cold War: Negotiating Tourist Experiences Across the Iron Curtain*, London and New York: Routledge, 2020; Nikolaos Papadogiannis, 'Political Travel Across the 'Iron Curtain' and Communist Youth Identities in West Germany and Greece in the 1970s and 1980s', *European Review of History*, 2016, 26:3, 526–553.

[17] Radina Vucetic, *Coca-Cola Socialism: Americanization of the Yugoslav Culture in the Sixties*, Budapest: CEU Press, 2018.

But, as already mentioned, Yugoslav psychiatry was not only global, non-aligned and partly Westernised: it was also an explicitly and self-avowedly socialist profession, whose practitioners functioned under authoritarian and often politically repressive conditions. Yugoslavia's 'psy' professionals and institutions thus also got involved in violent and repressive projects, which primarily targeted political dissidents or potential opponents of the regime. This book aims to offer one of the first in-depth studies of East European punitive psychiatry outside the Soviet Union.[18] It zooms in on two different ways in which 'psy' disciplines were mobilised for coercive political purposes. In the immediate aftermath of Yugoslavia's break with the USSR, the government organised an exceptionally violent experiment in Goli Otok, which aimed to 're-educate' suspected pro-Stalinists in the Yugoslav society and communist party. The Goli Otok camp's policies and measures demonstrated how psychoanalytic concepts of 'expanding consciousness' and progressive concerns with personal liberation and emancipation could go hand in hand with extremely oppressive ideas about compulsory psychological re-education. Then, in the second half of the socialist period, some 'psy' professionals and institutions took part in a much more conventional practice of punitive psychiatry, using exceedingly broad and vague psychiatric diagnoses to pathologise social and political non-conformity, and to delegitimise political critique by forcing dissidents into psychiatric hospitals. Even though these techniques seemed to have much in common with Soviet punitive psychiatric strategies, the Yugoslav context was still quite different, and the more liberal overall political framework allowed for a more involved and complex discussion about such psychiatric abuses. In following this psychiatric-political debate and especially the responses of those deemed mentally ill due to their political activity, the book explores how such challenges to punitive psychiatry drew on anti-psychiatric ideas and tested the limits of Yugoslav psychiatry's political progressivism.

It will become clear over the coming chapters that Yugoslav socialist psychiatry was fundamentally shaped by its engagements with the

[18] On punitive psychiatry in socialist Eastern Europe, see Maria Cristina Galmarini-Kabala, 'Psychiatry, Violence, and the Soviet Project of Transformation: A Micro-History of the Perm Psycho-Neurological School-Sanatorium', *Slavic Review*, 2018, 77, 307–332; Nanci Adler et al., 'Psychiatry Under Tyranny: A Report on the Political Abuse of Romanian Psychiatry During the Ceausescu Years', *Current Psychology: A Journal for Diverse Perspectives on Diverse Psychological Issues*, 1993, 12:1, 3–17.

concepts of primitivism, modernity and revolution. Well before socialism, the Yugoslav psychiatric profession aimed to carve for itself a central role in the process of modernising the country and its population. This aspiration was based on the profession's claimed expertise in the intricate mechanisms of human psychology and, by extension, their unique capability to intervene in shaping the collective national mind. From the beginning of the twentieth century, Yugoslavia's fledgling 'psy' disciplines actively involved themselves in discussions around 'civilising' and enlightening the country's largely agricultural population.[19] The terms of these discussions did not change in any fundamental way after 1945: socialist psychiatric civilising missions were more therapeutically optimistic and less concerned with 'catching up' with the West, but Communist-era 'psy' discourses were haunted by the figure of a 'primitive patient' (and primitive families and mentalities). This longstanding concern with eliminating backwardness and primitivism—as the final obstacles to achieving both modernity and socialism—permeated psychiatric, psychotherapeutic and psychoanalytic clinical practice and research. In the socialist period, the persistence in Yugoslavia of hierarchical and authoritarian social relations was ultimately blamed on such primitivism, and it was the role of the 'psy' disciplines to make their patients aware of these harmful political-psychological patterns so that they could be unravelled and transformed. In the end, only those citizens who managed to emancipate themselves from traditional authoritarianism and conformity to socio-political hierarchies would be able to complete the revolution and build a truly self-managing workers' society.

In that sense, there were striking similarities between twentieth-century East European psychiatry and West European colonial psychiatry.[20] Even though Yugoslav practitioners nominally shared language and cultural background with the people they treated, in terms of social class, privilege and educational experiences they had much more in common with their Western colleagues than with the majority of their peasant or working-class patients. Given the sustained psychiatric focus on the modernisation project and the civilising mission, it was very difficult for socialist 'psy' disciplines to overcome the profession's colonially inflected analyses of the

[19] See Heike Karge, *Der Charme der Schizophrenie. Psychiatrie, Krieg und Gesellschaft im serbokroatischen Raum*, Berlin: De Gruyter, 2020.

[20] See, for comparison, Richard Keller, *Colonial Madness: Psychiatry in French North Africa*, Chicago: University of Chicago Press, 2007.

behaviour and mentalities of Yugoslavia's own population. This tendency to apply civilisational scales and view progress in exclusively linear terms determined Yugoslav socialist practitioners' engagement with transcultural psychiatry, and limited their ability to provide a genuinely anti-colonial critique of global psychiatry.

In the end, a particular vision of 'revolutionary personality' emerged as the most appropriate solution for overcoming backwardness (see, in particular, Chapters 3 and 5). As this book demonstrates, Yugoslav psychiatry was fundamentally affected by Marxism and the communist ideology, but it was not merely 'tainted' by them. To the contrary, psychiatric and psychoanalytic professionals engaged profoundly with the concept of political revolution, and often used their research and clinical practice to reflect on their own role in a revolutionary society and in the state project of socialist revolution. Indeed, the experience of the revolution radically transformed the nature of Yugoslav 'psy' disciplines, and those disciplines were certainly aware of the revolution's disruptive and volatile potential. But in the course of the socialist period, psychiatrists gradually integrated narratives of revolution and revolutionary politics into the broader modernisation project, and offered their own profession and practice as indispensable tools for completing the revolutionary project on both individual and collective planes.

In terms of its structure and chronological span, this book is primarily focused on the socialist period in Yugoslav history. Chapters 3, 4, 5 and 6 all deal with a particular aspect of the complex relationship between Yugoslavia's version of socialism and its 'psy' disciplines. Chapter 3 explores the development of an innovative revolutionary discipline of psychotherapy and psychoanalysis, in line with Yugoslavia's experimentation with an alternative form of Marxism and workers' self-management. Chapter 4, on the other hand, demonstrates that Yugoslav psychiatry and psychotherapy engaged in repressive and authoritarian practices and political projects, despite the fact that the country's leading 'psy' institutions and individual researchers were increasingly concerned with notions of personal freedom and emancipation, and with dismantling social hierarchies. Chapter 5 describes how Yugoslav psychiatrists and psychoanalysts engaged with the global South and debates about decolonisation, and how their global clinical and ethnographic efforts shaped their research and practice at home. Chapter 6 aims to step beyond the consulting room, and argues that psychoanalysis, psychotherapy and psychiatry informed a variety of non-medical public discussions and discourses, becoming a site for formulating cultural and political criticism, as well as for thinking through the political challenges of the Yugoslav socialist experiments. However, the history of socialist psychiatry cannot be properly understood if it is not placed in a broader historical and chronological context. For those reasons, Chapter 2 spans the entire twentieth century in order to explain how socialist psychiatry engaged with, and was shaped by, a variety of pre-WWII concerns with modernity and modernisation, primitivism, backwardness and 'civilisational' development. Finally, Chapter 7—the epilogue—focuses on the immediate post-socialist period—the wars of Yugoslav succession of the 1990s—and examines how the Yugoslav 'psy' disciplines grappled with the breakdown of communism, and the profound psychological and political effects of the extremely violence and bloodshed that marked Yugoslavia's demise.

CHAPTER 2

Primitivism, Modernity and Revolution in the Twentieth Century: The Case of Psychiatry

In 1959, following a presentation at a medical conference in Sarajevo, Israeli psychiatrist G. R. Tamarin, a close collaborator of several Yugoslav 'psy' professionals, published an important and unusually honest article in a Yugoslav medical journal, in which he focused on the complications that psychiatrists and psychotherapists faced when dealing with uneducated, 'backward' and mentally 'undifferentiated' patients whose possibilities for self-reflection were limited. His article emphasised the multiple meanings of the word 'primitive': it could refer to those socio-economic strata considered uncultured in a European or Israeli setting, as well as to those with 'pre-logical' and 'fantastic' thought patterns hailing from the tribal depths of black Africa. Tamarin drew attention to the possible links between these two meanings. He was primarily concerned with the former group, with whom he regularly engaged in his daily clinical practice. These were Israeli patients with little education and no 'broader interests or ambitions', who struggled to get involved in any meaningful therapeutic interpersonal dialogue.[1] But Tamarin articulated very clearly this linguistic confusion regarding the exact connotation of the concept of 'primitivism', which was particularly important for Yugoslav psychiatrists

[1] G. R. Tamarin, 'Primitivna Licnost i Mentalna Higijena', *Medicinski Glasnik*, 1959, 50:2–2a, 55–56.

A. Antić, *Non-Aligned Psychiatry in the Cold War*,
Mental Health in Historical Perspective,
https://doi.org/10.1007/978-3-030-89449-8_2

as well. Throughout the twentieth century, Tamarin's Yugoslav colleagues tended to move between the two meanings of the word without reflecting on the transition. In psychiatric discussions, 'primitive' mentalities of European (or Israeli) populations were often associated with civilisational 'primitivism' of the non-European world, and this implicit connection affected the profession's engagement with both domestic and global concerns.

The article certainly resonated with Yugoslav postwar psychiatrists. 'Primitive' patients plagued Yugoslav psychiatry throughout the twentieth century. On the one hand, their problem was very similar to Tamarin's: the 'backward' and unsophisticated personalities of such patients made the practice of psychotherapy, let alone psychoanalysis, very difficult, and complicated the therapeutic potential of mental health techniques. But the problem was even more complicated than these clinical concerns: the reported 'primitivism' of the majority of psychiatric patients had deeper implications, as they were taken to represent the cultural status of the Yugoslav population as a whole. Yugoslav psychiatrists worried about how their own country and society were perceived by the developed — 'civilised'—Western world, and carved an important social and political role for themselves as they sought to ensure a place for Yugoslavia in a European family of modern nations.

Therefore, these psychiatric discussions were tightly related to the issues of cultural and political modernity and modernisation: following WWI and the creation of the first Yugoslav state, the political and intellectual elites embarked on a complex project of modern nation-building and 'Europeanisation' of a country made up of territories with very different historical traditions. As a result, the psychiatric profession received significant investment, as new university departments and hospitals and clinics were open.[2] In such a political context, and as a strategy for their own discipline's advancement, psychiatrists began presenting themselves as vital in the process of 'remoulding' the mind of the nation and fighting the widespread 'backwardness' of Yugoslavia's largely rural population. In the course of the twentieth century, this self-perception of the psychiatric profession would not change in any fundamental way, and would

[2] Srdjan Milovanovic, 'Prvi srpski psihijatri,' *Istorija Medicine,* 134: 9–10, 2006, 457–465; Nikola Peršić, 'Povjest psihijatrije u Jugoslaviji,' *Socijalna psihijatrija*, 15, 1987, 225–236; Ana Antić, *Therapeutic Fascism: Experiencing the Violence of the Nazi New Order*, Oxford: Oxford University Press, 2017.

continue across the great divide of 1945: 'primitivism' remained one of the core medical and clinical topics, and heated psychiatric debates around the discipline's self-appointed mission to modernise and 'civilise' the patient population served as a site to discuss a variety of related social and political topics, such as class relations and hierarchies, the effects of the social revolution, as well as the international 'civilisational' position of Yugoslavia.

The core of this debate consisted of the question to what extent social and cultural 'primitivism' could be overcome in the Balkans, and under what circumstances. The psychiatric profession considered the modernisation and civilisation of the 'backward' masses to be among its main tasks, and its core political leverage, whether in the context of interwar state- and nation-building, or within the framework of post-WWII revolutionary social and political transformations.

When discussed in psychiatric circles, 'primitivism' was often pathologised, as the discussion moved back and forth between socio-cultural and medical planes. In that sense, as I will argue in this book, Yugoslav (and broader East European) psychiatry shared some important intellectual and clinical frameworks with colonial psychiatry—in the way it conceived of its own 'civilising mission', in how it perceived itself, and how it conceptualised its own patient population and its relationship with it. When Yugoslav psychiatrists encountered their patients, they shared with them the same language and similar cultural background, but they found the patients' lack of education and low social rank deeply alienating, and often quickly translated those 'unmodern' characteristics and beliefs into medical disorders and psychiatric diagnoses.

Following the constitution of the Kingdom of Serbs, Croats and Slovenes in 1918, both the political and medical elites embarked on a project of wholesale modernisation and Westernisation of the society, which was tightly linked to the development of a new, unified national consciousness. Not only psychiatrists, but also anthropologists, ethnologists and medical doctors of all brands joined forces to propose the creation of a new European nation, to be forged out of three different 'tribes'.[3] The new progressive and 'civilised' nation of Yugoslavs was to result from a synthesis of the best and noblest attributes of the three

[3] Vedran Duancic, *Geography and Nationalist Visions of Inter-War Yugoslavia*, Palgrave Macmillan, 2020; Rory Yeomans, 'Of "Yugoslav Barbarians" and Croatian Gentlemen Scholars: Nationalist Ideology and Racial Anthropology in Interwar Yugoslavia', in Marius

groups; this novel 'Yugoslav consciousness', based on modern civic virtues and rational, 'enlightened' principles, would be on a par with Western nations, and would do away with the 'primitive' baggage of 'tribal' differences.[4] In order to achieve this, the health, hygienic and civilisational standards of the rural and urban populations had to be elevated. The psychiatric special mission primarily relied on the expectation that psychiatrists would be exceptionally capable of affecting the national psyche— keeping it safe from the pernicious influences of insanity and mental degeneration, and at the same time forging a modern national consciousness. In the Kingdom of Yugoslavia's search for national identity, psychiatric discussions regarding the nature, constitution and forms of development of the national character played a particularly significant role. This was especially true in the context of the Yugoslav intellectual and political elites' need to prove that the country truly and legitimately belonged to the society of modern, 'civilised' nations.

The first half of the twentieth century saw an upsurge of publications on the theme of ethno-psychiatry, and Eastern Europe participated in this increased academic production in a number of ways. After 1918 in Yugoslavia, deliberations and evaluations of the national character became even more salient, especially in the context of the new state's dual project

Turda and Paul Weindling, eds, *"Blood and Homeland:" Eugenics and Racial Nationalism in Central and Southeast Europe*, Budapest: CEU Press, 2007, 83–122.

[4] On political and cultural discussions regarding the meaning of interwar Yugoslavism, see Andrew Wachtel, *Making a Nation, Breaking a Nation: Literature and Cultural Politics in Yugoslavia*, Stanford: Stanford University Press, 1998; Dejan Djokic, *Elusive Compromise: A History of Interwar Yugoslavia*, New York: Columbia University Press, 2007; Marko Bulatovic, 'Struggling with Yugoslavism: Dilemmas of Interwar Serb Political Thought,'in John Lampe and Mark Mazower, eds, *Ideologies and National Identities: The Case of Twentieth-Century Southeastern Europe*, Budapest: CEU Press, 2004, 254–276; Christian Nielsen, *Making Yugoslavs: Identity in King Alexander's Yugoslavia*, Toronto: University of Toronto Press, 2014

of nation-building and Westernisation.[5] The new Yugoslav national character would be as far from the Ottoman cultural and historical legacy as possible; in fact, throughout the 1920s and 1930s, a group of anthropologists and ethnologists set about proving the biological proximity of the 'Dinaric' and 'Nordic races;' Vladimir Dvorniković and Branimir Maleš argued that the 'Dinaric race', to which a majority of the Yugoslav population arguably belonged, was closer to the 'Nordic race' than to any other 'race' in Europe. The entire Dinaric debate directly countered the Central and West European anthropological, psychiatric and ethnographic arguments regarding the 'primitivism' and 'brutality' of eastern Slavs.[6]

Psychiatrists (and psychoanalysts) found themselves in the midst of this heightened attention to questions regarding the nature and characteristics of the Yugoslav, Serbian or Croatian national mentality: What were the nations' or ethnic groups' qualities and shortcomings and how did they come to be? What marked the South Slavs' uniqueness and historical individuality? Answers to these questions were considered vital to working out the content, the meaning of the new Yugoslav nation. The end of WWI and the establishment of the Kingdom of Serbs, Croats and Slovenes marked a new start in the long-time search for the 'national essence;' the 'liberation' and final unification of the South Slavic lands offered an opportunity to re-mould and perfect the national mind, weed out the imperfections and symptoms of 'backwardness', 'primitivism', centuries of 'foreign enslavement' and ultimately join the family

[5] A number of studies have explored the history of the idea of national character in both Western and Eastern Europe, and probed its psychological-political meanings: R. Romani, *National Character and Public Spirit in Britain and France, 1750–1914*, Cambridge: Cambridge University Press, 2002; Peter Mandler, *The English National Character: The History of an Idea from Edmund Burke to Tony Blair*, New Haven: Yale University Press, 2006; M. Beller and J. Leerssen, eds, *Imagology: The Cultural Production and Literary Representation of National Characters*, Amsterdam: Rodopi, 2007; Balazs Trencsenyi, *The Politics of 'National Character': A Study in Interwar East European Thought*, New York: Routledge Studies in Comparative Political Thought, 2012.

[6] At other times, Maleš contended that the 'Dinarics' were indeed superior to their West and North European counterparts, and that the Balkan or Slavic racial type could infuse the decaying European West with virility, force, energy, and racially revive it, prevent it from degeneracy. See Branimir Males, *Antropoloska ispitivanja: Prilog ispitivanju telesnih osobina crnogorskih i susednih plemena*, Belgrade, 1932;Males, *O ljudskim rasama*, Belgrade, 1936, Vladimir Dvornikovic, *Karakterologija Jugoslovena*, Belgrade: Kosmos, 1939; Dvornikovic, *Psiha jugoslovenske melanholije*, Zagreb: Z. i V. Vasica, 1925.

of 'civilised nations'.[7] But the exuberance of the immediate postwar years quickly waned, when ethno-psychiatry began asking whether the population was truly reformable, and whether the highly unsatisfactory core traits of the national character were alterable at all. The task related to potential reform and modernisation of the national character gave the psychiatric community an opportunity to be directly involved in a straightforwardly political project, one that decisively pulled it out of psychiatric hospitals and asylums.

For Zagreb psychiatrist Nikola Sučić, the unification of 1918 represented a realisation of the long-time liberation dream of all Yugoslav 'tribes', but he warned that the ingrained negative and backward traits of South Slavs might prove to be a serious obstacle to national prosperity. As a result of centuries of subjection to foreign rulers, wrote Sučić in the introduction to his textbook on nervous and mental illnesses, South Slavs grew some highly deleterious national characteristics: having no other choice but to adjust to constant humiliation, exploitation and suppression, to the spiritual as well as material poverty, bearing and internalising the mark of inferiority in comparison to other, free nations, the South Slavic collective mind inevitably developed in pathological directions. They turned 'envious, arrogant, lazy, overly passionate, selfish, unreliable, careless to the point of affect'; moreover, the long-term experience of political and cultural oppression bred feelings of shame, collective dishonour, fear and anxiety, which were 'the source of all forms of mental freezing and backwardness, and an obstacle to cultural advancement of individuals and masses'.[8]

Sučić in fact described these historically conditioned collective traits as forms of 'affective disorders', treating the 'South Slavic race' as a psychiatric patient: 'There lay the consequences of that awful period, in the course of which South Slavs had been spiritually suppressed and as if under a spell again any positive work with no hope for a better future. A defeat after a defeat left them terrified and apathetic, for centuries on the level of mental poverty and cultural backwardness, from they still haven't awoken'.[9]

[7] Olivera Milosavljevic, *Savremenici Fasizma 2: Jugoslavija u Okruzenju, 1933–1941*, Belgrade: Helsinski Odbor za Ljudska Prava u Srbiji, 2010, 47–84.

[8] Sucic, *Bolesti zivaca I duse*, 12.

[9] Ibid., 13.

But within the rigid organicist framework of interwar biological psychiatry, it would take many generations and several centuries for pedagogues to alter a nation's character traits or mentality, and to erase such 'primitive' culture traits from the psychological picture of a collective. In his article titled 'Limits of education', pedagogue and psychologist Krsta Jonić argued that 'one should not expect deep changes to occur in one individual or one generation as a result of educational influences. That requires a much more *long-duree* perspective, and only over the course of many generations exposed to [proper] educational influences can one count on transformations and perfecting of instincts'.[10] Even more disturbingly in the context of the Yugoslav psychiatric mission, '[t]here have been many known examples when members of some primitive people, even though they had been introduced to civilization very young and seemingly got used to a cultured life, still under certain circumstances turned their backs on the new life and returned to their old uncivilized ways'.[11]

Sučić and his colleagues grew ever more pessimistic about their daunting task, especially given the profound distrust of the value of education and pedagogy among traditional psychiatrists and the frustrating everyday reality of hospital work. Sučić implored his readers to compare the grandiose architecture of Munich, Rome, Paris or Berlin to the meagre cultural institutions of their own country: 'We have not got such museums like other nations, we do not have such artwork either – and what we do have is scattered, unsystematic, with no determination of time and space'. What was needed was local and locally trained psychiatric professionals, who could lead the people out of the 'darkness of ignorance, the worst poverty and difficulty of all European peoples'.[12]

There was thus never any doubt that this was a mission for psychiatrists, that deliberations and evaluations of pluses and minuses of the national character fell squarely in the psychiatric professional domain. Their conclusions could often be unsettling: Belgrade's leading neuropsychiatrist Laza Stanojević noted that, as a result of centuries of cultural and spiritual impoverishment, 'the Oriental and Slavic races' were particularly

[10] Krsta Jonic, 'Granice vaspitanja', *Ucitelj*, 1933, 14 (48):1, 291.

[11] Ibid., 289.

[12] Nikola Sucic, *Psihologija i Psihopatologija covjecanstva: Psihologija i Psihopatologija Nagona i Ljubavi*, Zagreb, 1939, preface.

prone to superstition and superstitious beliefs. Moreover, the line between harbouring superstitious beliefs and exhibiting signs of a full-fledged mania was a thin one. Therefore, in addition to being symptoms of 'primitivism' and an 'enormous spiritual poverty', superstitious convictions could easily evolve into insanity: 'they [superstitions] hide in themselves nothing ill as long as they do not undergo a sick twist, i.e. as long as they do not begin to spread and build a system of irrefutability... in and of themselves they might not be signs of illness unless they tend towards such processing and systematization that turns them into a core around which kindred, maniacal ideas spread and build'.[13] In other words, superstition was in an important way akin to mania and insanity, a dangerous reservoir of blunders, prejudices and mistaken ideas of enormous power, which appeared extremely resilient and difficult to extinguish. This was yet another sign of cultural primitivism and a sad consequence of centuries lived in retrograde, medieval darkness; hospital psychiatrists faced the problem on a daily basis, and regularly lamented their patients' tendency to understand mental illness and its treatment in terms other than those of modern science.

In fact, Yugoslav medical practitioners as a whole seemed to wage an all-out war against the rural population's conceptions of health, illness, and hygiene. One report from the late 1920s objected to what was perceived as the peasant population's overwhelming and enduring distrust of physicians and modernity: 'people only see the [political] authority in the official doctor and rarely seek his help, turning instead to priests, imams and sorcerers'.[14] As one Bosnian peasant testified, the last time a doctor visited his village was twenty-three years ago, and people mainly healed themselves with the help of herbs and fortune-tellers.[15] In the interwar years, aggressive attempts at medical 'enlightenment' achieved notable results, but they also produced bitter conflicts with local populations in underdeveloped areas: the Central Hygiene Institute complained of many Yugoslav villagers' extremely reluctant cooperation with health authorities, their refusal to follow medical advice, report diseases, or subject themselves to prescribed treatments, noting that the population

[13] Sucic, *Bolesti zivaca I duse*, 50.

[14] Mihailo Avramović, *Nase seljacko gazdinstvo*, Belgrade: Stampa Sveti Sava, 1928.

[15] Vera Erlich, *Family in Transition: A Study of 300 Yugoslav Villages*, Princeton: Princeton University Press, 1966, 52.

was not informed about even the 'most elementary hygienic conditions.' Yugoslavia's leading social medicine and public hygiene expert Andrija Štampar and his colleagues demanded and administered harsh penalties against recalcitrant and 'unenlightened' peasants during epidemics.[16]

In the countryside as well as in the recently urbanized areas, moreover, fortune-tellers emerged as the psychiatric profession's rivals for popular attention and trust. They offered alternative, supernatural interpretations of psychological malaise, provided specific advice for resolving mental problems, and even served as a particular kind of psychotherapist, in the context in which no psychotherapy was practiced in clinics or hospitals. Consequently, since the late nineteenth century, the state attempted to eliminate or at least restrict and control their practice, but those efforts proved largely unsuccessful. Yugoslav psychiatrists, trained in Western Europe and deeply involved in broader European professional networks, thus likely had more in common with French or German doctors than with their illiterate peasant patients.

It was unsurprising then that psychiatrists presented the consequences of superstition—this potentially pathological national trait—as extremely serious, even life-threatening. In his article in a Belgrade medical journal, Stanojević related a disturbing story of a female patient obsessed with paranoid ideas of a superstitious nature, who compelled her husband to kill two women because she suspected them of casting evil spells on her and her family. After her two children died, she had had several miscarriages and suffered 'continuously from an unknown disease'. The patient grew convinced that her long-time misfortune was a result of the two women's magic; during her stay at the psychiatric hospital in Belgrade, she confirmed several times that the women often clearly told her that they were purposely throwing curses so that 'there would never be a healthy baby crying in my house'.[17] When they finally threatened her that they were working to bring about the deaths of both the patient and her husband, she reportedly could not endure any longer and convinced her husband to get rid of them. Stanojević cleared the husband of any guilt and responsibility: his mental state was understandably labile after listening to his wife's pathological paranoid ideas for a very long period.

[16] Centralni higijenski zavod, *Godisnji izvestaj za 1936.* g., 34.

[17] Laza Stanojevic, 'Dvostruko ubistvo nad dvema zenama, izvrseno od strane jednog seljaka pod uticajem sumanutih ideja gonjenja dusevno mu obolele zene (slucaj indukovanog ludila)', *Srpski arhiv za celokupno lekarstvo*, sv. 3, 181.

Although at first he had been very sceptical towards the entire narrative of spells, curses and magic, the husband finally caved in when the patient continuously intimidated him with stories of their impending death. Stanojević strongly emphasised the pathological effect that such powerful and frightening superstitious convictions had on an otherwise healthy and intelligent man.

This tragic case served as a perfect illustration of Sučić's arguments regarding the potentially disastrous consequences of popular beliefs in black magic: it demonstrated how a powerful system of paranoid pathological ideas developed from a strong superstitious seed, and it highlighted the broad impact of such beliefs—in Stanojević's interpretation, the husband, although not superstitious and 'primitive' himself, proved unable to resist the attraction of the wife's explanations simply because he was raised and lived in such an environment. Stanojević concluded that the single most important cause for the murders was the 'oriental' races' extraordinary predisposition to gullibility and superstitious misconceptions. There was no doubt in Stanojević's mind that superstition equalled and bred mental pathology. The patient, quite expectedly, was an illiterate peasant woman, whose 'blunders' and prejudices were deeply ingrained and seemingly could not be corrected by psychiatrists.

However, this concern with the potentially pathological 'primitivism' in Yugoslavia's peasant population in particular continued in a strikingly unchanged fashion after 1945 and the socialist revolution. In the newly communist country, Nenad Bohaček, a Zagreb-based psychiatrist, seemingly unaware of Stanojevic's above-described exploration of induced psychosis, undertook to present a very similar case—*folie a trois* this time, which involved a grown-up daughter convincing both of her parents that their entire family was persecuted and endangered. This case, recorded in 1951, was not nearly as tragic as the first one—nobody was murdered, but the three family members were taken to the Vrapce hospital in Zagreb because they had behaved disruptively and barricaded themselves in a room in a friend's house, where they reportedly broke furniture and sang loudly, 'mainly church songs'.[18] They had previously escaped their own house because they believed it haunted by ghosts and devils: the divorcee daughter, who had been exhibiting psychotic traits for years already, succeeded in persuading her (healthy and previously non-psychotic) father

[18] Nenad Bohacek, 'Slucaj inducirane psihoze – Folie a trois', *Neuropsihijatrija*, 1953, 1:2, 128–134.

and mother that her former husband's family had cast evil spells on her and 'tried to deliver her to the devil'. Interestingly, the psychiatrist who treated them in Zagreb was seemingly in full agreement with his interwar colleague Stanojević regarding the origins of the pathological outbreak: 'superstition... we consider exceptionally important for the development of induced psychosis in the parents. If [their psychological profiles had not provided] such a fertile ground, full of superstitious nonsense, the parents probably would not have succumbed so easily to the influence of the daughter, whose psychotic content was brimming with ghosts, demons, sorcery, and magic'. More straightforwardly, 'primitivism' figured as the vital factor: the father, who was described as more intensely affected by this psychotic episode than the mother, was 'primitive', 'crass' and a psychopath (the lines between primitivism and psychopathy remaining exceptionally blurry)—unlike the mother—and was consequently more difficult to dissuade even when separated from the daughter. It was this 'increased gullibility and primitivism' that functioned as the core preconditions for psychotic outbreaks and ideas to be shared in such a manner.[19] As Bohaček concluded, psychosis and pathology clearly thrived on the primitive and superstitious mental constitution of this peasant family, in which the daughter, ill as she was, was still deemed the most intelligent one.

Still, the tone of this postwar article was significantly different: unlike Stanojević's patient who could not be reached and transformed by modern medicine's civilising influence, the family discussed in Bohaček's case study seemed to have undergone a full recovery, and were returned to their village where their neighbours confirmed that they 'came to their senses'. The optimism of this outcome was telling: while socialist psychiatrists continued to rely on a surprisingly similar set of concepts to define their struggle with cultural 'backwardness', they did develop a therapeutic paradigm which enabled them to conceive of progress, education and their own 'civilising mission' in much more hopeful terms.

[19] Ibid., 131–134.

Psychiatry, Progress and ‘Primitivism’ After the Socialist Revolution

Writing after World War II ended, Dezider Julius, the then head of the Vrapče psychiatric hospital in Zagreb, accused Yugoslav interwar psychiatry of purposely ignoring the socio-economic context of mental illness for ideological reasons: for Julius, this was the central characteristic of ‘bourgeois psychiatry’, which was ‘in its entire structure an example of a non-dialectical manner of thought, because it view[ed] the phenomena of patients and illnesses as isolated, static, separate from their environment, and not dynamically, in their development and changes, keeping in mind their relationship with the environment and their mutual influences’.[20] Julius’ accusation suggested that the interwar paradigm was not only medically but also ideologically flawed. He may well have been right: delving deeply into the socio-economic and cultural context of madness and mental pathology could produce some quite unsettling answers regarding the need for radical social and political transformations.

The overall psychiatric paradigm changed in the aftermath of the Second World War, with the onset and development of the socialist revolution in Yugoslavia, but the profession’s preoccupation with ‘primitive’ patients continued in the context of socialist psychotherapy and psychoanalysis. In some ways, the immediate postwar presented the profession with even more demanding challenges, with its large-scale social dislocation, radical political transformations and the increasing social and political visibility of the peasant population. Already in 1945, the reportedly widespread outbreak of a unique type of war neurosis among resistance partisan soldiers tested the psychiatrists’ abilities as well as their shifting paradigms.

Towards the end of the war, the victorious Yugoslav People’s Army, which grew out of the Communist-led resistance movement, was plagued by a particular and reportedly uniquely Yugoslav form of soldiers’ neurosis, which was often referred to as ‘partisan neurosis’ or ‘partisan hysteria’. Unlike other forms of neurosis such as battle fatigue or shell shock, more common in Western armies, this disorder consisted of violent epileptiform seizures which re-enacted and simulated wartime battle situations and attacks. As the involved psychiatrists testified, there was no urge among affected Yugoslav partisan fighters to withdraw from the frontlines

[20] Dezider Julius, ‘Pitanja socijalne psihopatologije’, *Narodno zdravlje*, 1949, 6, 1.

and flee from battles. Quite to the contrary, partisan neurosis demonstrated the resistance army's extraordinary 'fighting spirit' and military and ideological commitment.[21] On the other hand, its disruptive and often theatrical nature caused major political and psychiatric concern in the immediate aftermath of the war, and served as a symbolic reminder of the chaos, confusion and social dislocation caused by the revolutionary changes. The psychiatric profession's involvement with and theories of partisan neurosis were directly and explicitly tied to their long-standing struggle with 'primitive' patients.

Very importantly, it was almost exclusively uneducated, often illiterate, politically unsophisticated, young and psychologically 'immature' peasant soldiers who were diagnosed with this illness, usually after they were given (or promised) important political responsibilities but experienced severe trauma and anxiety due to their own inadequacy and unpreparedness. Both psychoanalysts and traditional military psychiatrists remained firmly within the interwar paradigm of belated modernisation, and soon began discussing the partisan neurotic in terms of 'primitivism' and a lack of cultural, political or social sophistication. Their core yet unspoken concern was, of course, that the victorious partisan soldiers were considered to be the socialist republic's new military and political elite in the making, the main agents and beneficiaries of the most comprehensive, far-reaching and revolutionary elite turnover the Yugoslav society had ever seen. Their mental breakdowns attracted attention precisely because they could be seen to point to the inadequacies of the new order, as well as to the extremely disruptive and volatile potential of the revolutionary changes. Yugoslav psychiatrists in particular saw the partisan neurotic disorder as a sign of these soldiers' unpreparedness for taking over their new social responsibilities, and regularly warned of the psychological perils of entrusting the immature, the uneducated and the primitive with leading political, social and military roles.

Virtually all psychiatrists dealing with the problem agreed that these partisans' psychological problems demonstrated the core social and cultural difficulties of Yugoslavia's postwar revolutionary transition. The constructed psychological profile of the partisan neurotic thus exemplified a number of troubling socio-political tendencies of the immediate postwar era. Witnessing a true social revolution outside the hospitals,

[21] Hugo Klajn, *Ratna neuroza Jugoslovena*, Belgrade: Tersit, 1995 (reprinted—originally published in 1955).

Yugoslav psychiatrists found it very difficult to shed their long-time beliefs about the volatile nature of the 'backward masses', and pathologised the very upward mobility and other revolutionary societal changes of the new Yugoslav socialist republic. Unsurprisingly, by criticising dangers of the revolutionary chaos, psychiatrists recommended themselves as the optimal actors to resolve the tension, adjusting their pre-revolutionary 'enlightenment' mission to the new circumstances.

Hugo Klajn, a prominent prewar psychiatrist and psychoanalyst who treated large numbers of partisan hysterics at the very end of the war in Belgrade, made it clear that in his opinion it was 'likely that the unenlightened nature of our peoples contributed to the spread of hysterical reactions in this war'.[22] The correct attitude of the broader society to the patients should be that 'of a mature educator towards an immature pupil'.[23] The upwardly mobile illiterate peasant or unqualified worker was constructed as an unruly student, whose behaviour needed to be put in order by a sympathetic yet firm and authoritative teacher-psychiatrist. Therefore, if the newly emerging social elite was lacking a proper upbringing and education and needed to be enlightened, the psychiatrists reserved that role for themselves from the outset.

It was in the discussion around partisan hysteria that Yugoslav psychiatry demonstrated some of its most pronounced similarities with colonial psychiatric frameworks, primarily in its infantilisation of the partisan war neurotics. Because they were primarily very young—often teenagers or young adolescents—as well as of rural background and with little formal education, these patients were regularly constructed as unreasonable children—just as West European colonial psychiatrists developed the 'infantilism thesis' to construct 'primitive' African societies as stuck in the childhood stage of humanity and in need of superior Western leadership. Klajn opined that the illness was a 'sign of a certain slowdown in development, certain infantilism', or an 'underdevelopment of character'. In Croatian military psychiatrist Josip Dojč's opinion, the most common war neurotic was a 'young infantile and primitive' person; their neurotic seizures could be compared to 'some sort of infantile reaction of spite, similar to those by ill-bred small children, if parents don't fulfil their wishes. In the same way, these children throw themselves on the floor,

[22] Hugo Klajn, *Ratna neuroza Jugoslovena*, 149.

[23] Ibid., 151.

cry, scream, hit around with their hands and legs, in order to provoke pity, compassion or concern of those around them and achieve their goals in that way'.[24] Klajn's psychoanalytic colleague Betlheim agreed: 'it is known that the psyche of a hysteric is in many ways similar to the psyche of the underdeveloped, that there are many infantile traits in it. Our war neurotics are mostly youngsters, people with unfinished puberty ... similar to spiteful children, who throw themselves down, bite themselves and others, pull themselves and others for the hair etc.'. Furthermore, they were 'full of theatricality in a primitive way', and their urges were 'egocentric' and 'autistic'.[25] Therefore, 'primitivism' and childlike qualities went hand in hand in these diagnoses, as the doctors wrote with increasing alarm about the immature and incompetent yet overly ambitious 'primitives' taking over the new state and benefiting from revolutionary upward social mobility. Moreover, those psychiatrists who took a tougher line conflated primitivism and intellectual underdevelopment with psychological pathology and illness, referring to ill soldiers as 'psychopaths' as well as the 'weak-minded' or the 'intellectually insufficient'.

The main psychiatric focus was then to explore how to overcome this explosion of hysterical seizures, and how to contain the 'primitive' urges of their patients. As we saw above, Klajn emphasised a rather original 'pedagogical therapy', aimed at re-educating and enlightening the core of the patients' personalities. He spoke in favour of not only the need to educate the broadest social sectors about mental health and genesis of psychiatric illness, but also to engage in a much more all-encompassing agenda for popular edification.[26] Furthermore, the problem of partisan neurosis was primarily socio-political rather than medical or psychiatric. Medical attention needed to be accompanied by 'intensive political, cultural-educational and military work according to a special plan', and it was the latter that was truly vital as a therapeutic strategy.[27] To fight the aggressive mental condition, medical doctors needed to eliminate the educational, cultural and political backwardness of the up and coming peasant soldiers. The patient—unruly, disruptive child—stood in a subordinate position

[24] Josip Dojč, 'O biti zivcanih napadaja u ratu (ratna neuroza)', *Vojno-Sanitetski Pregled (VSP),* 1946, 3, 118.

[25] Stjepan Betlheim, 'Samoostecenja kod ratnih neuroticara', *VSP*, 1946, 3, 331–333.

[26] Klajn, *Ratna neuroza Jugoslovena*, 149–151.

[27] Arhiv Sanitetske sluzbe Ministarstva odbrane, R-19, Dr. Šalek, "Neuropatija (slicna histeriji)", 2.

to the psychiatrist-teacher, who now assumed the role of a social and cultural enlightener, or was in any case to be vitally involved in devising the plan for an ambitious educational elevation of the masses. Other, more pessimistic psychiatrists, such as Dojc or even Betlheim, insisted on much broader psychological testing to weed out the 'incompetent' and the psychopathic or neuropathic.[28] In both cases, psychiatrists were to play a vital role in addressing the most serious political crisis since the end of the war. Their own 'civilising mission' did not seem to change in any fundamental conceptual or clinical way, now that 'primitive' patients who suddenly overwhelmed psychiatric hospitals with their violent 'hysterical' seizures had a much higher political and social standing on account of their wartime contributions.

And while 'partisan hysteria' proved to be a relatively short-lived crisis—by 1955, a group of psychiatrists determined that a majority of the patients succeeded in 'outgrowing' the condition without serious consequences—some of the issues raised in these debates continued to influence the psychiatric discourse for decades to come. In the period after the break with the Soviet Union in 1948, Yugoslav psychiatrists increasingly focused on the traditional Balkan family, as a social institution in need of urgent reform in a socialist society and as a symbol of the Yugoslav society's persistent cultural backwardness. However, criticisms of family and family relations first appeared in relation to partisan hysteria. In his December 1944 report from the front on war neuroses in his division, military doctor Šalek interpreted 'partisan neurosis' as a problem of flawed upbringing quite literally. Namely, since the first instances of neurotic seizures appeared in the area of the Kozara mountain in Bosnia and later spread from there, Šalek averred that the cause for this could be found in the collective psychological character of the region, whose 'people are oversensitive, proud, touchy, ambitious, impulsive and explosive. Children are very spoiled, and spoiled children have a lot of difficulties facing disappointments when they grow up'.[29]

In other words, the poor upbringing of these partisan soldiers resulted in their destructive and pathological reactions to criticism and feelings of

[28] Stjepan Betlhaim, 'Samoostecenja kod ratnih neuroticara', VSP, 3:7–8, 1946, 331–333; Ruth Betlheim and Gordana Lerotic, *Stjepan Betlhaim: Radovi, pisma, dokumenti, 1898–1970*, Zagreb: Antibarbarus, 2006, 100.

[29] Arhiv Sanitetske sluzbe Ministarstva odbrane, R-19, Dr. Šalek, 'Podaci o ratnim neurozama', 246.

failure and injustice, and, by extension, demonstrated that both psychiatric and political interventions in family relations were necessary. Šalek zoomed in on the deficiencies of personal upbringing (characteristic for the peasant communities in the area) and the consequent lack of intellectual, political and cultural sophistication of his patients. He reportedly mostly observed neurotic conflicts in those persons whose general sociocultural awareness was low and self-love and egocentrism powerful: 'the only thing that could have helped was proper upbringing, and that was lacking....Mothers adore their children and precisely for that reason they don't raise them with enough discipline', which resulted in frequent violence and self-will.[30] The spread of hysterical reactions was thus going to be interrupted when psychiatrists succeeded in implementing appropriate corrective measures to reverse the loose, unruly manners that the patients had adopted as a result of their undisciplined childhood upbringing in a mountainous peasant community.

For Yugoslavia's thriving psychiatric and psychotherapeutic community in the 1950s and 1960s, the issue of family relations and in particular the upbringing of children became a vital professional as well as political concern. As we will see in the next chapter, the psychiatric profession took active part in discussion around the role of families in the creation of democratic and humanist socialism. Child psychiatrists and psychotherapists in particular became increasingly critical of the most prevalent form of parent–child relationships in Yugoslavia, arguing that such traditional and authoritarian family models might have deleterious psychological consequences and could actively prevent the formation of responsible and assertive socialist citizens. Unsurprisingly, these later generations of psychotherapists were less concerned about undisciplined or disruptive children and agitated for more democratic families, although they certainly shared Salek's belief that overly spoiled children were rather problematic, primarily because they remained unprepared for independent life and autonomous social and political engagement in adulthood.

According to Vojin Matić, family remained one of the core social institutions tasked with instilling conformism and practicing violence and coercion, the 'last bastion of state violence' even in an advanced democratic society. Even in the context of socialist workers' self-management in Yugoslavia, individual and discrete 'areas of coercion' were allowed to

[30] Ibid., 2.

continue existing unaffected, so that everyone 'had a tacit opportunity to play the role of a dictator in their own sphere, allegedly for "common good."' It was within families that such impulses for perpetrating violence and aggression were at their most potent, as the 'aggressive believed that their goal had to be achieved regardless of means'.[31] In the Yugoslav case, the persistent patriarchy of the 'archaic' family model further fed this violent cycle. As it transpired, the 'primitive' traits of psychiatric patients and the society at large now threatened to endanger the revolutionary project of building a truly free Marxist community.

Child psychiatrists and psychotherapists focused their critical attention on those parents who saw a threat in their children's 'healthy tendencies to emancipation and expansion' and who actively sought to 'throttle impatiently and radically any impulses for independence and spontaneous activity' in their children.[32] Such behaviour on the part of parents tended to have dire psychological as well as political consequences, and produced children who 'never opposed anything' and became insecure, unspontaneous, permanently indecisive, passive and subordinated, lacking independence. Psychiatrists wrote critically of those parents who were 'conservative and lacked culture', and were, as a result, unable to create a healthy environment for raising children.[33] Such disciplinarian approaches were common in traditional hierarchical and patriarchal families, which reportedly had little respect for children's independent thought and activity, and little interest in strengthening children's autonomous personalities. In Yugoslavia, parents often 'beat their children venting their own personal dissatisfaction on them. For the smallest thing, they insult children using most appalling expressions, terrify them with unspeakable threats. In other words, they lose control. Then they forget that, but the child never forgets'.[34]

But Yugoslavia's traditional families could swing from aggression and emotional detachment to material and emotional overprotectiveness. Indeed, Yugoslavia's leading child psychiatrist Nevenka Tadic argued that, in addition to overt authoritarianism of Yugoslav 'primitive' and

[31] Vojin Matić, 'Izmene dinamike odnosa prema autoritetu i njene posledice u klinickoj psihologiji', *Psihologija*, 1977, 13:2.

[32] Ibid., 8–9.

[33] Ljiljana Milosavljevic, 'Neka zapazanja o ponasanju bolesnog deteta', *Psihologija*, 1977, 10:2, 89–93.

[34] Tadic and Matić, 'Psihoterapija dece', *Psihijatrija Danas*, 1976, 1–2, 65–82.

archaic families, another cultural specialty was the parents' tendency to overprotectiveness: preventing the child's individualisation and emancipation, harming the process of gaining social independence, prolonging the dependent and indebted status of children into late childhood or even puberty and adolescence.[35] This tendency, although at first glance the exact opposite of the emotional coldness of authoritarianism, was rooted in the same phenomenon: the parents' lack of awareness of and respect for the child's individuality as a human being/citizen, their reluctance to give up their traditional, even conservative ('ossified') value systems in their relations with their adolescent child, or even their hidden hostility to and rejection of the child. Moreover, the two phenomena characteristic of the Yugoslav family had the same result: they failed to raise an independent and self-assured personality who had the confidence to find and express his or her own voice in social and personal issues.

It was clear that Yugoslav families were changing dramatically in the second half of the twentieth century, and the psychiatric profession, now thoroughly internationalised and closely acquainted with the most recent trends in child psychoanalysis as well as Western radical psychiatry, were prepared to act as supervisors of the transformation. Weeding out the lingering authoritarianism, patriarchy and backwardness in Yugoslavia's increasingly urbanised families had an explicit political value, and child psychiatrists and psychotherapists in particular used the consulting room to redraw traditional family relations and defend their child patients' right to equality and respect. Throughout the postwar decades, they sided with children as the 'oppressed' and taught 'uncultured' parents how to recognise and react to their children's finer emotions, sensibilities and inner struggles. Most importantly, in this new phase of the struggle against primitivism, the Yugoslav population was meant to reform its relationship to authorities and hierarchies, which had to be initiated in families first as it was in these crucial social institutions that children learnt obedience, dependence and helplessness. Again, child psychiatrists were to play a major role in this far-reaching social transformation: while definitions of the concept of modernity might have been significantly different under socialism, the psychiatric (and psychoanalytic) profession once again positioned itself at the helm of modernisation and emancipation, and considered itself vital to creating a functioning society based on

[35] Nevenka Tadic, personal email to author, 7 February 2014.

workers' self-management. The project of building 'new socialist men and women' depended on this struggle against (psychological) backwardness.

Peripherality, Global South and European Civilisation: Non-aligned Psychiatry

In the international context, the peripheral position of Yugoslavia remained a tremendously important factor for psychiatric discussions throughout the twentieth century. If Yugoslav 'psy' professionals adopted some of the core concepts and frameworks of colonial psychiatry when they treated and wrote about their own patients, they were acutely aware that they themselves belonged to a society which most of their Western colleagues considered to be lagging behind scientifically and culturally. In the interwar years, this position was logically difficult to sustain: while patients were often dismissed as well as pathologised because of their inability or unwillingness to partake in the discourses of modern medicine, in the international arena Yugoslav psychiatrists' efforts were focused on proving that the South Slavs did after all belong—biologically or civilisationally—to the European family of nations, and that they should not be compared to colonised non-European subjects and cultures. The paradox still remained, however: the profession's growing pessimism regarding their ability to implement their own civilising mission and modernise their patient population clashed painfully with their attempts to muster scientific evidence that Yugoslavs were indeed no different from Europeans in any fundamental sense. Interestingly, psychiatric epidemiological information could be and was regularly used as an indicator of cultural and civilisational progress, alongside other types of public health data. Therefore, this conditional Europeanness of the Balkan region significantly complicated the interwar psychiatric theories and, to an extent, clinical practices.

On the other hand, following 1945 and the constitution of a socialist government in the country, international links, exchanges and collaborations of Yugoslav medical scientists, including psychiatrists, changed quite dramatically. After 1948, the swift removal of Yugoslavia from the auspices of the Soviet bloc meant that the country was looking for its own alternative model of socialism as well as of conducting international relations without joining either of the two blocs.[36] The rather ingenious politics of non-alignment emerged as a solution which did not undermine Yugoslavia's political and cultural relationships with the Western world but also brought it much closer to the Global South.[37] Within the framework of non-alignment, Yugoslav practitioners got an opportunity for the first time to engage directly with colonial medical and psychiatric theoretical legacies and practices, as Yugoslav psychiatrists and medical doctors took part in a variety of East-South collaborative projects and exchanges, in the course of which they travelled to the former colonial territories to offer their expertise. This was indeed a unique historical moment for psychiatrists: for the first time, they were offered a possibility to compare their 'primitive' Yugoslav patients with those from societies characterised in colonial contexts by an altogether different kind of 'primitivism.'

These extraordinary encounters—between formerly colonised subjects and white doctors coming from the anti-colonial world—were supremely complex, not least because the official political condemnation of colonialism on the Yugoslav side did clash with psychiatrists' often fairly Eurocentric conceptualisations of development, modernity and backwardness. At the same time, the peripheral position of Yugoslavia (the perpetual problem of its conditional belonging to the 'European civilisation') and its leading role in the Non-Aligned Movement did seem to move the country to the South, closer to African and Asian societies, so that the Balkan region could now to some extent be compared (and comparable) to the decolonising territories.

This complicated political-psychiatric balancing thus marked the profession's exploration of primitivism and Yugoslavia's road to modernity in the socialist era. As we already saw, the socialist revolution did not radically alter Yugoslav psychiatrists' attitudes towards their own mission of modernisation of their patients, and their attempts to engage critically with colonial psychiatry in the global South while retaining the predominantly colonial ideas about 'primitivism' and underdevelopment produced

[36] Svetozar Rajak, 'No Bargaining Chips, No Spheres of Interest: The Yugoslav Origins of Cold War Non-alignment', *Journal of Cold War Studies*, 2014, 16:1.

[37] Vladimir Kulic, 'Building the Non-aligned Babel: Babylon Hotel in Baghdad and Mobile Design in the Global Cold War', *Architecture Beyond Europe*, 2014, 6; Ljubica Spaskovska, 'Constructing the "City of International Solidarity": Non-aligned Internationalism, the United Nations and Visions of Development, Modernism and Solidarity, 1955–1975', *Journal of World History*, 2020, 31:3, 137–163.

some surprising results. Indeed, Yugoslav psychiatry used the concept of primitivism to refer to 'uncultured', unsophisticated and uneducated European (or East European) populations, but the term, of course, had a significantly different meaning when it applied to 'civilisational' primitivism of the non-European world. In fascinating ways, the non-aligned engagements of Yugoslav psychiatrists forced them to reflect more systematically on the difference between the two meanings, and on the possible implications of that difference for the position of socialist Yugoslavia on the global axis of modernity.

In the interwar years, Yugoslav psychiatrists found it deeply unsettling that such deeply ingrained backwardness and primitivism of the society meant that the South Slavic population was considered culturally and biologically inferior by the Western nations. Sučić was particularly concerned that 'the South Slavs had stopped being a nation – they became common people [raja], despised by the cultured world'. Moreover, 'being a Slav, a Serb, a Croat or a Bulgarian meant being – uneducated, poor, oppressed … being: filthy and tattered'.[38] From Sučić's and Stanojević's points of view, it would thus prove understandably difficult to conform collectively to what was perceived as the norms of the civilised world, and ultimately win full acceptance into the European society of nations. This was one of the burning questions posed and debated by Yugoslavia's interwar intellectual and political elite: whether the Yugoslav peoples truly belonged to the civilised European West, or whether their geographical location or historical experience permanently tainted their mentality and national character. Psychiatrists once again established themselves as the most competent participants in the discussion.

Moreover, they had long perceived psychiatric illness as an indicator of sorts of socio-cultural modernity or otherwise of national and ethnic groups. The 'psychopathological index' of a culture also defined what position that culture occupied along the axis of civilisation. Such reasoning necessarily presupposed an essential link between modernity and pathology, and suggested that the pattern and character of 'racial psychoses' could reveal salient information about a nation's mental and cultural set-up. This was, in turn, based on one of the core assumptions of colonial psychiatry—that 'primitive' colonised societies suffered lower rates of mental illness because of the reported inherent simplicity of

[38] Sucic, *Bolesti zivaca i duse*, 10–11.

their communal and undifferentiated minds, which were then incapable of developing complex psychopathologies. Therefore, in the early twentieth century, Yugoslav psychiatrists engaged in a dialogue with their Western and Central European colleagues regarding the value and viability of comparative psychiatry, agreeing with colonial psychiatrists that qualitative and quantitative differences in patterns of mental pathology were directly related to the core features—and 'primitivism'—of national, racial or ethnic groups. If biological psychiatry could prove the 'racial' or 'genetic' closeness of the Yugoslav (or East European) peoples to their German or Western counterparts, then the problems stemming from historical backwardness or cultural primitivism might not present such an enormous obstacle to advancement and reform: the common 'racial' core of all the European peoples, expressed through commonalities in the distribution and frequency of various types of psychiatric illnesses, could conceivably override the weight of retrograde historical experiences.

In an instructive series of articles published in Serbia's most important medical journal of the time, neurologist Vladimir Vujić rejected and protested the research findings of those foreign scholars—most famously Eugen Bleuler—who placed Yugoslavs alongside 'North Africans, Abyssinians,... Turks, Australian blacks' because of their reported particular resilience to general (progressive) paralysis, in spite of a high incidence of syphilitic infections.[39] Vujić countered these claims with the hospital statistical data which confirmed syphilitic dementia to be one of the most common psychoses for Yugoslavs—in fact, the rate of progressive paralysis in the Belgrade psychiatric hospital conformed to, or even exceeded, that of the Leipzig and Freiburg hospitals. To him, this meant that Yugoslavs took part in the modern, civilised distribution of this disorder, which set them firmly apart from the 'primitive' groups mentioned above, even if this meant many more people in Yugoslav hospitals diagnosed with an apparently irreversible degenerative lethal illness. The same results Vujić ascertained with regard to two psychoses—schizophrenia and manic-depressive psychosis (bipolar disorder), except that 'schizophrenia was more frequent among Slavs and Jews than among Germans and Hungarians, but those differences were not considerable'.[40]

[39] Vladimir Vujic, 'Prilog uporednoj psihijatriji naroda o psihozama kod Srba I', *Srpski Arhiv*, 1934, sv. 9, 742.

[40] Ibid., 744.

As long as the general rates and patterns conformed to the Western findings, certain inconsistencies, dissimilarities and unevenness were allowed; in fact, they were, in Vujic's opinion, most probably a result of a particularly unfortunate set of historical circumstances and the consequent cultural backwardness: the lower rate of depressive and melancholic disorders (in comparison with manias) among the Serbian population, for instance, Vujić saw as a function of primitive popular beliefs and superstitions, which abounded in furious witches and other aggressive fantasies. These in turn shaped the collective consciousness and expressions of mental pathology.[41]

Vujić also vehemently disagreed with Viennese psychiatrist Emil Mattauschek, who claimed that Bosnians and Herzegovinians suffered extraordinarily frequently from epilepsy and hysteria, which indicated a higher incidence of hereditary degeneracy, and with Kraepelin, who echoed Mattauschek's views with regard to the Slavic propensity to hysteria. In fact, Vujić documented that the rates of both epilepsy and hysteria in Serbia and Yugoslavia never exceeded those calculated in Dutch, German and Swiss clinics.[42] In other words, Yugoslavs were European biologically but backward historically and, according to the distribution and rates of mental illnesses in Yugoslavia, biology did after all succeed in overpowering the negative historical experiences, a conclusion that allowed a modicum of optimism and professional self-confidence, especially in the organic framework of the interwar European psychiatry. It was, however, still unclear how the transition from primitivism to civilisation would occur.

In this regard, socialist psychiatry had a distinct advantage over its interwar predecessor in its wholesale embrace of psychotherapeutic and psychoanalytic methods as educational strategies, and in its focus on social aspects of mental health and illness. Moreover, the very civilisational superiority of the West was not unquestioned and unconditional anymore: the socialist East proposed a different, more ethically conscious and ultimately more worthy form of modernity This did not automatically translate into any fundamental changes in the psychiatric discourse of 'catching up' with the West, as we will see below, but at least the Western ideal

[41] Ibid., 745.

[42] Ibid.

was not constructed and defined in an uncritical and uniformly positive way anymore, and both psychiatrists and other intellectuals could discuss the (supposedly hierarchical) cultural relationship between Eastern and Western Europe in more flexible and innovative terms. Moreover, Yugoslavia played a critical role in the creation of the Non-Aligned Movement, and this dramatic restructuring of its international links and alliances bred a new political language of anti-colonialism, anti-racism and solidarity with the decolonising world. This new orientation influenced psychiatric thinking as well, especially when the psychiatric profession was involved with the Global South. Still, the socialist conceptualisation of progress and development remained firmly linear, and the notions of 'primitivism', backwardness and underdevelopment continued to be used regularly in both political and psychiatric parlance. In that sense, Yugoslav socialist psychiatrists were in a complex intellectual position, and were often hard pressed to reconcile their theories of modernisation and 'primitive' patients with the fierce political anti-colonialism of the non-aligned movement.

Quite surprisingly, socialist psychiatry was often quite slow to shed some important colonial tenets and conceptualisations. Vladimir Jakovljević, who was Eastern Europe's most prominent and prolific transcultural psychiatrist, tended to agree with John Collin Carothers' that the 'civilised world' was generally characterised by higher frequencies of 'complex' mental pathology, and concluded that Yugoslavia certainly belonged to the culturally and socially advanced European family of nations.[43] Even in the 1960s, a Yugoslav psychiatrist found it vital to emphasise that the country was on a par with Western Europe—a thesis which guided his prewar colleagues and which clearly survived the dramatic ideological transformations of 1945. During his long stay in Guinea in the early 1960s, where he helped develop local psychiatric services, he regularly referred not only to his Guinean patients but also to Guinea's social and cultural structures as 'primitive' and 'oriental'. At the same time, and despite Jakovljević's pronouncements regarding Yugoslavia's civilisational 'Europeanness', the conditionality and peripherality of his own country's position still haunted his writings, and so did his descriptions of his Yugoslav patients.

[43] John Collin Carothers, 'A Study of Mental Derangement in Africans, and an Attempt to Explain Its Peculiarities, More Especially in Relation to the African Attitude to Life', *East African Medical Journal*, 1948, 25:4, 142–166.

In the southernmost parts of Yugoslavia, for instance, the rate of neurosis among the general population was reportedly less than a half of the neurotic morbidity in 'civilised countries'. This was one of the more incontrovertible indicators of the society's comparative civilisational position; moreover, it was the more 'primitive neurotic disorders' which prevailed in the Yugoslav society over more complex and intellectualised ones commonly found in countries like France. Yugoslav patients expressed their mental pathology in more primitive, non-verbal and psychosomatic ways; by contrast, West European neurotics were characterised by complex psychopathological mechanisms and advanced abstract forms of thinking.[44] Even though Jakovljević insisted that such differences were ultimately of a merely quantitative type, and were superseded by the overall similarity of (civilisationally conditioned) clinical symptoms, he still made it abundantly clear that Yugoslavia (and Macedonia) were marked by 'extreme forms of backwardness' in certain important social and cultural aspects. According to his own clinical-anthropological observations, this was a 'primitive society experiencing rapid advancement', and his Yugoslav patients' levels of cultural education and modernity were by all accounts comparable to those of the Africans whom he encountered and treated.[45] Somewhat surprisingly, it was this uncertainty about Yugoslavia's own cultural identity that made socialist psychiatrists' transcultural musings much more complex and ultimately more progressive than those of both their Western colleagues and their interwar counterparts: as they engaged in clinical work and ethnographic research, Jakovljević and his collaborators could not but draw indirect parallels between the Yugoslav and African experiences and hardships as both regions embarked on revolutionary paths of liberation and faced comparable challenges of rapid, highly disruptive modernisation.

Precisely because of this, as we will see in Chapter 5, Yugoslavia's transcultural psychiatry constructed a more dynamic and optimistic image of 'primitive' decolonising societies. While Yugoslav psychiatrists' ideas of modernity and progress remained inflexible, they could not accept one of colonial psychiatry's core tropes—that non-European colonised societies, with their simplistic and underdeveloped minds, were static

[44] Jakovljević, 'Doprinos Proucavanju Uloge Psiholoskih Uticaja Sociokulturne Sredine u Patogenezi Neuroza', *Neuropsihijatrija*, 7, 1–2 (1959).

[45] Jakovljević, 'Prilog Proucavanju Sociopsihogeneze Neurotickih Poremecaja Licnosti', *Sociologija*, 2 (1959).

and largely incapable of development and modernisation, which regularly caused extraordinarily high rates of mental pathology in the 'native' population. This approach was part and parcel of the colonial 'infantilism thesis', which proposed that African cultures were permanently stuck in the 'childhood stage of humanity', providing an insight into the nature and state of the human race before 'civilisation'. First and foremost, such a static and pessimistic approach would not have boded well for Yugoslavia, which faced its own developmental psychological and cultural hardships following the revolutionary social transformations after 1945. But equally importantly, Jakovljević and his collaborators were primarily social psychiatrists. While the interwar psychiatric profession searched for biological proofs of Yugoslavia's civilisational status, their postwar Marxist colleagues focused instead on complex socio-economic structures and developments, and their largely positive effects on 'backward' and modernising societies. Even though he could not get away from a hierarchical framework of thinking, Jakovljević still believed in the ability of 'primitive' societies to overcome such difficulties in the context of modernisation, learn and transform quickly, and ultimately construct complex and progressive cultural, political and social institutions. It was this rejection of purely biological and organicist frameworks that made socialist psychiatrists more convincing as they criticised colonial practices: Yugoslavia and Guinea must both 'catch up' with Western levels of modernity and civilisation, but they were supremely capable of doing so and doing it successfully—perhaps as demonstrated by the partisan hysterics of 1945, who were all declared cured with no consequences within a decade.

This, of course, raises much broader questions about Yugoslavia's and Eastern Europe's cultural identity. In terms of their political self-perceptions, socialist Eastern Europe and Yugoslavia still remained centrally attached to the idea of 'Europe' as a benchmark of civilisation. Not only transcultural psychiatrists but also a host of other intellectuals and political commentators often relied on orientalising, racist, Eurocentric and essentially colonial discourses of the white West. This was qualified by the experience and ideology of socialism, as well as, in the Yugoslav case, by the practices and discourses of non-alignment. But it remains unclear how influential the NAM was in transforming socialist Eastern Europe's orientalising tendencies. At times, it did appear that official political declarations related to the importance of non-alignment aimed to take Yugoslavia outside of Europe altogether, and in the very least, they portrayed Yugoslavia as a particularly understanding and compassionate partner to the decolonising world.[46] The introduction of a 1979 special issue of the communist youth journal *Nase teme*, dedicated to the African continent, referred to Yugoslavia and Yugoslavs as having a 'particular African vocation', emphasising the country's close links with Africa and longstanding commitment to Africa's independence.[47]

Furthermore, even though the Balkan region might have seen itself as politically, geographically and civilisationally European (even under socialism), its historical legacy was one of imperial subjects rather than imperial rulers, and the attachment to a 'European identity' was accompanied by narratives of cultural inferiority and experiences of rejection by Europe. In that sense, non-aligned Yugoslavia's geopolitical and civilisational status was permanently unstable.[48] The psychiatric profession engaged in lengthy comparative discussions of socialist, Western and African psyches, and such discussions, which were thus far left entirely unresearched, offer a unique insight into the nature and complexity of non-aligned Yugoslavia's political and cultural vacillation in the triangle between the East, West and South.

Yugoslavia's discourses of non-aligned solidarity have been criticised harshly by some scholars. Jelena Subotić and Srdjan Vučetić refer to Yugoslavia's NAM-inspired anti-imperialism as an exercise in 'performing solidarity' with the Third World for the purposes of advancing the country's international political status but without any fundamental understanding of the problem of racism and racial relations in the Cold War world. Subotić and Vučetić focus on political discursive practices of the Yugoslav leadership as well as on some aspects of the 'lived experience' of non-alignment in Yugoslavia to argue that the country's embrace of the language of non-aligned solidarity was primarily opportunistic and did not reflect a truly emancipatory ideological orientation.[49] This was mainly because, as the authors write, Yugoslavia cherished its cultural identity as a white European state, and developed a 'superiority complex' in its relationships with its African and Asian partners. Moreover, Yugoslav

[46] Rajak, 'No Bargaining Chips, No Spheres of Interest', 179.

[47] *Nase Teme*, 1979, 23:3.

[48] Catherine Baker, *Race and the Yugoslav Region: Post-Socialist, post-Conflict, Postcolonial?*, Manchester: Manchester University Press, 2018.

[49] Jelena Subotic and Srdjan Vucetic, 'Performing Solidarity: Whiteness and Status-Seeking in the Non-aligned World', *Journal of International Relations and Development*, 2019, 22, 722–743.

leaders themselves often expressed dismissive, even racialised opinions about the decolonising countries (and their understanding of socialism),[50] while African and Asian students in Yugoslavia regularly faced physical and verbal abuse from the local population, and were systematically ostracised.[51] Therefore, the Yugoslav political leadership's arguments that their solidarity with the decolonising world was based on their country's comparable experiences of colonial oppression (in the Habsburg and Ottoman empires) and its successful war of liberation/independence in WWII were constantly undermined by the Yugoslavs' failure to reflect on their own 'white privilege' in a thoroughly racialised world.

This lack of reflection was often obvious in public and political representations of African societies and individuals (and of Yugoslav leaders visiting African countries)—such images tended to exoticise 'distant' cultures and relied on well-used colonial tropes, symbols and interpretations, even though they officially promoted messages of anticolonialism, solidarity and anti-racism. As Sladojević has convincingly argued, the Yugoslav narrative of anticolonial solidarity between Eastern Europe and Africa might have contributed to this limited reflection. The Yugoslav leadership and intellectual insisted that Yugoslavia was capable of developing a special understanding of and relationship with its NAM partners primarily because, despite being white and European, it was never the coloniser and never engaged in imperial oppression.[52] However, this position seemed to release Yugoslavia from any need for a critical reconsideration of its own contributions to the old colonial order, or the perpetuation of racialised discourses of Africa and the Global South after decolonisation.

In some ways, these criticisms were undoubtedly founded, and applicable to the psychiatric profession's experiences. For instance, Yugoslav psychiatrists' relationship to their African colleagues and hosts was one

[50] Rajak, 'No Bargaining Chips, No Spheres of Interest', 146–179.

[51] Milorad Lazic, 'Neki problemi stranih studenata na jugoslovenskim univerzitetima šezdesetih godina XX veka, s posebnim osvrtom na afričke studente [Some problems of foreign students at Yugoslav universities in the 1960s, with special focus on African students]', *Godišnjak za društvenu istoriju* 2009, 2, 61–78.

[52] Ana Sladojevic, 'Beyond the Photographic Frame: Interpretation of Photographs from the Museum of Yugoslavia's Collection in a Contemporary Context', in Radina Vučetić and Paul Betts, eds, *Tito in Africa: Picturing Solidarity*, Belgrade: Museum of Yugoslavia, 2017.

of (benevolent) hierarchy as much as of solidarity—they were there to teach and guide, export an original socialist model of modernisation and offer an alternative to the failed colonial project. Even though they could detect similarities between African and Yugoslav (or Balkan) experiences and historical structures, they (and other experts who travelled southward from Eastern Europe) still considered themselves to be self-evidently in a superior position and significantly more advanced along the axis of modernisation.[53] Furthermore, their repeated references to the Guinean society's both economic and cultural 'primitivism' and underdevelopment indicated that the Yugoslav psychiatric profession divided the world into 'civilised' and 'uncivilised' parts, and thereby established a fundamental distinction between 'European' Yugoslavia and 'backward' Africa (see Chapter 5).

On the other hand, NAM-related practices and languages of solidarity went well beyond political discourses and international students' complaints. While at times references to the Balkans' and Africa's shared past as victims of colonial oppression rang hollow, narratives of solidarity fundamentally shaped a variety of aspects of Yugoslavia's collaboration with its NAM partners. Such narratives also played a major part in different fields of knowledge and art production in Yugoslavia. These expressions of solidarity were, of course, directly linked to the country's immediate political goals, but they were not entirely cynical or superficial. The shared experiences of fighting resistance wars and handling dramatic consequences of rapid social and political transformations further reinforced the political and cultural bonds which developed between Yugoslavia and its NAM partners.[54] African history and contemporary politics, and in particular African socialism, became important fields of research, and a lot of space was dedicated to these topics in Yugoslavia's public discourse as well as in more specialised scholarly journals. Moreover, different sections of the Yugoslav society became deeply committed

[53] For a similar argument regarding the broader political and cultural discourse in Yugoslavia, see Sladojevic, *Images of Africa*, Belgrade: Museum of Contemporary Art, 2015.

[54] Paul Betts, 'A Red Wind of Change: African Press Coverage of Tito's Visits to Decolonizing Africa', in Vucetic and Betts, *Tito in Africa*, 46–77.

to spreading the message of anti-colonialism and solidarity, often without any ulterior motives or hidden selfish interests.[55]

The psychiatric profession contributed significantly to this increase in the production of more sophisticated knowledge about the decolonising world. And because their research was often explicitly comparative, it shed important light on the reconceptualisation of the relationship between the Balkans and Africa. As we will see in Chapter 5, Jakovljević's involvement in the Guinean mental health scene was complex, both problematic and much more progressive than that of his Western colleagues. In many ways, Yugoslav psychiatrists' and medical experts' engagement with the Global South were influenced by their collaboration with Western European institutions as much as by the Yugoslav non-aligned political orientation. It was his involvement with French psychiatry which originally sparked Jakovljević's interest in the decolonising world, largely because such transcultural research was gaining supreme importance in 1950s and 1960s Western Europe.

But as we saw above, it was precisely these comparisons between Yugoslav and French patients that threw in sharp relief the insecure position of Yugoslavia (and the Balkan region) as European entities. After he started his clinical and ethnographic work in Guinea, Jakovljević's descriptions of his Macedonian and his Guinean patients occasionally became virtually indistinguishable even though he never acknowledged these similarities explicitly—both groups reportedly characterised by comparable degrees of individual and collective backwardness, and confusion in the face of rapid modernisation and change—while most of the French patients he encountered during his specialisation in Paris seemed to come from an altogether different civilisation despite some broad pan-European structural similarities.[56] It was such psychiatric work more than any other political or intellectual discourse that emphasised the deep ambivalence of Yugoslavia's cultural status. In terms of socio-cultural relations,

[55] Leo Mates, *Nesvrstanost: teorija i savremena praksa [Non-alignment: Theory and Contemporary Practice]*. Belgrade: Izdanje Instituta za međunarodnu politiku i privredu, 1970.

[56] Jakovljević, 'Doprinos Proucavanju Uloge Psiholoskih Uticaja Sociokulturne Sredine u Patogenezi Neuroza'; see also Jakovljević, *Kulturna sredina i psihički poremećaji ličnosti: transkulturno-psihijatrijsko proučavanje u Afričkoj Gvineji* (PhD thesis), University of Zagreb, 1967.

psychological profile, family structures and other social institutions, clinical and anthropological research demonstrated that Yugoslavia's largely rural population perhaps had a lot in common with the 'primitives' of the decolonising world. The two meanings of 'primitivism' finally came together.

But socialist non-aligned psychiatry was still based on radically different ideological premises, and could not fully adopt the colonial psychiatric framework of 'primitivism', even though it tended to use some of the same concepts. In that sense, the psychiatrists' first-hand discovery—even if it was never stated explicitly—that the Yugoslav population's 'backwardness' was not fundamentally different from the civilisational 'tribal primitivism' of 'native' African populations in fact worked to produce original transcultural psychiatric approaches, which at times challenged the colonial framework. In an important way, socialist psychiatrists failed in the project bequeathed to them by their interwar predecessors: to prove the Yugoslav people's civilisational affinity with Europe over other underdeveloped and 'backward' societies. However, in the context of socialist psychiatry, this failure was not so damning, and it enabled the development of a more inclusive discourse about the human psyche and its cross-cultural universality.

Postwar global transcultural psychiatry was based on the idea of universality of the core mechanisms of the human psyche irrespective of cultural or social differences. In their attempts to decolonise the profession and its intellectual paradigms, postwar psychiatrists embarked on a search for a new definition of common humanity and a global model of the human mind.[57] The universalism of immediate post-WWII transcultural psychiatry seemed to be taken for granted in the Yugoslav context: psychiatrists and anthropologists often emphatically insisted that Africans were as capable of logical and analytical thinking as Europeans.[58] In the 1970s, in an article on the notions of change and development in Africa, one of Yugoslavia's leading researchers in development studies and cross-cultural communication Nada Svob-Djokić ironically commended Western European researchers for finally concluding, decades after the end of colonial regimes, that 'the mental mechanism of Africans was no different than

[57] Heaton, *Black Skin, White Coats.*

[58] Biserka Cvjeticanin, 'Kontinuitet i dinamicnost africkih kultura', *Nase Teme*, 1979, 23:3, 785–795.

ours'.[59] But Yugoslav psychiatry's universalism rested on a unique idea of solidarity between the East European and African regions, and insisted on the comparability of their respective social and political experiences. Partly because of that and partly due to their Marxist focus on socio-economic determinants of mental health, Yugoslav clinicians avoided the exoticisation of cultural differences and narrowly defined cultural factors, a trend common in Western transcultural psychiatry.

In the early stages of decolonisation in particular, both psychiatrists and policymakers in the Western world were primarily concerned about the predicted psychological toll of cultural change and cross-cultural mixing. For some of the leading transcultural psychiatrists, dangers of 'acculturation' were tremendous, and they principally applied to less developed societies, who were experiencing fast-paced social, political and cultural transformations. As US psychiatrist Ari Kiev noted, acculturation and cultural change were only guaranteed to have harmful mental effects on underdeveloped and developing societies, while any pathological potential of similar cross-cultural influences in Western societies was not considered worthy of exploration.[60] The situation was rather unusual: while transcultural psychiatry, as a relatively new discipline, sought to establish a role for itself as a facilitator of harmonious cross-cultural communication, its West European representatives still viewed cross-cultural contact as a major source of mental pathology and worried about the ability of 'primitive' decolonising nations to adjust to rapid changes.

Marxist psychiatry, on the other hand, worried much less about the ability of 'primitive' societies to integrate and adapt to progressive cultural, political and technological transformations. Beyond the rigid organicist framework, socialist non-aligned psychiatry focused on the extraordinary developmental potential of 'primitive' societies, emphasising the possibility of successful social, cultural and psychological transformations in both Balkan and African societies. This ability to 'catch up' thus promised to erase the difference between 'backward' and 'civilised' societies in the near future. The therapeutic optimism of socialist psychiatry further reinforced the belief that progress and development could be achieved through cross-cultural exchange and

[59] Nada Svob-Djokic, *Nase Teme*, 1979, 23:4.

[60] Ari Kiev, *Transcultural Psychiatry*, New York: Free Press, 1972.

collaboration. In fact, Jakovljević's most important theoretical contribution—his concept of 'revolutionary personality'—emphasised the productive, creative and constructive, rather than pathological, potentials of dramatic social and cultural conflicts, which always accompanied revolutionary change or modernisation projects. In Jakovljević's reading, both the Yugoslav and the Guinean social revolutions were driven by such revolutionary personalities, whose ability to overcome unhealthy psychological influences and to thrive in their rapidly changing societies boded well for the second and the third worlds' ambitious developmental plans. In that sense, the idea that cross-cultural exchange and transformation were primarily pathogenic was certainly not dominant in East European transcultural psychiatry, perhaps precisely because the socialist profession did not prioritise cultural over social, political or economic factors and differences.

Furthermore, it was only in Eastern Europe that the notion of 'acculturation' in the specific context of decolonisation and rapid globalisation was interpreted in an explicitly positive way. For Yugoslav commentators and psychiatrists, for instance, it was of foremost importance to insist on the dynamic nature of African cultures and societies: writing against the idea that (sub-Saharan) African societies were static, ahistorical and marked by 'unchangeable traditions and tribal exoticism', Jakovljević's anthropologist colleague Biserka Cvjetičanin emphasised their dynamic history and their current creative grappling with large-scale changes. Before colonial conquests, during colonial regimes and after decolonisation, different African groups and societies experienced constant change both within the confines of their own borders and in contact with other cultures, so that their capability of dynamic development and transformation was in no fundamental way different from that of Western societies.[61]

Cvjetičanin introduced Marx's definition of acculturation—as a process of 'creation under the pressure of novel circumstances and by no means as a simple dissolution of a culture which suffered a blow from outside'. Moreover, Cvjetičanin was one of the very few voices who insisted that acculturation was a two-way process, which changed Western societies as well. It was no coincidence that this voice came from Marxist Eastern Europe: this intervention argued that the influence of African

[61] Cvjeticanin, 'Kontinuitet i dinamicnost africkih kultura'.

(non-Western cultures) on the Western world was not minuscule or non-existent.[62] Cvjetičanin warned that acculturation was not assimilation or a mechanical transplantation of certain traits and mores from a more developed society to a less developed one, but it meant 'transformation and creative integration'. In the course of this process, the receiving culture demonstrated its own dynamism and ability not only to adopt new elements but also to change them and ensure the authenticity and continuity of its own identity. In that sense, African cultures were neither mere imitators of more developed traditions nor unchangeable/ahistorical: just like all other societies, they chose which foreign elements and cultural aspects to adopt, adapt and fit in their own existing structures, thereby producing novel (dynamic and modern) creative totalities.

Finally, even those African groups or societies which proved more impervious to change and external influences were not static and paralysed in their rigid traditions: traditional culture was not necessarily an obstacle to progress but it should also be seen as a 'dynamic factor of development. It is natural for tradition to resist change. But that resistance in itself could cause change... Transformations are therefore resisted but such a conflict gives birth to new initiatives'.[63] African societies were not simply catching up, in other words, but producing authentic and valuable cultural contributions in the process of their rapid development and transformation. This was an insight crucially relevant for East European societies and their prospects.

Such optimistic takes on development, modernisation and progress, however, were not universal, even among the most prominent representatives of Yugoslavia's socialist academic elite. In fact, Yugoslav anthropological and psychological discussions of the global South produced one of the most forceful articulations of the idea of unbridgeable cultural differences between European and African 'minds'. Despite her general acceptance of the universality of psychological mechanisms of all human groups irrespectively of their cultures, even someone like Svob-Djokić could argue that Africans were indeed fundamentally, civilisationally (if not biologically) different from 'us'. Her approach demonstrated that the overall universalist framework and socialist anti-colonial rhetoric could easily coexist with essentialising and reifying interpretations of African

[62] Ibid., 789.

[63] Ibid., 790.

socio-cultural traditions. In fact, it was mainly because of this fundamental difference, marked by African cultures' specific relationship to individual as well as history, that, in African societies, changes and development were so difficult, slow and potentially harmful and pathological. As a result, 'we cannot say that African cultures witnessed a scientific model of thinking, nor developed any kind of philosophy'. Moreover, the African 'worldview' was mythological rather than scientific and historical, and 'did not accept a future, but was primarily oriented towards the past'.[64]

Even though Cvjeticanin, Jakovljević and many others argued against seeing Africa as a continent outside of history (or existing without history), Svob-Djokić came dangerously close: she concluded that, from the point of view of an African person, history was not 'a progression of human acts developing from the past towards the future' (i.e. linear) but a rhythmical 'series of events without a beginning and an end'—no progress was possible. Without any clear sense of future (or past), and without a workable concept of human agency, African societies as a whole struggled to accept foreign innovations and modernising trends. In this much more pessimistic view, 'change' and development could not mean creative integration and synthesis—the elements and cultures were simply too distinctive, and African societies' attempts at modernisation and progressive changes were often incompatible with traditional mores, which sometimes had catastrophic consequences, such as extreme turmoil, 'genocides of entire nations and tribes… and bloody repression of revolutions'.[65] And while for many Yugoslav intellectuals Africa's ability to progress and develop was unquestionable (just like Yugoslavia's was), Svob-Djokić's reading demonstrated that this could be constructed as a much more uncertain process. In 1979, this pessimistic take was not particularly surprising, but what was unexpected was the author's reading of the origins of the numerous economic, political and social problems faced by African countries several decades after decolonisation: instead of focusing in some detail on the negative effects of neo-colonialism (which she mentioned in passing), she essentialised Africa's 'traditions' and broad cultural patterns and blamed them for the continent's escalating crises.

[64] Svob-Djokic, 523.

[65] Ibid.

In insisting on the fundamental difference between Africans and 'us', Svob-Djokić left no doubt as to which of the two she considered a superior 'civilisation'. Here again, the civilisational and geopolitical instability of Yugoslavia's international position manifested itself in what Subotić and Vučetić termed the Yugoslav society's 'superiority complex' vis-à-vis the decolonising world, and Africa in particular. Just like in West European discourses of acculturation and cultural difference, the universalist framework, discussed in Yugoslav psychiatric and social sciences, could also incorporate hierarchical thinking, exoticising assumptions about cultural differences, and lingering colonial paradigms. In that sense, socialist psychiatric and anthropological articulations of the concepts of primitivism and civilisation remained complex and ambivalent. While the post-1945 development of new approaches and discourses often marked a departure from the interwar elaborations of civilisational hierarchies, the socialist psychiatric profession continued to construct the struggle against 'primitivism' within the Yugoslav society as its central task. This internal 'civilising mission' then largely determined how Yugoslavia's transcultural psychiatrists and anthropologists interpreted their own country's—and region's—position in relation to the non-European world. In an important way, their tendency to draw historical parallels between Eastern Europe and the global South could produce an alternative articulation of anti-colonial universalism, based on a unique narrative of cross-cultural solidarity. But as we saw above, this by no means guaranteed that socialist Yugoslav discussions of the global South and its development would be decolonised in any fundamental way.[66]

[66] Mark, Kalinovsky and Marung, *Alternative Globalizations*.

CHAPTER 3

Psychotherapy as Revolutionary Praxis

Somewhat surprisingly, the establishment of socialist revolutionary governments throughout Eastern and South Eastern Europe did not automatically translate into a support for psychodynamic approaches, even though all countries of the emerging socialist bloc shared the orientation toward social medicine, prophylactic public health policies and a heightened awareness of the role of socio-economic factors.[1] In the field of psychiatry, the effects of Soviet medical ideologies were in fact much more conducive to the continuation of the biological paradigm, and, in the immediate aftermath of World War II, the attempted Pavlovisation of psychiatry largely prioritised neurological, biochemical and reflexology research and approaches. As Ari Kiev noted on Communist world psychiatry, 'the approach to treatment in these countries [was] by and large [a] somatic one in which constitutional, genetic and physical factors [were] all stressed'.[2] In the other countries of the

[1] On the importance of prophylactic medicine and social(ist) hygiene in the Stalinization of the Eastern bloc, see Bradley Matthys Moore, 'For the People's Health: Ideology, Medical Authority and Hygienic Science in Communist Czechoslovakia', *Social History of Medicine*, 2014, 27:1, 122–143.

[2] Ari Kiev, 'Introduction', in Ari Kiev, ed., *Psychiatry in the Communist World*, New York: Science House, 1968, 16; on Soviet psychiatry, see also Julie V. Brown, 'Heroes and Non-heroes: Recurring Themes in the Historiography of Russian-Soviet Psychiatry',

A. Antić, *Non-Aligned Psychiatry in the Cold War*,
Mental Health in Historical Perspective,
https://doi.org/10.1007/978-3-030-89449-8_3

Eastern Bloc, partial attempts at the Pavlovisation and Sovietisation of psychiatry initially resulted in predominantly biological and hereditarian conceptual frameworks, and somatic research and treatment orientations. Recent research has convincingly countered the view that Soviet and East European psychiatry were ideologically monolithic, intellectually static and dominated exclusively by reductionist interpretations of the Pavlovian framework.[3] However, such non-dogmatic experimentation generally did not start before 1953, or even 1956. Throughout the Soviet bloc, the 1950s were largely marked by physiological theories, organicist therapeutic work and an institutional merging of psychiatry with neurology, while psychiatric 'materialism' came to denote physiological and neurological approaches. It was only after Stalin's death that explorations of psychotherapeutic possibilities began in earnest, although even those could be threatened by official condemnations and suspicion of psychoanalysis and psychodynamic theoretical frameworks.[4]

In the period between the liberation and falling out with the Soviet Union, Yugoslavia too was being increasingly drawn into the East European network of professional and medical associations, although it still kept a fairly lively exchange with West European and US institutions, mainly through the United Nations Relief and Rehabilitation Administration (UNRRA) mission in Belgrade. However, the growing impact of Soviet medical, public health, and psychiatric approaches was evident. Calls for the 'Stalinisation' of Yugoslav health care and medicine tended to reinforce organic, 'materialist' approaches to psychiatric theory and treatment, and those psychiatrists and mental health researchers who worked within the biomedical paradigm and had little interest in exploring the psychological effects of human cultural or emotional experiences were likely to gain the upper hand, despite the blow that the war had dealt

in Mark S. Micale and Roy Porter, eds, *Discovering the History of Psychiatry*, Oxford: Oxford University Press, 1994, 297–310; George Windholz, 'Soviet Psychiatrists Under Stalinist Duress: The Design for a 'New Soviet Psychiatry' and Its Demise', *History of Psychiatry*, 1999, 10:39, 329–347.

[3] Sarah Marks, 'Ecology, Humanism and Mental Health in Communist Czechoslovakia', in Mat Savelli and Sarah Marks, eds, *Psychiatry in Communist Europe*, 134–152.

[4] Sarah Marks and Mat Savelli, 'Communist Europe and Transnational Psychiatry', in Marks and Savelli, *Psychiatry in Communist Europe*, 1–26; Boris M. Segal, 'The Theoretical Basis of Soviet Psychotherapy', *American Journal of Psychotherapy*, 1975, 29:4, 503–523.

them.[5] As Vladimir Jakovljević aptly noted, the Stalinisation impulse offered an opportunity to 'the bearers of the prewar psychiatry' who had been educated in the organicist tradition 'which they endeavoured to proclaim dialectical-materialistic.'[6] Yugoslav physicians, psychiatrists, and public health functionaries regularly participated in congresses and completed medical specialisations in different fields of medicine and neuropsychiatry in the USSR, Czechoslovakia, Hungary or Poland.

This orientation affected medical and psychiatric theories and approaches, and psychiatric debates regarding the relative influence of heredity, psychological processes and environmental factors on the development of mental illness were increasingly couched in terms of the core influences in Soviet medical research. During the visit of Czech physicians and medical workers to Slovenia, Brno neurologist Dr. Hrbek discussed with his Yugoslav colleagues different ways in which the field of neuropsychiatry in the new East European people's republics could incorporate the core assumptions of dialectic materialism, while Slovene psychiatrist Dr. Kanoni insisted on the importance of Lenin's theory of reflection for the completion of that immense task.[7] Leading paediatricians embarked on the Ministry of People's Health-funded research on the importance of Pavlov's insights for child psychiatry and disability studies.[8] Talented young psychiatrist Ante Pavković attempted to resolve the contradiction between organicist psychiatry and Marxism's socio-economic awareness by applying Lysenko's theory of heredity of acquired diseases to the field of psychiatry.[9] As late as 1949, the conclusions of the second postwar congress of Yugoslav neuropsychiatrists urged the profession to organise

[5] See, for instance, Nikola Nikolić, 'Vladimir Iljić Lenjin i Zaštita Narodnog Zdravlja', *Medicinski Glasnik*, 1947, 1, 5; G. Nikolić, 'Oktobarska Revolucija i Razvoj Sovjetske Medicine', *Vojno-Sanitetski Pregled*, 1947, 4, 11–12; V. Stojanović, 'Velika Oktobarska Revolucija i Zaštita Narodnog Zdravlja u SSSR', *Medicinski Glasnik*, 1947, 2, 2, Nikola Nikolić, 'Razviće Sovjetske Medicine', *Medicinski Glasnik*, 1947, 1, 9.

[6] Vladimir Jakovljević, 'Yugoslavia', in Kiev, *Psychiatry in the Communist World*, 96.

[7] Zapisnik naučnog sastanka neurologa i psihijatara FNRJ odrzanog od 6. do 8. X 1949. u Opatiji, Narodno zdravlje, 1949:4, 302.

[8] Archive of Yugoslavia, Fond 36, Savet za narodno zdravlje i socijalnu politiku, file 27-566, 'Socijalno suzbijanje mucanja u decjem dobu'.

[9] Ante Pavković, 'Nasledjivanje duševnih i nervnih oboljenja u svetlu Lisenkove teorije naslednosti', *Narodno zdravlje*, 1946, 3, 62–99. On the role of Lysenko in the development of Soviet science, see David Joravsky, *The Lysenko Affair*, Chicago and London: The University of Chicago Press, 1986; Ethan Pollock, *Stalin and the Soviet Science Wars*,

a committee for researching the issue of heredity in the field of neuropsychiatry through the lenses of Lysenko's theory, even though at the same time the participants of the congress sent an official telegraph to Josip Broz expressing their 'consternation with the activities of the leaderships of the USSR and the other Informbureau countries' and their 'monstrous attacks, defamation and lies' against Yugoslavia.[10] The project was soon dropped, unsurprisingly, and its appointed coordinator Pavković instead left for Switzerland on a medical specialisation fellowship.

It was already clear at this meeting, however, that postwar Yugoslav psychiatry would develop in a radically different direction. The congress proposed that the psychiatric institutions of the country insist on sending mental health professionals abroad in order to train in the fields of psychotherapy and child psychiatry/psychoanalysis in particular, lamenting that those two areas had been profoundly neglected in 'capitalist Yugoslavia', and also indicating the future orientation of the profession as a whole (especially as the congress identified 'psychoneuroses' rather than schizophrenia or organic psychoses as the most important mental health problem of socialist Yugoslavia).

After 1948, the Yugoslav foreign policy underwent a radical shift, and consequently by 1951 Yugoslavia was firmly integrated in Western medical academic and professional networks, while these early tendencies and interests in Pavlovian science were soon marginalised; in the decades after 1948, they were primarily represented by an older, more conservative generation of Yugoslav psychiatrists, who remained suspicious of psychoanalysis. As Jakovljević concluded in his analysis, such Pavlovian approaches were often championed by practitioners of an organicist bent, whose interest in reflexology was dictated less by political commitment and more by their rather apolitical suspicion of 'modern' psychodynamic approaches. The situation in Yugoslav psychiatry was significantly different in that respect than in many other left-wing mental health professions—unlike their Cuban or Argentinian counterparts,[11]

Princeton, NJ and Oxford: Princeton University Press, 2006; and Nils Roll-Hansen, *The Lysenko Effect: The Politics of Science*, Amherst, NY: Humanity Books, 2005.

[10] Zapisnik naučnog sastanka neurologa i psihijatara FNRJ odrzanog od 6. do 8. X 1949. u Opatiji, Narodno zdravlje, 1949:4, 313.

[11] On the other hand, there were notable Yugoslav attempts to combine and integrate behaviourism (or reflexology) and psychoanalysis, most notably by Belgrade psychologist Milenko Karan. He made a thinly veiled reference to Soviet psychiatry by noting his

for instance, Yugoslav psychiatrists and psychotherapists rarely attempted to articulate direct connections between Pavlovian psychiatry and social revolution (or revolutionary clinical practice), and seldom focused on the politically progressive potentials of the Pavlovian theory and practice.[12] In the remainder of this chapter, we will explore how the theoretical and clinical framework of Yugoslav psychiatry got transformed in the aftermath of this radical political shift, and how the profession's involvement in transnational 'psy' networks across the Iron Curtain produced a unique brand of revolutionary Marxist psychotherapy and psychoanalysis.

* * *

In 1948, Vojin Matić, who would go on to become Yugoslavia's first trained child psychiatrist and the most important postwar psychoanalyst, was still a confused recent neuropsychiatry graduate, employed at Belgrade's Neuropsychiatric Clinic under the supervision of—and in perennial conflict with—leading neurologist Vladimir Vujić. According to Matić's own memories, this was a difficult period for a young professional who was uncomfortable with the dogmatic tenets of Yugoslavia's Sovietising psychiatry, as well as with the theories and therapeutic strategies of Central European organic psychiatry, which both insisted on neurological and physiological foundations of the human psyche: 'It was universally accepted that everything is inherited, according to the rules of genetics, which was still in its infancy as a science and often abused, sometimes unconsciously by physicians themselves, at other times by politicians, who saw it as a political tool against their opponents'. In the context of building a new socialist psychiatry under the Soviet auspices, Matić felt obliged to constantly perform a 'magician's trick' of 'grafting human mental life onto what physiologist Pavlov ascertained in relation to dogs'

opposition to any 'dogmatic-materialist interpretations of reflexology', but still insisted on deconstructing the Freud-Pavlov binary and developing an integrated approach, in which reflexology was to provide an 'organic basis' for psychoanalysis (Milenko Karan, 'Ivan Pavlov I Sigmund Frojd: Prikaz jednog pokusaja refleksoloske verifikacije nekih psihoanalitickih stavova', *Psiholoski bilten*, 1959, 3:3–4, 277–298).

[12] Marco Ramos, '"Psychotherapy of the Oppressed": Anti-Imperialism and Psychoanalysis in Cold War Buenos Aires, and Jennifer Lambe, 'Revolutionizing Cuba psychiatry: The Freud wars, 1955–1970', in Anne-Emanuelle Birn and Raul Necochea Lopez, eds, *Peripheral Nerve: Health and Medicine in Cold War Latin America*, Duke University Press, 2020.

stomach glands, i.e. the so-called conditional reflexes', and to invoke Oparin and Lysenko regularly in psychiatric discussions at the clinic. Moreover, everyday realities of hospital work frustrated him, and he was particularly bothered by his neurologist colleagues' casually derogatory attitude towards psychiatric patients, who were not considered human and were not to expect a humane treatment: 'provoking and mocking [mental hospital patients] was often justified and viewed as a successful joke', especially if they suffered from paranoia or were undereducated.[13]

Matić started his medical studies in 1930s Vienna with Julius Wagner-Jauregg, but the Viennese academic and intellectual setting was additionally important for Matić's professional development because this was where he first got in contact with and grew interested in psychoanalysis. In 1937, following his return to Yugoslavia, he started his psychoanalytic training in Belgrade and joined Nikola Sugar's Belgrade psychoanalytic society. Unfortunately, the outbreak of the war interrupted Matić's psychoanalytic involvement, and in the immediate postwar years, it seemed unlikely that he would be able to pursue his former interests in Freud, hypnosis and the concept of the unconscious. In the summer of 1948, he was scheduled to go to an unspecified clinic in Leningrad for a neuropsychiatric specialisation.

However, by mid-1948, that prospect was rendered impossible due to the dire political relationship between Russia and Yugoslavia. Instead, when, in that same year, a WHO representative visited the Yugoslav Ministry of Health and asked interested young physicians to apply for fellowships to pursue medical specialisations in Western Europe, Matić submitted an application for Georges Heuyer's clinic in Paris, outlining his intention to work on child psychiatry. The application was soon approved and Matić received WHO funding to travel to Paris the following year.[14] At Heuyer's clinic, Matić completed his habilitation, developed a lifelong interest in child psychoanalysis and made contacts which would determine his own career as well as the development of child psychiatry in Yugoslavia. Matić, a member of Šugar's prewar kruzhok, educated an entire postwar generation of psychoanalysts (and

[13] Vojin Matić, *Moji zivoti* (Novi Sad, 1985), 86–87.

[14] Archive of Yugoslavia, Fond 31, Komitet za zastitu narodnog zdravlja, f. 65–92, 'Spisak lekara predloženih za specijalizaciju u inostranstvu'.

child psychiatrists) in Yugoslavia, and maintained close professional relationships with leading French psychoanalysts such as Rene Deatkine and Serge Lebovici. In the 1950s and 1960s, Yugoslavia became an experimental site for some of the newest and most progressive forms of child psychotherapy, while many of Matić's students and younger colleagues subsequently developed rich contacts with not only French but also British, American, Scandinavian as well as Soviet psychiatrists and psychoanalysts.[15] Outside the narrow field of child psychiatry, Yugoslavia's leading psychiatric institutions formed long-lasting collaborations and designed joint projects with partners from across the Iron Curtain, which permanently transformed the landscape of the country's psychiatric research and practice.[16]

The turbulent professional trajectory of Vojin Matić—and in particular his sharp change of direction away from Sovietised mental health frameworks towards psychodynamic and explicitly psychoanalytic theory and practice—was thus paradigmatic of the complex cultural and political influences to which Yugoslav psychiatry was subject at this time. Yugoslavia was the only socialist country in which psychoanalysis positively thrived and, despite a rocky start, developed into the dominant theoretical and clinical approach.[17] Moreover, while Yugoslav psychiatrists and psychoanalysts quickly became well integrated in West European and American medical and professional networks, they still worked in a socialist country which searched for an alternative form of Communist democracy. Therefore, the 'Westernisation' of Yugoslav psychiatry

[15] Ksenija Kondić, 'Vojin Matić and Filozofski Fakultet', in *Legende Beogradskog Univerziteta: Vojin Matić: 1911–1999*, Belgrade, 2008, 12.

[16] The Institute of Mental Health's rising international profile serves as an excellent and typical example here. Under the leadership of the indomitable Slavka Moric-Petrovic throughout the 1960s and 1970s, it conducted a series of ground-breaking research projects—in methods of rehabilitation of psychiatric patients, treatment of alcoholics, and diagnosis and treatment of psychological disorders in university students—in collaboration with the US Department of Health, Education and Welfare (Social and Rehabilitation Service), which offered generous funding support. See Institute of Mental Health, *Development of a Screening Method for the Early Identification of Psychological Disorders in University Students*, Belgrade, 1973, grant number: 19-P-58413-F-01; *Ispitivanje rehabilitacionog potencijala i metodologija rehabilitacije psihijatrijskih bolesnika*, Belgrade, 1972, VRA-4-63; *Metodi lecenja i rehabilitacije alkoholicara*, Belgrade, 1973, VRA-YUGO-8-68.

[17] For an overview of the development of Yugoslav psychoanalysis under socialism, see Mat Savelli, 'The Peculiar Prosperity of Psychoanalysis in Socialist Yugoslavia', *Slavonic and East European Review*, 2013, 91:2, 262–288.

was a complex and layered process, and Matić and his many colleagues and disciples often re-framed the concepts and techniques of British and French psychotherapy and psychoanalysis to respond to the pressing social and cultural problems of building democratic socialism.

This chapter explores how West European psychiatric, psychotherapeutic and psychoanalytic experiences and insights were used to help construct proper Marxist citizens and families in Yugoslavia, and how Yugoslav psychotherapists hoped to employ a psychoanalytic approach both inside and outside the clinic to revolutionise patriarchal, authoritarian and hierarchical social relations. This was then to be a revolutionary and activist psychoanalysis, which was meant to contribute to a broad political and cultural discussion in Yugoslavia about constructing a society based on genuine Marxist collective and individual emancipation, an alternative to both Stalinist state socialism and Western capitalism/liberal democracy.

This was truly unique: while psychoanalysis was far from banned and exterminated in socialist Eastern Europe, in most countries it was confined to various degrees of underground existence, and informally integrated in a series of therapies and approaches labelled as 'dynamic' or 'psychotherapeutic'.[18] Moreover, both psychology and psychiatry played an important role in the project of producing a new, socialist personality across the region, but, as Christine Leuenberger pointed out with regard to GDR, in such circumstances psychoanalysis was more likely to be perceived as 'politically subversive' and to '[offer] an alternative conception of human nature' to the one promoted by orthodox Marxism-Leninism or Pavlovian approaches.[19] It was arguably only in Yugoslavia that the clinical and theoretical aims of psychoanalysis aligned quite closely with the political revolutionary agenda of workers' self-management, so that psychoanalysis became directly involved in the process of overhauling the social and psychological conditions in order to build a democratic socialist person.

In her recent book on post-WWII psychoanalysis, Dagmar Herzog argues that the postwar period was marked by an exceptionally close relationship between psychoanalysis and politics, and that, more than being simply an influential clinical technique or 'therapeutic modality',

[18] See Eghigian, 'Was There a Communist Psychiatry?'

[19] Leuenberger, 'Socialist Psychotherapy and Its Dissidents'.

Western psychoanalysis of the 1960s, 1970s and 1980s evolved into a very prominent 'toolbox for cultural criticism', and ultimately deeply affected a variety of other political, cultural and intellectual fields. Herzog traces the trajectory of psychoanalytic controversial involvements in non-medical areas of life, and documents its development into an 'integral part of twentieth-century social and intellectual history'.[20] This willingness on the part of leading Western psychoanalysts to engage with broader social, religious and political issues, claims Herzog, enabled the discipline to experience its second 'golden age' in the 1960s, following its gradual decline in the United States. In fact, these later psychoanalytic practitioners openly defied the early postwar injunctions of some of the most senior psychoanalysts to refrain from discussing any extra-psychological factors and stay away from political or sociological conceptions.

And while Herzog's argument is convincing and very useful for reframing the study of Cold War psychoanalysis, it maintains an almost exclusively Western focus. However, it was in a small socialist East European country that some of the most radical ideas regarding an activist psychoanalysis developed as early as the late 1950s, well before comparable developments, described by Herzog, ensued in Western Europe. Moreover, Yugoslav psychoanalysts styled themselves not only as perceptive social critics and politically subversive intellectuals, but also as direct revolutionaries in their everyday clinical practice. Even though they participated in broader social and political discussions, their primary field of political action and involvement was the consulting room, in which they proposed to directly transform archaic social relations and promote self-management by undoing traditional Yugoslav patriarchal and authoritarian families.

In socialist Yugoslavia, therefore, psychiatry and psychotherapy opened up and became directly engaged in discussing crucial questions about shaping and reshaping political minds, experimenting with new political ideas, and building, as the Communist Party called it, a genuine democracy. Psychoanalytic and psychotherapeutic theories became increasingly important for understanding and developing the notions of individual enlightenment and self-management that underpinned Yugoslavia's reform Communism. In turn, various philosophical and sociological interpretations of self-management shaped the Yugoslav, Marxist version of

[20] Dagmar Herzog, *Cold War Freud: Psychoanalysis in an Age of Catastrophes*, Cambridge, 2019.

psychoanalysis and encouraged its practitioners to think in more activist and politically engaged terms. As we will see below, Yugoslav psychiatrists and psychotherapists made explicit references to the politics of workers' self-management as well as to the importance of Marxism for their clinical practice. But even when they did not openly discuss these connections between politics and socialist psychiatry, their language, concepts, analytical categories and narratives often resembled the most important political debates of the time, and directly addressed some of the most pressing concerns from those debates. Moreover, Yugoslav socialist psychiatry's aims and preoccupations were often closely aligned with radical politics and with the clinical-political tenets and goals of the Western radical psychiatry movement.

Raising Self-Managing Marxists: Socialist Psychiatry and the Pursuit of Freedom

After 1949 the Yugoslav political system saw itself almost exclusively as an ideological antithesis to the USSR, a 'really existing negation of the concept of state socialism' and central planning.[21] It began searching for an alternative ideological and political basis for legitimation, which would move away from Stalinist totalitarianism without endangering the socialist essence of the Yugoslav revolution. In 1949, the Communist Party's leading ideologue Edvard Kardelj suggested that socialism meant 'such an organization of a people's community which would represent a mutual cooperation of equal, free people' and would eliminate 'a uniformity imposed from above and hierarchical subordination to the centre'.[22] Already by the early 1950s, the most important ideologues of Yugoslav Communism developed their doctrine of socialist workers' self-management, which was partly based on Engels' notion of the 'state that withers away', on Marx's early writings and analysis of the Paris Commune, and on Gramsci's theories and partly inspired by the Yugoslav Communists' wartime experiences of popularly elected and popularly responsible committees/councils.

[21] Marie-Janine Calic, *Geschichte Jugoslawiens im 20. Jahrhunert*, Munich: C.H. Beck Verlag, 2010, 240.

[22] Radovan Radonjic, *Sukob KPJ s Kominternom I drustveni razvoj Jugoslavije, 1948–1950*, Zagreb: Narodno sveučilište grada Zagreba, Centar za aktualni politički studij, 1979, 281.

The state soon implemented a set of legislative measured aimed at economic and political decentralisation and 'de-bureaucratisation' through workers' councils and gradual democratisation of cultural and social life. Such reforms, of course, stopped well short of introducing a multiparty political system and disbanding the political monopoly of the Communist Party, but they did de-Bolshevize Yugoslav socialism and ultimately helped build a more pluralistic society. The political image of an ideal citizen of this novel and experimental system, consequently, changed quite significantly. The new Yugoslav self-managing worker needed to possess robust assertiveness, independence of mind and a host of other critical psychological and intellectual qualities in order to sustain the political experiment; he or she would also need to leave behind dogmatic, authoritarian or subservient frames of mind which characterised previous models of social relations. The emergence of such a revolutionary personality was going to be an exceptionally complex and difficult process, and the budding and ambitious psychiatric and psychotherapeutic professions in Yugoslavia wholeheartedly offered to take active part in this fundamental political project.

When Yugoslavia began forging closer political, social and cultural relations with Western Europe and the United States, it was psychiatry, psychotherapy and psychoanalysis in particular which profited the most from this exchange, and these professions became thoroughly Westernised and firmly integrated in these alternative networks.[23] In the course of this transformation of the Yugoslav mental health professions, psychiatrists and psychoanalysts became primarily concerned with the issue of authoritarian family relations, aiming to liberalise and democratise society through democratising family.[24] In fact, Yugoslavia offered an excellent site for social experimentation in this regard: through the combination of the country's more open version of socialism and Western psychoanalysis, psychoanalysts hoped to achieve a more humane society, neither capitalist nor Stalinist, a society deeply committed to human emancipation and autonomy which invoked early Marx as its ideological beacon. That sort of self-realisation of the individual was to be achieved only in a self-managing society—in which truly free, authentic, diversely educated

[23] Interview with dr Nevenka Tadić, 7 February 2014, Belgrade, Serbia; Interview with dr Dusan Popovic, 13 February 2014, Belgrade, Serbia.

[24] Nevenka Tadić, *Psihijatrija detinjstva i mladosti*, Belgrade, 1989 (reprinted), 18–19.

workers and citizens took part in making all important decisions regarding their political, social, economic, cultural lives.[25]

In other words, Yugoslav 'psy' professionals wanted to create a society devoid of hierarchies, patriarchy and social and political authoritarianism. A combination of psychoanalytic psychotherapy and self-managing socialism was the key, and the experience of psychoanalytic treatment as well as the political conditions of anti-authoritarian self-management were supposed to transform the 'primitive' and dictatorial Yugoslav psyche. While Yugoslavia's most well-known political dissidents, philosophers and sociologists gathered around the group Praxis, complained that workers' self-management failed to reach its full potential, psychoanalysts made that very same point, but were never persecuted. In that sense, self-management remained the mark of originality of Yugoslav psychiatry and psychoanalysis—it provided the basis on which the postwar psychiatric understandings of the human psyche and its possible transformation rested.

Child psychiatrists and psychoanalysts in Yugoslavia were particularly concerned with the great demands of modernity and of the new democracy in Yugoslavia, which asked for growing personal responsibilities and exceptional mental stamina. Matić, for instance, articulated a very telling understanding of the nature of socialism and the role of individuals in a socialist society. He conjured up a memorable image of experimental direct democracy and emphasised the supreme role of psychiatry in preparing the population for it: 'We are entering a society in which every individual carries his share of responsibility, in which awareness, pleasure derived from labour, and true personal dedication are more necessary than ever, in which every individual will make decisions about economic, foreign, internal policies, about war and peace. In such a society, every individual should be raised in such a way as to be able to be involved in a community without fear or aggression, keeping the originality of his personality and feeling of personal freedom'.[26] This utopian vision drew directly on Marx's 'German ideology', which also served as the ideological foundation of the new platform of workers' self-management: compare to Kardelj's contemporaneous injunction that socialist Yugoslavia should 'constitute a free and courageous man whose worldviews and concepts

[25] Vojin Matić, *Kada pocinje vaspitanje deteta*, Belgrade, 1955, 61–62.

[26] Ibid., 62.

were broad and diverse, and who was foreign to bureaucratism and narrow formalism of thinking.'[27]

And indeed, in socialist Yugoslavia the issue of massive social and individual restructuring was high up on the political agenda. In particular, it was the elimination of patriarchal families that was to be at the core of the social revolution and of achieving the true emancipation of self-managing socialism. This patriarchal psychodynamics generated the authoritarian father, obedient and inconsequential mother, and highly hierarchical, disciplinarian relationships with children. Socialism, on the other hand, was to bring about the (political, social, personal) emancipation of women, and to introduce egalitarianism in family relations. However, in Yugoslavia the entrenchment of traditional family authoritarianism belied the achievement of such lofty democratising aims within families, and it also fatally harmed the process of raising self-managing citizens. Moreover, if Yugoslav psychiatrists looked east, they could see a very traditional and authoritarian, custodial psychiatry, which could not provide any meaningful guidance when it came to re-educating parents. Paradoxically, it was in Western psychoanalytic and psychiatric ideas that Yugoslav child psychiatrists discovered a set of guidelines for eliminating Yugoslav family and child pathologies, and for creating a more humane version of socialism. It was, in particular, psychoanalysis which was to become the intellectual tool for making families and parent–child relationships more socialist and more self-managing: in the 1950s and 1960s Yugoslav child psychiatric circles, psychoanalysis was seen as 'a democratic, liberating psychotherapy, which stands for independence and personal liberties of individuals'.[28]

As psychotherapist Vladeta Jerotić later confirmed, psychoanalysis coupled with self-analysis presented a unique way to achieving unsurpassed human autonomy, self-actualisation and educational growth: unlike traditional psychiatry, it educated without relying on authoritarianism, and, by increasing patients' self-knowledge, 'created pre-conditions for the constitution of a mature and autonomous personality' and for attaining the 'freedom of self-development'. For Jerotic, the ethics of psychoanalysis required that practitioners shun any attempts at manipulation or indoctrination, and focus on advancing a democratic dialogue with

[27] Kardelj, *Borba*, 14 January 1950.

[28] Tadić, *Psihijatrija detinjstva i mladosti*, 20.

the patient.[29] For these reasons, a society of true socialist self-managing workers was in fact impossible without psychoanalytic guidance. As Jerotić elaborated in the discussion following his presentation, 'psychoanalysis needed to be accepted... in a broader sense' in the Yugoslav society, as it provided methods and strategies not only for dealing with mental pathologies but also for 'widening the consciousness'.[30]

Marxism, Revolution and Psychoanalysis

Yugoslav psychoanalysts and psychiatrists tended to draw direct parallels between psychoanalysis and Marxist revolution, and even between Freud and Marx themselves, as personalities who intervened in modern history in comparably forceful ways. In an extremely laudatory article about Freud's legacy, on the occasion of the hundred and twentieth anniversary of his birth, Zagreb-based therapist Muradif Kulenović focused on the intellectual kinship of Freud and Marx, two exceptional thinkers, linked by their fate as émigrés in London, whose subversive ideas remain in equal measure dangerous and fascinating to contemporary audiences. Moreover, in Kulenović's reading, both Freud and Marx contributed to the same revolutionary historical project: of courageously 'shaking up the world of human illusions', and striving relentlessly to induce humanity to understand 'the deepest, the unknown in itself, that which had always been repressed, and which served to create mythologies or to be rationalised with notions and ideas far removed from people's genuine desires'.[31] Both Marx and Freud, the ultimate believers in Reason as the substitute for God, drew attention to the core conflicts and struggles: between the conscious and the unconscious in the case of Freud, and between different social structures in a historical process in the case of Marx. In that sense, Freud's theory was in fact for Kulenović a conversion of Marx's interpretation of historical conflicts in a societal context to the language of individual psychology, while Freud's *Interpretation of Dreams* was a continuation of sorts of the Communist Manifesto, coming exactly fifty years later. They both insisted on self-knowledge and the discovery

[29] Vladeta Jerotic, 'Psihoanaliza, autoanaliza i autonomija licnosti', *Psihoterapija*, 1975, 2, 215–217.

[30] Ibid.

[31] Muradif Kulenović, 'Izgnanstvo i smrt u tudjem gradu', *Psihoterapija*, 1976, 6:2, 196.

of unconscious yearnings before any social and psychological liberation or revolution could be achieved. In this way, psychoanalysis yet again became a tool for Marxist praxis in the sphere of individual consciousness, which Yugoslav mental health specialists seemed to embrace wholeheartedly as much for therapeutic as for political reasons.

In 1967, the Yugoslav audience had an extraordinary opportunity to witness a Yugoslav psychiatrist's impassioned defence of psychoanalysis, its clinical and political values, from a harsh attack by an American Pavlovian psychologist. In his preface to the 1967 translation of US psychologist and philosopher Harry K. Wells' well-known monograph *The Failure of Psychoanalysis*, Vladimir Jakovljević decided to offer an in-depth evaluation of the author's arguments and assess the overall achievement of psychoanalysis in the context of contemporary mental health sciences. In this unique case, an openly Marxist psychiatrist (who regularly quoted Marx's writings in his own clinical publications) set out to demonstrate the incompatibility of Marxist humanism and Pavlovian conditional reflex theory (and, by extension, behaviourism) to an American colleague, and to re-assert the importance of the legacy of psychoanalysis for both Western and East European humanist psychiatry.[32]

Jakovljević did not shy away from critiquing psychoanalysis and its Freudian origins, nor did he in any way approve the mainstream private practice version of psychoanalysis in the United States, which he thought had been hijacked by the most reactionary section in the American society—the middle class—and heavily adapted to its narrow needs and interests. Moreover, he outlined what he thought were the most negative societal influences of psychoanalysis, most notably its reluctance to 'comprehend the complexity of social and personal problems, viewing them from the point of view of individual maladaptation' and seeking often purely individualistic solutions to such difficulties through therapy. On the other hand, Jakovljević recognised that the core contribution of psychoanalysis, from a socialist point of view, had to do with undermining the social, ethical and cultural value system of the bourgeois society: 'exposing the bourgeois hypocrisy and helping construct more open moral relations in families and other social communities'.[33] In that sense, Jakovljević

[32] Jakovljević, 'Preface', in Harry Wells, *Neuspeh psihoanalize: Od Frojda do Froma*, Belgrade: Kultura, 1967, 1–51.

[33] Ibid., 13.

confirmed, psychoanalysis had a social and cultural revolutionary potential which was difficult to overlook.

Even though Jakovljević critiqued psychoanalysis at the very outset for its lack of clarity regarding the overwhelming importance of socio-economic factors for understanding mental pathology, in his own brief account of the discipline he emphasised broader social environment, offering an idiosyncratic interpretation of the core psychoanalytic theories. Writing about 'normal personality' in a psychoanalytic sense, Jakovljević noted that a healthy person's development 'primarily depended on the balanced nature of a social setting in which the person grew up and lived, and which would enable the creation of satisfactory interrelations within the personality structure'. On the other hand, even though he criticised Freud for focusing too much attention on internal psychological factors, Jakovljević still declared that, in classical psychoanalysis, 'every mental disturbance… is caused by a disrupted personality development which stems from an adverse social environment'.[34] Therefore, Jakovljević adjusted his reading of the psychoanalytic notions of normality and pathology in order to factor in the predominant significance of broader societal (and economic) factors, which will also be crucial for his contributions to global transcultural psychiatry.

Furthermore, Jakovljević's defence built an even stronger case for psychoanalysis (and against Pavlovian science and behaviourism) by returning to original Marxist writings. For him, psychoanalysis was more than just abstractly revolutionary in its subversive and destabilising effects on middle-class Central European families; it was also directly linked to some of Marx's core concepts. In his materialist critique of psychoanalysis, Wells dismissed the notion of the unconscious as a 'mythological construct', explaining it away through references to sensory and verbal signal systems, and reducing it, in Jakovljević's interpretation, to the mechanisms of remembering and forgetting. But for Jakovljević, the concept of the unconscious had a much more fundamental meaning, and was vital to understanding the human psyche as well as human nature. In particular, he related the unconscious to the Marxist notion of alienation: Jakovljević claimed that even Marx accepted, if indirectly, the existence of the unconscious when he emphasised the primary importance of one's 'social being' and the 'objective socio-economic forces

[34] Ibid., 22–23.

[which] determined man's thinking and action despite his [sic] will'. In other words, Jakovljević interpreted the preeminent significance of socio-economic historical circumstances in Marx's theory as a direct link to the Freudian unconscious, quoting Rosa Luxembourg's statement that the 'logic of the historical process always came before the subjective logic of human beings'.[35] In this discussion, the effects and influences of 'the logic of the historical process'—a force that determined human consciousness in any particular context—stood for the unconscious, which functioned outside human volition and awareness, and shaped identity and agency. In his own defence of the notion of the unconscious, Kulenović put forward a very similar reading of Marxism and alienation through a psychoanalytic key, arguing that the 'influence of the unconscious on human life' was very clearly demonstrated in Marx's theory of historical materialism.[36]

Beyond this, psychoanalysis had further meaning for Jakovljević as a social-scientific tool for understanding alienation (in its Marxist meaning), and for unpacking and addressing broader problems in the human condition identified in humanist Marxism. In fact, from such a humanist perspective which predominated among Yugoslav psychiatrists, psychoanalysis became the most appropriate intellectual framework for furthering 'human self-knowledge' and for constructing 'a more complete freedom of personality without external and internal inhibitions'. In that sense, the contribution of psychoanalysis to Marxist human emancipation was immense, and primarily through the analytical concept of the unconscious, which offered a unique framework for tackling and resolving alienation (and self-alienation). Here, then, was where the true revolutionary repository of psychoanalysis lay—in its ability to contribute to a range of humanities disciplines, such as philosophy, sociology or anthropology, in order to 'help them construct a more comprehensive understanding of the nature of modern human existence' and psychology.[37] Only such a full and rounded understanding of the complexity human condition could then enable (revolutionary) changes in social circumstances as well as human psyche.

The core problem of Pavlovian reflexology and its American offshoots, on the other hand, was their mechanistic model of the human psyche

[35] Ibid., 28–29.

[36] Kulenović,'Psihoanaliticki koncept nesvjesnog', *Socijalna Psihijatrija*, 1974, 2, 25–39.

[37] Jakovljević, 'Preface', 49–51.

and, in particular, of the relationship between society and individuals. This interpretive framework contributed very little to a holistic understanding of human potential and creativity in their sociological as well as psychological meanings, and of the complexity of human experience. In Jakovljević's Marxist interpretation, psychoanalysis was both non-conformist as a discipline and primarily focused on non-conformist, potentially revolutionary or disruptive personalities: 'from Freud to Fromm, … psychoanalysis always viewed individuals as potential rebels of sorts, who strove to overcome dominant models of the society in which they had developed'.[38] On the other hand, American psychology, as represented by Wells and his 'pragmatism', could not account for the emergence of novel ideas and revolutionary pathways (or personalities), and could never explain how such original modes of thinking developed which challenged and transformed existent social paradigms. This was because this strand of psychology 'identified normality with perfect achievements in accordance with a given's society's values and norms', and was therefore by default conservative. In this reading of psychoanalysis, therefore, the discipline became a handmaiden of revolutionary thinking: an intellectual framework which could both explain and enable/encourage the development of rebellious personalities, and sow the seed of social revolution.

In his commentary on Marxist psychoanalyst Igor Caruso's work, Jakovljević put forward the concept of 'engaged psychoanalysis', and treated it as identical—or at least highly comparable—to revolutionary Marxism in its emancipatory potential: 'just like revolutionary Marxist praxis, engaged psychoanalytic practice aims to help individuals become freer creators of their own and social history, shedding light on the conditions and forms of their alienation and on possibilities for overcoming it'.[39] According to Jakovljević, it was a natural mission of psychoanalysis—in its 'anthropological' and activist guise—to play a central role in developing authentic personalities and deepening their consciousness: the discipline's potentials for constructing such authentic citizens and a free society were virtually unlimited, and this form of Marxist and anthropologically minded psychoanalysis was indispensable for achieving socialist revolution on both personal and societal levels.

[38] Ibid., 47.

[39] Jakovljević, 'Predgovor za knjigu I. Karuza: Drustveni aspekti psihoanalize', in *Prilozi sa socijalnu patologiju*, Belgrade: Sloboda, 1984, 257–259.

But once a society underwent socialist transformation, psychoanalysis in its classical form might appear too pessimistic: while Freud, due to his own socio-cultural context, 'erroneously considered that every civilisation was in and of itself repressive', the neo-Freudians of the second half of the twentieth century revised this aspect, and moved away from the idea that all societal factors must have a negative, frustrating effects on human creative impulses. In fact, these later renditions of the psychoanalytic theory allowed for progressive and non-repressive civilisations/societies, in which individuals could develop their creativity through social inclusion and participation. Such a fully humanist society could, of course, only come into being if all forms of 'man's exploitation of man' were done away with, so that authentic human creativity became a source of pleasure rather than a product of need and coercion. Jakovljević generally agreed with Erich Fromm's understanding that only 'capitalist and totalitarian-socialist societies were completely ill', while seeds of truly healthy humanist societies existed in Yugoslavia, India and Egypt, the leaders of the non-aligned world. In the final analysis, for both Fromm and Jakovljević, it was solely a self-managing society—'decentralised democratic socialism' based on 'free associated producers'—which allowed and 'enabled a full development of human creative forces'—this was impossible in any 'bureaucratised system'.[40]

Still, healthy individuals could exist in unhealthy societies—but they had to be 'rebellious personalities', in constant conflict with non-progressing forces in their own societal environment. Jakovljević thus heavily criticised Karen Horney, another leading neo-analyst, for her definition of normality as harmony, balance and absence of conflict: 'a man only develops and gets humanised through overcoming conflicts' and difficulties. In fact, if we accept that certain social and political structures are ill, individuals who live in harmony and accordance with such pathological systems cannot be considered normal. This, as we will see later, would form the basis of Jakovljević's theory of revolutionary personality, who is in constant struggle with the backward norms and values of his or her society.

In addition, other Yugoslav psychiatrists emphasised that the discipline of psychoanalysis was particularly significant in a revolutionary society

[40] Ibid. 257–259.

precisely because it allowed them to move away from the reductive organicism of traditional psychiatry, and to take into consideration—systematically and analytically—the role of sociological, cultural and political factors in their patients' personal histories. For Marxist practitioners, as Stjepan Betlheim pointed out, this was of utmost ideological as well as clinical importance: a psychiatric framework which reduced psychological conflicts to biological, chemical or neurological explanations removed any potential for social critique or engagement, and undermined Marxist psychiatrists' ability to relate their work to broader socio-political trends and objectives.[41] Psychoanalysis, as practiced in socialist Yugoslavia, made such a link eminently possible.

Stamping Out the Authoritarian Family

A comprehensive transformation of family relations and structures was officially high on the list of priorities of most socialist regimes in Eastern Europe: at least in their formal legislative activities and public political campaigns, the people's democracies sought to involve women in the labour force in order to undermine the reactionary patriarchal attitudes, relations and practices which predominated within family settings.[42] The socialist regimes' actual record in this regard was, of course, very chequered, and their support for women's emancipation at home and in the workplace was not always consistent or even entirely genuine.[43] Still, in socialist Eastern Europe—and in Yugoslavia—the equality of women in the private and public spheres was fully legalised, and their access to universal (and free) education and healthcare significantly affected their social position, self-perception, and, at times, even their role within the family. These massive social and economic changes 'offered opportunities for educational and occupational advancement, cultural and material enrichment, and social engagement'; for many, the new socialist public

[41] Stjepan Betlheim, 'Kakav je stav lekara prema psihoanalizi', *Nas Vesnik*, 1956, 3, 204.

[42] Donna Harsch, *Revenge of the Domestic: Women, the Family, and Communism in the German Democratic Republic*, Princeton: Princeton University Press, 2007; Jill Massino, 'Something Old, Something New: Marital Roles and Relations in State Socialist Romania', *Journal of Women's History*, 2010, 22:1.

[43] Katherine Verdery, *What Was Socialism, and What Comes Next?*, Princeton: Princeton University Press, 1996.

discourses of equality and related policies also meant that new concepts of womanhood, motherhood and fatherhood suddenly became available.[44]

With regard to family structures, however, the socialist policies of emancipation and 'liberation' of women and families often led to the 'double burden' issue, and the formal and legal changes could not fully challenge the persistence of patriarchal mindsets, so that socialist families frequently remained hybrids of progressive and traditional beliefs, arrangements and practices—a problem compounded by a dizzying pace of urbanisation and a large influx of rural population which brought its own family mores to socialist cities.[45] It was precisely this problem of a slow and painful transformation of socialist family relations that Yugoslav psychoanalysts attempted to address in their clinical practice. In this regard, this clinical aim was fully aligned with the state's official political, ideological and legal commitments.

The Yugoslav version of socialism, moreover, seemed to dictate an extraordinary set of criteria for child-rearing, and the 1948 split played an enormous role in transforming the state's understanding of childhood and its core characteristics. Already in 1949, Milovan Djilas, one of the Communist Party's leading ideologues, instructed the existing children's organisations in Yugoslavia to avoid raising children 'whose minds will be cropped [and moulded] in the same way', but instead called on them to encourage the creation of 'free, socialist people, people who think and work courageously and fearlessly, whose opinions are broad and diverse'.[46] Furthermore, the socialist youth association of Croatia proclaimed a year later that children should grow up as 'decisive, intrepid, enterprising'. The Third Plenum of the Communist Party of Yugoslavia, dedicated to discussing the tasks of socialist education, fully supported Djilas's condemnation of schools which excelled at instilling 'uniform thinking', and throughout the 1950s, Party documents insisted that the

[44] Shana Penn and Jill Massino, eds, *Gender Politics and Everyday Life in State Socialist Eastern and Central Europe*, Basingstoke: Palgrave Macmillan, 2009.

[45] Hilda Scott, *Does Socialism Liberate Women? Experiences from Eastern Europe*, London: Beacon Press, 1974; Sonia Kruks, Rayna Rapp, and Marilyn B. Young, eds, *Promissory Notes: Women in the Transition to Socialism*, New York: Monthly Review Press, 1989.

[46] Igor Duda, 'Djeca socijalističke domovine. Izgrađivanje pionirske tradicije u Hrvatskoj 1950-ih godina' in Lada Duraković and Andrea Matošević, eds, *Socijalizam na klupi: Jugoslovensko društvo u očima nove postjugoslovenske humanistike*, Pula and Zagreb: Srednja Europa, 2013, 75–101.

creation of 'free creative personalities' was the core aim of Yugoslavia's policies on children. In addition to rigid, traditional schools, patriarchal families presented a fundamental obstacle to the fulfilment of such ambitions.

The state's new thinking about childhood undermined patriarchal assumptions in yet another crucial way: it expected children to assume serious political roles and responsibilities from a very early age. Already at seven, by joining the Pioneer Organisation, socialist children exited the period of 'political innocence' or 'neutrality', and began the process of becoming ideological and political agents in their own right.[47] Instead of seeing children as passive, deferential, politically oblivious and dependent—as they were socialised to be in authoritarian and traditional families—the socialist state viewed them as the future pillars and protectors of the legacy of communism, and active, conscious and equal contributors to the political process.

The new socialist family in Yugoslavia was supposed to raise future self-managers and liberated workers—and it had the greatest responsibility in effecting this grand transformation of psychological consciousness and social practice. As one treatise argued in the 1950s, the family remained the first school of human emotions and of new, revolutionary social relations, which prepared both children and parents for their new social and productive roles, and which therefore had to rest on the ideals of independence and lack of exploitation.[48] Moreover, distinguished anthropologist and sociologist Zagorka Pesic argued that patriarchal morality prevented people from becoming active participants in self-managing systems, because it discouraged initiative and control from the bottom, and produced personalities who tended to wait passively for orders and directions rather than taking the lead themselves. The current society in Yugoslavia demanded 'conscientious and well developed personalities who

[47] Ildiko Erdei, '"The Happy Child" as an Icon of Socialist Transformation: Yugoslavia's Pioneer Organization', in Lampe and Mazower, *Ideologies and National Identities*, 154–179.

[48] Branka Savic, 'Porodica i drustvo (porodica i vaspitanje dece)' (Belgrade: Izdavacka kuca Rad, 1958), 28.

will be prepared to lead the process of societal transformation', and families could not raise such personalities if they insisted on patriarchal mores and fought against children's 'stubbornness'.[49]

Throughout psychiatric discussions, patriarchy and authoritarianism were marked as the authentic cultural traits of the Yugoslav family (and social) structure, which set it apart in a broader international context. One of the central characteristics of the Yugoslav family structure was that 'expressions of disobedience and resistance to parents, teachers and other adults, especially if they were higher up on the hierarchical scale, were condemned and punished, while obedience and submissiveness were encouraged. Parents and adults were sacred beings who may not be called in question or disputed'.[50]

In their quest to instil in their children blind obedience and subordination to higher authorities, patriarchal parents became guilty of producing automatons and weak personalities, who would only be capable to fulfilling other people's orders. On the contrary, the fledgling Yugoslav society of self-managers needed independent young people, 'who thought with their own heads'.[51] The dangers of family authoritarianism were well illustrated in a clinical case treated by Ksenija Kondić, a young psychologist at Belgrade's Consultancy for mental hygiene. Kondić treated a ten-year old girl, Gordana, who had persistent problems with enuresis although her family situation at first appeared stable and comfortable. Still, the psychologist soon noted that the relationship between the parents was fairly disturbed, but even more importantly, that the father's harsh treatment of the girl might be the core of the problem. According to Kondić's notes, the girl's mother confirmed that, unlike his gentle and open attitude towards their son, 'the father was very cold [to the patient], and rigidly stuck to the view that a female child was less important than the male one'. Moreover, 'he wouldn't let her play with other children because she belongs at home' as a girl. It was precisely this lack of concern for the patient's feelings, which was itself a result of an inflexible patriarchal worldview that produced timid, apprehensive children, unprepared for any autonomous decision-making. As Kondić concluded, the patient

[49] Zagorka Pesic, 'Sukob starog i novog u braku i porodici' (Belgrade: Izdavacka kuca Rad, 1958), 16–17.

[50] Tadić, *Psihijatrija detinjstva i mladosti*, 30.

[51] Pesic, 25.

was growing up to be the perfect image of submission: 'she speaks softly, fairly fearfully, with her hands in her lap, often looking down'. She was obedient, 'never said a word more than she was asked'. Moreover, 'she moves exactly as she speaks - silently, she is barely audible, careful not to touch or move any object'. Most damningly, 'she never does anything before asking for permission first'.[52]

Yugoslav child psychotherapists used explicitly political terms such as 'democratic' and 'undemocratic' families, and placed the idea of democratic family relations at the core of their professional ideology. In Matić's opinion 'a child who grew up in a democratic family acts in a free way, is not withdrawn, is normally cheerful. However, a child who grew up in a non-democratic family demonstrates in their social behaviour the exact opposite characteristics'.[53] For Vladislav Klajn, who openly declared his allegiance to both Marxism and psychoanalysis, lingering patriarchal attitudes in non-democratic families contributed to 'the slowing down of societal progress' in the direction of workers' self-management, because patriarchal organisations as such were remnants of past historical structures, whose gradual disappearance was inevitable in socialist Yugoslavia. In order for the 'new world' to be realised and for all the social and cultural sacrifices made for it to pay off, the future Marxist society would need to ensure that democratic families are based on and promote comprehensive 'social welfare': 'general wellbeing, feeling of safety, freedom from fear' as well as 'social justice for all, decreasing primitivism, end of slavery to anachronistic traditions… full emancipation of women, …increased sense of personal responsibility'.[54] Klajn, like many of his colleagues, referred to patriarchal or undemocratic families as 'primitive', and drew his readers' attention to the phenomenon of urbanisation, in which many rural inhabitants brought traditional family values to urban settings and potentially undermined the modernisation process in that realm. Instead, Klajn called for the 'newcomers' to 'accept the already achieved degree of family democratisation in [their new] environments,

[52] Ksenija Kondić, *Prirucnik za vezbe iz psihopatologije detinjstva I mladosti*, Belgrade, 1991 (reprinted), 18–19.

[53] Matić, *Mentalna higijena*, 49.

[54] Vladislav Klajn, *Ljubav, seks, porodica*, Belgrade and Novi Sad, 1981, 242.

and use their expansive youthful energy to further encourage that environment to take more steps towards attaining a new quality of free and democratic family'.[55]

In everyday dealings with patients and their parents, Yugoslav psychiatrists constantly collected evidence for what they perceived as the need to reform the structure of traditional families: at the Institute for neuropsychiatry of children and youth, for instance, a thirteen-year-old girl was treated, whose mental state deteriorated dramatically after her parents moved in with the paternal grandparents. The psychologist in charge of this paradigmatic case related the severe decline of the quality of nuclear family life to this decision of the parents to live in an extended family, and highlighted the pernicious effects that older and more traditional family members might have on the child's mental health as well as on the overall relationship between the child and her parents.[56] In an even more dramatic case, an eight-year-old boy was brought to see a therapist because he kept attempting to commit suicide. The boy lived with his parents and paternal grandparents, which seemed to reinforce a highly hierarchical family set-up: the mother was, according to the therapist, consistently patient with and submissive to her in-laws, their needs and demands, while at the same time being extremely harsh and intolerant towards the boy. In addition, the boy reportedly witnessed instances of family violence committed by the alcoholic grandfather.[57] Regardless of whether the child became insecure or aggressive, problematic family relations robbed the society and the state of valuable citizens.[58] Authoritarian, traditional and non-democratic families thus constituted an immense political problem, and an obstacle on the path to self-managing socialism.[59] Tadić shared her conclusion that a family's insistence on 'well tried and traditional value systems leads children to conformism and to political, religious, social infertility'.[60]

55 Ibid., 240.

56 Kondić, *Prirucnik za vezbe iz psihopatologije detinjstva I mladosti*, 38–39.

57 Ibid., 32–33.

58 Rahela Galevska, 'Poremecena porodica i deca' (public lecture), Belgrade: Izdavacka kuca Rad, 1958.

59 Ibid., 36.

60 Tadić, *Psihoanaliticka psihoterapija dece i omladine*, Belgrade, 1984 (reprinted), 82.

Moreover, patriarchal and traditional Yugoslav families were explicitly linked to severe, long-lasting and sometimes irreversible psychological damage. In the course of their research into the family conditions of a group of psychotic patients in the early 1970s, a team of Skopje-based Macedonian psychiatrists discovered that most of the families under scrutiny were characterised by an 'authoritarian' and undemocratic emotional climate. This was reportedly particularly true for the patients' childhood families, while their contemporary families exhibited 'democratising and individualising' tendencies. Such recent developments, however, were predominantly outward and superficial, affecting the form rather than the essence of family relationships—in reality, 'patriarchal attitudes were still persistent'. Furthermore, the key obstacle to healthy inter-personal relations in such families was their 'emotional rigidity' and a high level of social conformism, so that the established traditional values and hierarchical relationships were rarely challenged, and those challenges regularly led to serious intra-familial conflicts. In the majority of the psychotic patients' families, for instance, the core illness-inducing conflict revolved around the parents' uncompromising disapproval of their children's choice of profession (most commonly in the arts)—in such cases, the parents' lack of understanding for their children's desires, and their 'prohibition of the development of [artistic] talents' regularly caused acute psychotic breakdowns in the children. The psychiatrists concluded that 'family was the foundation of illness and health', and that traditional Balkan families could be fundamentally incompatible with robust mental health.[61]

The problem of rigid parents was, thus, placed at the core of this heated discussion, especially the personality and pernicious psychological and political influence of authoritarian, harsh and perfectionist fathers, who could reportedly be responsible for enormous pathological personality changes in childhood, and pre-determine a child's problematic relationship with law and state. In fact, in the context of psychoanalytic criticisms of the patriarchal structure of the family, Yugoslav child psychotherapists tended to pay relatively more attention than their Western colleagues to the role of the father in the development of the child's personality and pathologies. While the figure of the

[61] Bogoljub Mojsiev et al. 'Uticaj intrafamilijarnih odnosa na pojavu akutnih psioticnih stanja', *Socijalna psihijatrija*, 1974:2, 133–137.

father was generally theorised to a significantly lesser extent in European psychoanalytic circles, those psychoanalysts and psychotherapists concerned primarily with critiquing authoritarianism and patriarchal hierarchies seemed to focus on the role of the father to an exceptional degree, possibly because the father—more than any other family member—symbolised the undemocratic patriarchal social potential and power asymmetry within the family, and was a representative of a repressive society, carrier and implementer of its values.

In one of the most influential and systematically researched articulations of this emphasis, Kondić, whose doctoral dissertation explored the role of parents' mental pathologies in the emergence of children's neuroses, argued that fathers played a 'dominant role in exerting negative influence, both individually and in a dyad with the mother, on the development of neurotic disorders in their children'.[62] According to Kondić's research results, fathers of neurotic children regularly assumed an authoritarian stance within the family, or withdrew emotionally from that relationship so that they treated their children in an 'impersonal' way. At times, moreover, their attitude towards their children was primarily determined by their need to 'punish' the wife. Moreover, this figure of a fearsome authoritarian father transcended generations and apparently remained impervious to broader progressive social changes, shaping and reproducing problematic personality structures and family dynamics. One of the mothers who took part in Kondić's dissertation research shared her painful realisation that she was becoming frightened of her son: 'I was afraid of my dad, terrified of him.... for a long time now I've known that I have been afraid of my husband as well, that I have lived in constant fear of him.. and now I realise that I'm starting to fear my own son in a similar way'.[63] Consequently, Kondić called for a 'radical reconsideration of the actual role [of the father]... in the development of children's psychological life from the very beginning', as well as for 'a significantly more active and earlier inclusion of fathers in the care for and education of their children'.[64]

[62] Ksenija Kondić, *Povezanost decjih neuroticnih smetnji sa strukturom licnosti odnosno patologijom roditelja* (PhD dissertation), University of Belgrade, 1980, 406.

[63] Ibid., 302.

[64] Ibid., 406.

As Till Van Rahden has convincingly argued in the context of West Germany, the idea that democracy ultimately rested on egalitarian and antihierarchical family practices increasingly gained ground from the 1950s on. A broad range of intellectuals and other public figures insisted that 'patriarchal-authoritarian' understandings of fatherhood inhibited the development of democratic consciousness and fostered fascistic and militaristic political choices.[65] For many in Central Europe, then, the concept of political power was tightly related to ideas of fatherhood and familial authority, and attempts to democratise the social and cultural practices of the national public inevitably involved the promotion of new models of family relations.

In various case studies, the personal as well as social and political consequences of an inadequate father were portrayed as potentially daunting. Moving away from the concept of a 'schizophrenogenic mother', a group of Croatian psychiatrists explored the pathological role of fathers in families of adolescent schizophrenic patients—they discovered and described 'dictatorial' personalities, patriarchal and hierarchical relations, and emotionally cold families in which daughters were marginalised while sons bore the brunt of parents' ambitions and expectations.[66] In 1975, for instance, two physicians from the psychiatric department of Belgrade's elite 'Dragisa Misović' hospital discussed a young male student, whose identification with the father could have easily led to a 'psychotic dissolution of personality' and the patient's subsequent inability to become an autonomous being and take part in constructive social relationships.[67] The father was described as a 'dominant-narcissist' type, who 'submitted

[65] Till Van Rahden, 'Families Beyond Patriarchy: Visions of Gender Equality and Child Rearing Among German Catholics in an Age of Revolution', in Nancy Christie, Michael Gauvreau, and Stephen Heathron, eds, *The Sixties and Beyond: Dechristianization as History in North America and Western Europe*, Toronto: University of Toronto Press, 2013, 270–293, and 'Fatherhood, Rechristianization, and the Quest for Democracy in Postwar West Germany', in Dirk Schumann, ed., *Raising Citizens in the 'Century of the Child:' Child-Rearing in the United States and German Central Europe in the Twentieth Century*, Studies in German History 12, New York: Berhahn Books, 2010, 141–164.

[66] Vasko Muacevic, Ljiljana Bastaic, Leo Henig, and Ksenija Maslo, 'Nasa zapazanja o promjeni uloga u obitelji u toku obiteljske terapije psihoza, *Socijalna Psihijatrija*, 1974:2, 153–157.

[67] Djordje Bogicevic and Zoran Rakic, 'Uloga oca i pseudoseksualizam kao odbrana u klinickoj slici psihoze (prikaz slucaja)', *Psihoterapija: Casopis za psihoterapiju i granicna podrucja*, 1975, 5:1, 43–59.

and shaped the entire family according to his own needs', while the mother was weak, passive and rejected by the father. Moreover, the son idealised the father throughout his childhood, adolescence and early youth—stifling criticism of and dissatisfaction with various aspects of the father's behaviour. In the psychiatrists' opinion, this led to a 'pathological identification' with the father, which inevitably bred dependency and failure to develop as an autonomous social being. The patient testified that 'in order to describe my father, I'm actually describing myself, because he is constantly in contact with me, constantly watching my reactions. Sometimes I feel like going somewhere and experiencing something myself [on my own], because he is always present in everything'.[68] At other times, he confirmed that the 'son is his father's mirror', while the father himself appeared rather proud that his child had 'ninety-nine percent of his [the father's] traits'.[69]

For the psychiatrists treating the younger man, this was a supremely dangerous situation, and one they perceived to have been systematically planned by the father, who was afraid to allow the child (especially son) to grow up, become a rival and usurp or undermine the father's position within the family. The relationship between the father and the son thus turned into a political battle for power and dominance, in which the father's sense of safety was severely shaken. As a result, the son of a dominant or narcissistic father would find it very difficult to avoid fully adopting and imitating the father's concepts and value systems, and to develop as an independent, confident and self-actualised person. Instead, the patient tended to behave almost exclusively according to the father's directions, judgements and evaluations. In a situation like this, the younger man proved inadequate in his adult roles as a husband and father, and as a political activist. In fact, the psychotherapeutic treatment seemed to directly encourage the patient's disobedience and challenges to the parental authority, and those were deemed as signs of recovery and progress. The psychiatrists reported that, towards the end of therapy, the patient's father came in to complain about his son's 'insolence' and disrespect, asking if he was allowed to beat him up.[70] This dramatic change in behaviour, more than anything else, signalled to the psychiatrists a

[68] Ibid., 52.

[69] Ibid., 50.

[70] Ibid., 55.

possibility that the patient might be able to recover the autonomy of his ego.

Some psychoanalysts took their discussions of the issue of patriarchal families beyond their consulting rooms and into the public realm. In the second half of the 1970s, for instance, Vojin Matić agreed to write an advice column for a high-circulation Belgrade-based popular magazine *TV Novosti* (TV News), and his unusual yet long-term engagement with thousands of readers' letters illustrated many of the themes which marked this peculiar development of Yugoslav psychoanalysis. In his responses to readers of all ages (very often children and teenagers), Matić described challenging familial relationships and their harmful effects on children in particular; such families were characterised by the 'parents' incomprehension, brusqueness and rigidity' which frequently resulted in their children's serious psychological disturbances and dysfunctionality. One reader blamed his personal difficulties on the 'narrow-mindedness' of the society, in which 'a daughter does not dare approach her mother with her problems'. Certain problems reported to be typical for traditional patriarchal families often came to the fore, and the letters Matić chose to respond to publicly emphasised the gravity of psychological complications that such situations could cause in those family's most vulnerable members. As one reader stated, her inability to continue with school and her deep depression were due to the constant malicious arguments between her mother and paternal grandmother, who lived in the same household throughout her childhood. Another female reader complained of her sense of worthlessness and her inability to set up an independent life because her family's love and appreciation were always exclusively showered upon her brother, while her parents 'constantly silence[d] and [misunderstood]' her, and ignored her needs and desires.[71] Parents who were unnecessarily or incessantly harsh and dismissive in their communication with children, physically and verbally aggressive over the 'slightest of misdemeanours which for others would appear completely normal' paraded through Matić's column almost on a weekly basis—possibly a conscious choice of his in order to emphasise the social and political importance of 'democratic' and mutually respectful family relations, and the multiple and often irreversible negative consequences of everyday family brutality.

[71] Matić, 'Zelim da pitam: Briga za brata', *TV Novosti*, 736, 2 February 1979, 35.

Matić, of course, regularly supported children and young people when they complained of their 'old-fashioned' families and their expectations, and encouraged them to resist or, if possible, move away from such pressures. For instance, when a reader reported that the grandparents she was living with after her parents' divorce were extremely strict, only allowed her outside if escorted by her brother and constantly reprimanded her ('the grandfather, moreover, curses, screams at me, beats me'), Matić noted with regret that 'old people' in general found it hard to alter themselves and their 'archaic views' but commended the reader for managing to resist such demands successfully and defend herself against them.[72]

Interestingly, Matić's readers often seemed to be aware of the psychoanalytic discourse regarding the potentially profound psychological significance of such authoritarian family practices, and regularly established the link between harsh patriarchal upbringing and subsequent mental health issues. As one reader stated, her general 'strangeness' and inability to establish and maintain both friendships and emotional relationships clearly stemmed from her 'patriarchal family' and 'strict upbringing', which meant that she was 'often punished for slight transgressions' and her social relationships were closely supervised. The reader even maintained that her behaviour had been so tainted by her family experiences that she would have had to 'be born all over again in order to be more like the rest'.[73]

Activism in Psychotherapeutic Consulting Rooms

Emancipatory psychotherapy was by no means a socialist invention: left-wing groups across the world recognised its potential for aiding progressive political projects. In particular, the 1960s and 1970s demonstrated that psychological and psychotherapeutic theories and techniques could be mobilised for explicitly emancipatory political aims: for instance, while criticising the psychological profession's propensity to pathologise women's complaints and reinforce patriarchal authority as natural, American second-wave feminists utilised the language of humanistic psychology in order to push their own liberationist agenda, and to argue that women needed opportunities for personal growth, self-actualisation and

[72] Matić, 'Zelim da pitam: Nepoznata bolest', *TV Novosti*, 742, 16 March 1979.

[73] Matić, 'Zelim da pitam: Nevino optuzivan', *TV Novosti*, 728, 8 December 1978, 35.

for the development of 'their fullest human potential'.[74] But it was only in Yugoslavia that this radical political agenda of self-actualisation through psychotherapy became the primary purpose of the profession as a whole: in the American and West European cases, feminist consciousness raising groups existed on the margins of the discipline, and tried very hard to distinguish themselves from conventional psychotherapy. Political activists often adopted (and radicalised) the language of psychology, psychotherapy and psychoanalysis, but it was only in socialist Yugoslavia that this became the profession's (and state-funded) mainstream identity.

However, in the second half of the twentieth century, many worried that the strategy of forging an alliance between radical politics and psychotherapy carried the risk of de-politicising the women's liberation movement, and re-framing women's oppression as a personal, psychological problem with an individual 'solution' which precluded collective political action.[75] The Western feminist movement never fully resolved this paradox. Yugoslav psychoanalysts, on the other hand, addressed this problem squarely from the very beginning, emphasising that the dividing line between family therapy and political revolution was porous and increasingly irrelevant, and using explicitly political language and concepts to talk about family relations, children's mental health and the role of the parents. In the Yugoslav case, the sustained state investment in such a revolutionary brand of psychotherapy produced a unique situation in which a radical political agenda dominated the discipline of psychoanalysis, while psychoanalysts saw direct links between family and political structures, turning the very therapeutic encounter into a vehicle of revolutionary politics.

Many Yugoslav psychiatrists (especially those who underwent psychoanalytic training) proposed original ideas regarding an activist psychoanalysis, which might abandon its 'aristocratic' position in the cabinet and get involved in proper social change. They often criticised Western psychoanalysis for its failure to focus more on collective rather than individual freedoms, and to take detailed theoretical account of the numerous economic, political, racial or religious pressures in modern societies: 'the

[74] Ellen Herman, *The Romance of American Psychology: Political Culture in the Age of Experts*, Los Angeles: University of California Press, 1995, 292.

[75] Ibid., 298–299.

psychoanalyst... most frequently closes his eyes before the social and political issues of his time'.[76] What they had in mind for their profession was radically different, and it involved changing the society by revolutionising family relationships and structures through clinical practice—such an unusually activist stance might be one of the most defining features of East European (socialist) psychoanalysis, and it was founded on the ideas of self-management and its continuous implementation in both families and society at large.

In her book on psychopathology and youth, Tadić drew a direct parallel between a 'patriarchal family' and 'bureaucratised social' relations, equating non-democratic familial arrangements with dictatorial political structures, and concluding that the youth needed to liberate itself from both in order to realise its own authentic emotional, cognitive, social capacities (in socialist Yugoslavia, the Soviet political system was regularly characterised as 'bureaucratic' and 'bureaucratised').[77] Family thus became yet another experimental site in which hierarchical relations were to be gradually unravelled (de-Sovietised) and patients were to be induced to replace them with more egalitarian and self-managing structures. The psychotherapeutic process had immense repercussions for the reality outside the consulting room: the crucial experiences of liberation, free expression and decision-making, self-knowledge and increased consciousness which patients gained in the course of psychoanalysis would inevitably shape their actions and behaviour in everyday life.

For child psychoanalysts, it was particularly important from the very beginning of the therapeutic relationship to demonstrate their respect, authentic interest and curiosity, and pay painstaking attention to everything the patient said or did; the therapist thus assumed the role of a liberator, emancipator. The therapist, moreover, aimed to reduce the child's dependency on the parents, while an appreciation of the patient's opinion needed to be communicated and followed through consistently. Slovene analyst Meta Kramar noted that the 'therapist... enabled him [the adolescent patient] to become active in his own life and assume initiative, and above all to become autonomous in his decisions'. Moreover, the 'therapist's respect for the patient's autonomy should be even more firmly embedded in his relationship with the patient in child psychiatry, because

[76] Tadić, *Psihijatrija detinjstva i mladosti*, 19.

[77] Ibid., 18–19.

the patient, as a child, was used to assuming a more passive and subordinated position before adults'.[78] In fact, such psychoanalytic insights provided an excellent framework for political interventions: the therapist needed to help their young patients to 'fight for their true needs and independence', even if it meant encouraging children and adolescents not to accommodate to the demands of their—flawed—family environment.

Following the lead of Anna Freud, Franz Alexander and Virginia Axline, Tadić recommended that analysts and therapists behave as 'the good parent', correcting the mistakes of patriarchal child-raising, 'by accepting the [patient] exactly as they were, with their good and bad traits, by listening carefully and appreciating them without judging, devaluating and condemning them'. In this way, therapy could alter children's and young people's social potentials and abilities, and teach them to engage in social relations differently in the future.[79] Moreover, the therapist must 'maintain deep respect towards the child's ability to resolve their own problems if they are given an opportunity for that'. Following Axline's principles of non-directive play therapy, Tadić advised that, in the complex relationship between the child patient and the therapist, 'the child leads, the therapist follows'. In this way, a full-blown personal transformation would be allowed to occur: 'in the safety of the [therapeutic] room, where the child is the most important person, the master of the situation and of himself, where nobody tells him what to do, nobody criticises what he does, ... he feels at last that he can spread his wings. He can look at himself clearly as he is fully accepted. He can test his ideas, and express himself fully, because this is his world'.[80]

Matić also advocated a more humane and sentimental treatment of hospitalised children by general physicians, not only psychiatrists, and criticised the assumption that children were supremely resilient creatures who can easily forget even painful and ugly interventions: 'physicians often forgot a child's soul and proclaimed humane gestures to be sentimentalities which harmed children's discipline'.[81] However, a different, warmer

[78] Meta Kramar, 'Prikaz psihoterapije decaka sa govornim smetnjama', *Psihijatrija danas*, 1976, 1:2, 196.

[79] Tadić, *Psihoanaliticka psihoterapija dece i omladine*, 66–67.

[80] Ibid., 69–72.

[81] Vojin Matić, 'Dete u bolnici', *Medicinski Glasnik*, 1954, 7–8, 275–277.

approach was necessary for the support and maintenance of the hospitalised child's mental stability, while reliance on intimidation, threats, emotional harshness and even physical punishments were causing unimaginable harm and were to be abandoned at once. Matić curiously stated that 'a child, with his individuality, already attained the right of citizenship in medicine', and this attainment, a new realisation of the psychological essence of children's personalities, should now not only transform the relationship between children patients and their doctors, but also be the first step towards a transformed political subjectivity. This argument then also required a much greater level of respect for children patients as equals (e.g. Matić was resolutely against deceiving children and lying to them about their need to stay in the hospital, or about the length of such stay).[82]

Importantly, while in Western Europe or the United States such clinical experiences primarily aimed to advance individual transformation and emancipation of child patients, Yugoslavia therapists placed these personal psychological goals explicitly in a political context: the issue of human freedom and its relationship to authoritarianism came to the very centre of the psychiatric understanding of child and youth psychotherapy. Tadić used very peculiar terminology to describe the position of a child psychotherapist who was asked to treat a patient by parents or a state agency: 'a psychotherapist must be aware of a trap, in which they often fall, to become a protector and advocate of the interests of the family and of the society, and to serve their interests uncritically'. This was particularly important because it was most often the case that the decision regarding psychotherapy was not made by the patients themselves, but by their parents, schools, psychological centres, etc., who 'should take responsibility for their part in the development of mental disturbances in children and youth'. Furthermore, sending a child to a therapist could be 'the last and most decisive pressure and enslavement'. Clinical contexts thus turned into arenas for political experimentation and activism: 'The therapist should not act like a person who offers freedom to the enslaved while smiling at and encouraging the enslaver', but should

[82] For a similar take, see also Ljiljana Milosavljevic, 'Neka zapazanja o ponasanju bolesnog deteta', *Psihologija*, 1977, 10:2, 89–93.

instead increase the political awareness and liberation potential of the enslaved.[83]

According to Tadić's understanding of her profession's societal role, psychotherapists could not gift freedom, or 'serve it on a plate', to their passive patients—but they were central to enabling patients to attain consciousness of the core social and psychological conflicts which determined their psychological suffering. Only such a radically egalitarian therapeutic relationship allowed patients the freedom to design their own responses to a variety of internal and external pressures. In that sense, this progressive revolutionary psychotherapy was most certainly not about dictating troubled young people how to react to their regressive environments: even though parents were often 'aggressive or inhibiting', and social institutions 'exploitative, bureaucratic, unjust and violent', psychotherapists had no right to directly pressure children and adolescents into battling and rejecting such limitations. Psychotherapy was fundamentally about 'conquering freedom', which meant that patients, including children, needed to take responsibility for their own decisions—whether to fight, or surrender and withdraw. Therapists could not do that on patients' behalf—but they could guide them towards revolutionary consciousness and a radical interpretation of the most pressing social, political and personal conflicts.[84]

Although she did not directly refer to them, Tadić's critical proclamations about the role of psychiatry in perpetuating societal oppression echoed some of the most important principles of radical psychiatry, a contemporaneous and mainly Western-based movement which emphasised alienation, hierarchy, inequality and social coercion in modern societies as the core causes of mental suffering. As Claude Steiner, the movement's founder and one of its most prominent theorists, wrote in an influential 1971 article, '[p]sychiatry has a great deal to do with the deception of human beings about their oppression', and it is precisely this collusion that Tadić's vision of activist psychoanalysis attempted to unravel: by proclaiming their 'neutrality', psychiatrists in fact became

[83] Tadić, *Psihijatrija detinjstva i mladosti*, 20–21.

[84] Tadić, *Psihoterpija dece i omladine*, Belgrade: Naucna knjiga, 1984, 21.

'[enforcers] of the domination and [their] lack of activity becomes essentially political and oppressive'.[85] On the other hand, radical psychiatrists, (as well as Tadić and her colleagues) primarily sought to counter the deception, make patients aware of their own oppression, and enact liberation through an explicitly politicised therapeutic process.

Tadić and Matić appeared to closely follow Herbert Marcuse's injunction—that psychiatry should be a 'subversive undertaking' which would 'prepare the mental ground for [the struggle against society]', that any action to tackle psychological illness would need to take place on a political level, and that psychiatrists should act as political saboteurs of any oppressive elements within the social order, preventing their patients from '[collaborating] in their own repression'.[86] As per the advice of the Massachusetts-based Radical Psychiatry collective, Tadić's writings invited her colleagues to see their (child) patients 'as oppressed people who must be liberated' rather than 'sick people who [needed] "treatment"'.[87]

In the case of some analysts, the critique of authoritarianism and suppression of children's vital creative capacities extended to the school system quite naturally. Tadić's close collaborator Svetomir Bojanin wrote of the contemporary schooling system as a 'social disease', which merely aimed to produce docile servants of the ruling political regime and actively prevented individual emancipation and 'liberation of the spirit'. 'Creatively frustrated people', argued Bojanin, 'were often able to lead only limited existence, experienced neurotic difficulties, became prone to alcoholism, drug abuse, and even schizophrenic psychoses'.[88] But in addition to these individual psychological problems, the schooling system as it was reportedly led to even greater political dangers. By encouraging obedience and competitiveness, schools undermined children's and young people's solidarity, empathy and independence of mind, and, in addition to producing mental disorders, made societies vulnerable to both 'the deathly promoters of fascism with their Mathausens, Jasenovacs and pogroms and the deathly promoters of Bolshevism with their Gulags

[85] Claude Steiner, 'Radical Psychiatry: Principles', in *The Radical Therapist*, New York, 1971, 16–17.

[86] Herbert Marcuse, *Negations: Essays in Critical Theory*, Boston: Beacon Press, 1968.

[87] Rough Times Collective, 'Introduction', *The Radical Therapist*, London, 1974, 8–9.

[88] Svetomir Bojanin, *Škola kao bolest*, Belgrade: Plato, 1990, 146.

and Goli Otoks'.[89] In other words, the third way of self-management and personal liberation was not possible without a radical re-thinking of the educational system and its rigid—psychopathological—hierarchies, in which teachers were 'the absolute masters' in their classrooms.

Restoring Patients' Humanity

In general psychiatric hospital practice, this approach to psychotherapy called for the re-establishment and recognition of psychiatric patients' fundamental humanity. As we saw in the beginning, this was a rather ambitious project in the context of Yugoslavia's early postwar hospital psychiatry. The problem of the psychiatric staff's disdain towards or disinterest in psychiatric patients, which Matić commented upon as a young trainee psychiatrist, persisted in various mental health institutions despite the striking liberalisation tendencies in the psychiatric profession.[90] As late as 1969, Pavao Brajsa, a psychiatrist in the Medical Centre of the east Croatian town of Varazdin, reported his own personal and professional transformation which came about as a result of his close contact with a group of schizophrenic patients in remission. According to his own admission, Basic was initially very reluctant to dedicate much time to schizophrenic patients, choosing instead to focus his research and clinical energies on the issue of adult and child neuroses. In order to minimise the unpleasant task of interfacing with schizophrenic outpatients at the Medical Centre, he decided to see all of them (twenty to thirty people) only once a week, at an appointed hour, and restricted his engagement to brief, impersonal, detached conversations and writing prescriptions.

However, as a result of these forced and decidedly anti-therapeutic waiting room meetings, the patients reportedly developed a particularly productive, humane and therapeutic group dynamic, and started involving the medical staff in their conversations and mutual interactions. Over time, these spontaneous gatherings turned into proper group therapies, while the original medical approach, which Brajsa self-critically termed 'anti-therapeutic' 'train station psychiatry', evolved into a set of dynamic and analytic techniques ranging from individual talking therapy to family

[89] Ibid.

[90] See Ivan Simic, 'The curious case of Aleksandar Milivojevic: The Donja Toponica hospital and mental health in socialist Yugoslavia', *Social History of Medicine*, 2020, 33:4, 1350–1362.

therapies as well as therapeutic excursions outside Varazdin. According to Brajsa, this dramatic transformation was initiated and implemented by the patients themselves, who fought against the psychiatrist's own resistances, his own inability to see in them anything but 'psychiatric patients incapable of normal communication'. Instead, the rushed and dreaded weekly meetings with schizophrenic patients turned into a process of 'humanisation, deinstitutionalisation, de-psychiatrisation…a process of pressuring the psychiatrist, the psychologist and the nurse to get closer to their patient, to accept him as a human being'. Moreover, Brajsa admitted to having been surprised by this 'discovery in a [schizophrenic] patient of a human being capable of love and deserving to be loved': 'together we discovered that we had something to say to each other, that we could talk'. The entire experience helped erase the rigid boundaries between the psychiatrists and the patient, and bred a sense of togetherness, a truly humane, empathetic and solidary community of people who 'needed each other'.[91]

It is particularly important in this case that the process of creating a properly therapeutic and humanised psychiatry was credited entirely to the patients (with the most serious psychiatric diagnosis), and was reportedly completed in spite of the psychiatrist's intentions. This portrayed the patient as not only a fellow human worthy of psychiatric respect but also superior to the psychiatrist in their ethical qualities, potential for empathy and personal responsibility, and able to teach the medical establishment a crucial lesson.

This process of acknowledging psychiatric patients' humanity was certainly not straightforward and unproblematic. Everyday practices and relationships between inmates and psychiatrists in psychiatric hospitals were indeed difficult to change, especially because such institutions tended to house chronic patients whose hospital confinement often extended to several decades. Apparently unable to improve such patients' psychological state, hospital psychiatrists would often minimise their contact and therapeutic efforts, resorting to brief and increasingly repetitive summaries of the inmates' mental and physical deterioration in case files—just as Brajsa did at the beginning of his engagement with his group of schizophrenic patients. In pre-socialist Yugoslavia, the language of psychiatric patient case files was explicitly derogatory and exclusive:

[91] Pavao Brajsa, Jasna Ozimec, Jelena Baldauf, 'Otpori "novom" pristupu shizofrenom bolesniku na varazdinskom podrucju', *Psihoterapija*, IV: 2, 1974, 206–208.

psychiatric patients were not expected to have much to give to the therapeutic process, such as it was, and any contributions they might have offered were regularly dismissed as 'babbling' of 'primitive' and 'senseless' personalities. Moreover, such patients, usually diagnosed with schizophrenia or mental retardation, were described as less than fully human: 'empty' and intellectually and affectively 'obtuse', unable to maintain social contacts with or express any interest in their environment, they reportedly behaved as automatons, who could only pretend to think or feel.[92]

Many of these tendencies continued after the Second World War, and despite the broader ideological and theoretical transformations within the psychiatric profession. What remains of the socialist-era patient case files of Yugoslavia's largest psychiatric hospital, 'Laza Lazarević' in Belgrade, demonstrates precisely such continuities, especially in the early postwar years. Throughout the 1950s, at times psychiatric descriptions of patients' behaviour and personalities resembled the harshest of legal indictments, impatiently piling accusation upon accusation, and condemning patients' psychological limitations as if they were their own personal responsibility. For instance, in May and June 1950, prewar psychiatrist Nadezda Jevtić described a female patient as 'sleepy, cranky, obtuse, with a confused look in her eyes. Negative, doesn't answer any questions… she doesn't do anything, only rambles around the ward, "thinking", she is so obsessed with herself that she can't pay attention to anything else'. However, only a few months earlier, the patient was evaluated by another psychiatrist, whose narrative and tone indicated a notable transformation in approach, even in the case of chronic and 'incurable' inmates. In this psychiatrist's description, the patient was 'not fundamentally alienated from her environment' even though she was not particularly interested in it. Still, 'she remains connected to the circle in which she lives, but in which she doesn't feel well'. In a hitherto rarely encountered narrative move of solidarity, the psychiatrist seemed to understand and even justify the patient's increasing disinterest and separation from her immediate surrounding. In order to reinforce that solidarity and understanding, the psychiatrist concluded that the patient was 'very sensitive in her essence, and often

[92] Ana Antic, *Therapeutic Fascism: Experiencing the Violence of the Nazi New Order*, Oxford: Oxford University Press, 2017, 67–78.

hurt'.[93] Moreover, the psychiatrist clearly viewed the patient's behaviour, and her limited affect for her own family, as a consequence of her deteriorating psychological illness rather than some fundamental personal or ethical flaw. Such a significant change in the hospital psychiatric language within the same case file boded well for the future.

In the following years and decades, the structure of patient files changed quite importantly in the hospital, and patients were almost never described as 'babbling', 'primitive' or 'bizarre' anymore. Throughout the 1960s and later, Yugoslav psychiatrists' theoretical discussions about the humanity and integrity of their patients seemed to exert some slow and gradual influence on day-to-day hospital practice. For instance, if they were capable, 'Laza Lazarević' patients were now regularly encouraged to take up work, and their efforts were frequently noted by psychiatrists with appreciation—this might have been the first time the hospital's personnel had referred to their chronic patients with such straightforward respect.[94] There were other signs of change: patients now had much more regular access to social workers and psychologists, and these evaluations, included in the patient files, often demonstrated that a more humane approach was indeed possible and desirable.[95] Overall, as the example from the above file demonstrated, the very tone of the dominant psychiatric language was considerably transformed over time (in a process parallel to the one described by Brajsa in Varazdin) so that patients were not always described in dehumanising, dismissive and alienating terms. Instead, psychiatrists' expressions of solidarity grew more common, and even when they defined their patients as 'empty' or 'apathetic', they were often able to identify and comment on those patients' genuine emotional reactions.

The case of Nadia G. was particularly illustrative in this sense.[96] Admitted in 1949, Nadia underwent a series of somatic treatments, most notably the insulin coma therapy, and was first described (often by Jevtic herself) as 'bizarre', 'illogical', 'theatrical' and 'autistic', 'underestimating' everyone else around her and boasting of her own superior status. She was reportedly highly unpleasant and impatient with the personnel,

[93] Archive of the Neuro-Psychiatric Hospital 'Laza Lazarevic', F-1, file 24790, patient admitted 11 June 1949.

[94] Ibid., file 24856, patient admitted 5 July 1949.

[95] Ibid., file 28621, patient admitted 20 April 1949; file file 20413, patient admitted 11 December 1944.

[96] Ibid., file 24658, patient admitted 7 July 1947.

but even when she was kind and polite, this was dismissed, even mocked, as a further sign of her mental deterioration. Nadia was often 'irksome' to the hospital staff with her frequent inquiries about her hospital stay and therapy. In one of her early interviews, she indicated that her psychological problems might have been linked to wartime events and shock, but, in line with prewar Yugoslav psychiatric practice, such allusions to possible psychological traumatisation were never commented on, nor did they have any effect on Nadia's ultimate diagnosis—schizophrenia. Moreover, Nadia's references to and concern for her own family members in her initial interview were similarly ignored, while she continued to be discussed as emotionally empty and 'affectively obtuse'.

However, as Nadia's stay in 'Laza Lazarević' stretched on into the 1950s and 1960s, her treatment was entrusted to a younger generation of psychiatrists (Jakulić, Trpković and Marjanović), and her patient file started looking significantly different, even though almost every new psychiatric note insisted that there were no remarkable changes in her psychological state. A few years after her admission, Nadia began working in the hospital's workshop as a seamstress, and she was reportedly very successful and committed to her work—although it was not until January 1962 that she received the first commendation by a psychiatrist for her efforts. She was reportedly an 'efficient' and 'neat' worker, well respected among her hospital colleagues; moreover, 'she completes her work in an excellent manner, and is capable of replacing the full workload of one paid staff member'. Furthermore, Nadia's interest in her own family members now got acknowledged for the first time as relevant for understanding her overall psychological state—particularly her poignant concern for the health of her elderly mother, and her repeatedly expressed wish to reunite with her expat daughter: 'she states she is waiting for her daughter to return from Algeria, and then she could die, she cries on this occasion'. While Nadia's deteriorating intellectual abilities were noted, they were interpreted as an inevitable result of the progress of her illness, and Jakulic insisted that, in spite of this, 'we need to attempt to recuperate her damaged family relations'. When communicating with Nadia's family, her psychiatrists conscientiously made sure to obtain her consent for any decision about her future treatment and accommodation—a radical departure from previous, and particularly pre-socialist, psychiatric hospital practices.

It was this hitherto unfamiliar note of empathy that now often transformed the narrative tone of the hospital's patient files and psychiatric interventions. In their attempts to better grasp and illustrate their patients' complex mental universe, hospital psychiatrists now tended to write longer and significantly less mocking notes and 'check-ins'. Moreover, in their notes, it now happened regularly that patients' voices were allowed to take over the dialogue for significant periods of time, and events or developments were described largely from their point of view—their words and expressions reported without too many psychiatric intrusions or interpretive (and dismissive) comments, even when psychiatrists clearly did not think that they could improve their chronic patients' health in any fundamental way.[97]

This narrative empathy extended beyond the file, as in the case of Svetozar S., another long-term inmate diagnosed with schizophrenia, who was removed from his hospital employment in 1962 and protected by his psychiatrists because they thought that his working conditions under the supervision of a particularly problematic foreman 'amounted to exploitation of psychiatric patients'.[98] Svetozar, like Nadia and many others whose psychological state did not improve in the course of their decades-long hospitalisation, were some of the hospital's most challenging patients—their 'failure' to be cured belied the socialist psychiatric promise and served as a dispiriting reminder of the profession's limited therapeutic possibilities. But by the 1960s, even though hospital psychiatrists were not offering such patients very much in terms of therapy, the nature of their relationship with the psychiatric staff did transform in an important way. As we already saw in Matić's poignant description of his early hospital practice, his senior neuropsychiatrist colleagues regularly laughed at, dehumanised and deliberately provoked psychiatric patients whom they could not understand. In the immediate postwar years, moreover, psychiatric case files often read as painstakingly collected evidence of patients' inappropriate, irksome and unacceptable behaviour. But several decades later, in the country's largest psychiatric hospital, one was hard pressed to find similar examples of mockery, dismissal and dehumanisation, even though the material conditions and therapeutic opportunities available to chronic patients may not have changed dramatically.

* * *

[97] Ibid., file 24856; file 20413, patient admitted 11 December 1944.

[98] Ibid., file 24856.

In the second half of the twentieth century, radical and critical psychiatry became an extremely influential intellectual strand, inspiring philosophers, political thinkers and activists who critiqued and grappled with different forms of hierarchy, oppression and inequality. Street protesters in 1960s Western Europe relied on psychoanalytic theory to make sense of their environment and to frame their visions of a future society, while the intellectual 'new left' borrowed and adjusted psychoanalytic insights in order to analyse the socio-economic and cultural faultlines of modern society. In most of these places, psychoanalysis was often the ultimate subversive discipline, aiding the intellectual process of deconstructing the existing political power structures. In Yugoslavia, however, psychoanalysis became a tool for revolutionising society in line with the state's (official) political ideology. This did not mean that psychoanalysis was in fact not subversive in self-managing Yugoslavia: as we will see in Chapter 6, which details the discipline's intellectual cross-overs with Praxis, the language of psychoanalysis could certainly serve to criticise the failings and hypocrisies of Yugoslavia's political project. But the theory of workers' self-management and of alienation, as developed by Yugoslav Party ideologues, relied centrally on ideas of human emancipation and full creative development, individual freedom and autonomy. In their sustained attempts to carve out political space for themselves between Stalinist orthodoxy and Western capitalism, Yugoslav Party Marxists provided an opportunity for psychoanalysts to expand on their visions of individual emancipation and revolutionary society. As it happened, Yugoslav psychoanalysts' and psychotherapists' understanding of their own role in transforming traditional 'authoritarian' families aligned closely with the state's political project for tackling patriarchy, and family and gender relations.

In their professional discussions and clinical publications, many psychoanalysts used overtly political language to discuss their professional aims and experiences, showing that the goals of Marxism, workers' self-management and psychoanalysis/psychotherapy were fundamentally intertwined. Their involvement in the Western networks of knowledge production was central here. West European practices and theories of psychoanalysis and psychotherapy figured prominently in Yugoslav clinical discussions, but they were regularly linked to the broader goals of revolutionary politics, self-management or socialist struggle against patriarchy or 'bureaucratised' political relations. Yugoslav 'psy' professionals made a concerted effort to prove an ideological affinity between Marxism and psychoanalysis—Vladislav Klajn, Vojin Matić, Nevenka Tadić, Vladimir Jakovljević, Muradif Kulenović were some of the most prominent ones, and they debated the notion of activist psychoanalysis, which sought to get involved directly in the social and political overhauling of the country. In most cases, the consulting room was a revolutionary field, in which tensions and debates over broader social, cultural and political changes played out, and the psychotherapeutic project of transforming and democratising families was part and parcel of the more ambitious political aim to develop a democratic Marxist personality and society. In that sense, the Yugoslav experiment, in which a new activist psychoanalysis became mainstream and state-funded psychotherapy, remains central to understanding the role of psychoanalysis as a tool for socio-political critique and activism in the second half of the twentieth century.

CHAPTER 4

Authoritarian Psychiatry

As we have seen in the last chapter, in the aftermath of WWII and the political split with the USSR, Yugoslav psychiatry and psychoanalysis became the most liberalised and Westernised professions in the region. Of all the socialist countries, it was only in Yugoslavia that psychoanalysis thrived, receiving generous material and logistical support from the state, and intervening in the most important political debates of the time. From the early 1950s on, Yugoslav socialist psychiatrists gradually became full-fledged members of the Western European medical community, developing a rich culture of professional exchange with their Western European as well as American colleagues—as the case of Vojin Matić and his disciples illustrated very well. Moreover, Yugoslav 'psy' disciplines adopted an ambitious agenda of facilitating personal emancipation, aiming to support and counsel families and individual patients in their efforts to unravel oppressive social structures and shed authoritarian mentalities. In that sense, this new brand of internationalised socialist psychiatry strove to play an active role in the project of building a genuine Marxist democracy, and exploring the psychological and psychotherapeutic aspects of the concept of workers' self-management.

However, the history of Yugoslavia's 'psy' disciplines was not as straightforward as the last chapter might indicate. While many leading

A. Antić, *Non-Aligned Psychiatry in the Cold War*,
Mental Health in Historical Perspective,
https://doi.org/10.1007/978-3-030-89449-8_4

'psy' professionals' and institutions were clearly interested in experimenting with radical politics and revolutionary notions of human liberation, Yugoslav socialist psychiatrists were also involved in more authoritarian 're-education' projects, in instances of political abuse and manipulation, and in the subsequent Eastern European psychiatric and pedagogical networks.[1] In an important sense, therefore, these thoroughly Westernised revolutionary professions did belong to the socialist bloc as well, and shared clinical practices, ideas and aims with their East European counterparts. As we will see in the rest of this chapter, in the immediate aftermath of the 1948 break, the Yugoslav 'psy' disciplines contributed to the operation of the violent re-education program at the Goli Otok camp, the most authoritarian and repressive political project in the country's history, which primarily targeted Soviet supporters and sympathisers within the Yugoslav Communist Party. Several decades later, evidence started mounting that pointed to the psychiatric profession's involvement in the suppression of political dissidents and non-conformist, and a set of testimonies emerged which linked Yugoslav experiences to the notorious practices of Soviet punitive psychiatry.

Postwar psychoanalysis and psychiatry thus provide a useful lens through which to study the complicated and unexpected political alliances of the Cold War. While the Yugoslav socialist regime allowed freedoms and opportunities unmatched in the socialist world, it also devised exceptionally brutal and oppressive measures to deal with opponents it considered particularly dangerous. These complex and contradictory historical trends were clearly reflected in the character and development of Yugoslavia's psychotherapy. The Yugoslav state not only tolerated psychoanalytic and psychotherapeutic critique of lingering institutional authoritarianism, but also supported these disciplines and strengthened their influence. On the other hand, the authorities were from the very beginning equally interested in Soviet-style psychiatric experiments, and sent mental health professionals 'to the West' in order to gauge prison psychiatric practices in the Soviet Union.[2]

[1] Amnesty International, *Yugoslavia: Prisoners of Conscience*, London, 1985; British Medical Association, *Medicine Betrayed: The Participation of Doctors in Human Rights Abuses*, London, 1992, 64–82; Vladimir Markovic, *Za ljudska prava: Moje disidentske uspomene*, Belgrade: Slobodna Knjiga, 1999.

[2] Aleksandar Pavkovic, Pismo od 26.9.1998, quoted in Dragoslav Mihailovic, *Goli Otok 5*, Belgrade: Sluzbeni Glasnik, 2012, 355–359.

In socialist Yugoslavia, therefore, in every facet of society, psychiatry and psychotherapy became instrumental in shaping and reshaping minds, and experimenting with new political ideas. Psychoanalytic and psychotherapeutic theories became increasingly important for understanding and developing the notions of individual enlightenment and self-management that underpinned Yugoslavia's reform Communism. On the other hand, in Goli Otok, the project of individual reformation took on an exceptionally violent guise, but it was informed by the same principles that shaped the theory and practice of progressive child psychotherapy and psychoanalysis, discussed in the previous chapter. Moreover, psychiatrists were involved in these explicitly political enterprises, whether as liberal professionals or as contributors to the idea of violent re-education, and offered elaborate psychological interpretations of Marxist/Communist concepts and of the importance of self-management. Towards the end of the socialist period, testimonies of political prisoners demonstrated that liberal psychiatric institutions and professionals, committed to patients' emancipation and revolutionary struggle against political authoritarianism, could also be implicated in Soviet-style punitive psychiatric practices. In the 1970s and 1980s, therefore, it was confirmed yet again that very similar notions and ideological principles could be used within the same sociopolitical framework and by the same profession but for radically different purposes.

Goli Otok and Early Yugoslav Psychoanalysis

> The Romanian tanks are on their borders, the Bulgarian tanks are on the Bulgarian borders, on the Hungarian borders stand and wait the Hungarian tanks, and at that very moment, when the Party needed you the most, you stabbed it in the back. That's not nice, that's treason, and you need to realize that. We shall try to help you to get yourselves out of that quagmire.[3]

This is how, in 1950, Marija Zelić Popović, Yugoslav state police investigator, greeted one of the first groups of political prisoners who were about to undergo years of brutal physical torture and political

[3] Quoted in D. Simic and B. Trifunovic, *Zenski logor na Golom Otoku: Ispovesti kaznenica i islednice*, Belgrade: ABC Produkt, 1990, 228.

're-education' because they were suspected of pro-Stalinist ideological leanings and activity. In 1948, Yugoslavia, a newly socialist, revolutionary country which had just emerged from the most devastating conflict in its brief history, experienced yet another exceptionally turbulent international episode: its close military, political and ideological relations with the USSR crumbled within a few months, and Yugoslavia fell out of the Soviet sphere of influence. In June 1948 the Yugoslav Communist Party (CPY) was expelled from the Cominform (Communist Information Bureau, an international forum of communist and workers' parties, founded in 1947). This followed the Cominform's damning resolution which accused the CPY of deviating from Marxism-Leninism, and promoting openly anti-Soviet policies and viewpoints.[4] As we already saw, the Tito–Stalin split ultimately benefited Yugoslavia, and the Yugoslav regime's unique position within the Eastern bloc allowed its leaders to pursue experimental policies, and to encourage rich exchanges with both the Eastern and the Western worlds. However, this political break had serious social consequences; Yugoslavia's falling out with Moscow was further complicated by its dangerous geographical position: as Zelić Popović noted with great alarm, the state was surrounded by Soviet satellites, and the prospect of foreign invasion as well as internal treason was a real possibility for years. Moreover, the intimate ideological bonds between the Yugoslav and Soviet Communist Parties could not be broken off so easily, and many committed communists' loyalties remained hopelessly confused.

The country's dangerous departure from the increasingly oppressive Soviet zone sparked, in turn, the most authoritarian and Stalinist-like political episode in Yugoslavia's entire history. Afraid for its survival and fearing popular defection to the Soviet side in case of invasion, the Yugoslav regime embarked on a long and thorough purge of its most esteemed cadres.[5] Thousands ended up in political prisons, and the regime devised a programme of 're-education' for all those former

[4] Vladimir Dedijer, *Izgubljena bitka J. V. Staljina*. Belgrade: Prosveta, 1969; Leonid Gibianskii, 'The Soviet-Yugoslav Split and the Cominform', in N. Naimark and L. Gibianskii, eds, *The Establishment of Communist Regimes in Eastern Europe, 1944–1949*, Boulder, CO: Westview Press, 1997; Tvrtko Jakovina, *Americki komunisticki saveznik: Hrvati, Titova Jugoslavija i SAD 1945–195*, Zagreb: Srednja Europa, 2003; Rina Kullaa, *Non-Alignment and its Origins in Cold War Europe: Yugoslavia, Finland and the Soviet Challenge*, London: I.B. Tauris, 2012.

[5] Ivo Banac, *With Stalin Against Tito: Cominformist Splits in Yugoslav Communism*, Ithaca, NY: Cornell University Press, 1988.

comrades who 'failed' to understand the true meaning of the Soviet–Yugoslav split. The most notorious of the several 're-education' camps established was the Goli Otok labour and prison camp complex. Here, a brutal psychological experiment was conducted with tens of thousands of inmates incarcerated on a secluded island off the northern Croatian coast. While much has been published on Goli Otok, the psychiatric aspect of its regime remains completely unexplored. This section sheds light on how certain psychiatric as well as psychoanalytic ideas shaped the conceptualisation and realisation of this experiment, and discusses the central role of these disciplines more broadly in East European authoritarian political projects. In so doing it explores how elements of the psychoanalytic tool kit could be employed, along with certain behaviourist techniques, and put to use in the service of so-called political re-education, rather than as a therapeutic practice. In this respect, although the Goli Otok camp also relied on the input of individual analysts and therapists, this section is primarily concerned with how Freudian ideas and techniques were appropriated as a form of overt political control, where 'the patient' in fact had no choice but to participate in this 'talking cure'.

The history of the Goli Otok camp demonstrates that the concept of self-management could be combined with various psychotherapeutic and psychoanalytic theories both in violent camps and in Westernised psychotherapeutic consulting rooms, in order to achieve rather different results in the realm of re-education. But even when it was implemented in the extreme context of violence and coercion in the camps, it still retained the connotation of personal growth, development, and ultimate liberation—although at Goli Otok, that liberation was to be achieved through a complete destruction and unravelling of the inmate's 'treacherous' personality.[6] Psychoanalysis and psychotherapy were thus instrumental for both—unravelling and rebuilding.

Wartime Origins of 'Re-education' Experiments

In the aftermath of the unprecedented violence of the Second World War and the socialist revolution of 1945, psychodynamic and psychotherapeutically oriented approaches became quite influential in postwar psychiatry

[6] This peculiar combination of therapeutic self-reform and destruction has already been studied in the context of the Soviet Gulag; see Steven Barnes, *Death and Redemption: The Gulag and the Shaping of Soviet Society*, Princeton: Princeton University Press, 2011.

in Yugoslavia. This was quite unlike developments in other countries of the socialist bloc. Psychiatry underwent a radical transformation during the war, challenging an almost exclusively organicist, German-influenced, hereditarian scientific outlook and developing into a mental health discipline, notably shaped by psychoanalytic ideas, and with a new focus on environmental influences. However, the origins of this lasting change did not lie in the radical socialist overhaul of 1945 but in the war years themselves. When Yugoslavia's communist psychiatrists argued that a socio-economic transformation and psychological healing could free society of mental woes, they echoed views already promulgated by a unique institution in wartime Yugoslavia: the Institute for Compulsory Re-education of Communist Youth in Serbia. The latter, which had been founded and run by the Serbian collaborationist government (1942–1944) openly accepted various psychoanalytic principles, notably transference, and seriously considered the role of psychological and environmental factors in the emergence and therapeutic treatment of mental illness.[7] Moreover, the institute provided a model for the application, in a most peculiar form, of psychodynamic therapies. Its techniques aimed to erase the dire psychological effects of the 'national trauma' of the country's humiliating defeat and occupation in 1941.

The institute was important for postwar socialist psychiatry and served more specifically as a model of sorts for the labour camp which the Yugoslav state established for suspected pro-Stalinists in its own ranks in 1949 – the aforementioned infamous Goli Otok (*Naked Island*, or *Barren Island*). At the institute, sustained efforts were made to try to persuade the pro-communist young to abandon their ideological beliefs and support the pro-fascist government of Serbia. The institute combined elements of psychoanalytic thought with a behaviourist interpretation of human psychological development, accompanied by violent physical punishments. Goli Otok used the same approach but significantly increased the intensity of physical violence. In fact, one of the leading men of the wartime collaborationist Belgrade Special Police's Anti-Communist Section (which co-organised and co-ran the institute, and was otherwise under Gestapo auspices), Bozidar Becirevic, was co-opted by the postwar Yugoslav state police, and kept alive in order to share his 'expertise'

[7] Milan Borkovic, 'Zavod za prinudno vaspitanje omladine u Smederevskoj Palanci', *Istorijski Glasnik*, 1966, 1, 97–98.

regarding the techniques of questioning and 're-educating' communist prisoners.[8]

The head of the wartime institute, Milovan Popovic, believed that his educational philosophy was centrally informed by the theory and practice of psychoanalysis. In a statement that explicitly referred to Freud, Popović explained:

> it is necessary to establish between us and them a relationship full of closeness and trust. Freud could only use psychoanalysis to treat the ill if he succeeded to develop in his patients true love, of [a] sexual nature, towards himself. Only then did they open their souls to him and allowed him to see their wounds. We must observe similar rules. The children must first believe in us, that we will defend and protect them like the closest of kin, and only then can they reveal their souls to us.[9]

In other words, Popovic protested against the brutal police treatment of young political prisoners before they were sent to the institute, claiming that such violence and cruelty could only exacerbate the ideological delusions of the offenders. However, although there were important commonalities between the institute and the postwar Goli Otok prison camp, the latter integrated violence with certain psychoanalytic ideas and re-education techniques much more forcefully.

The continuity of expertise across 1945 ensured that there were important affinities between the two experimental projects. The wartime institute had developed an internal structure similar to the one at Goli Otok, and encouraged self-management among the inmates; young inmates were expected to participate in decision-making processes wherever possible. An internal spying structure was also fostered; inmates were incited to report on one another's suspicious or dissident behaviour to the instructors, and to view the latter as their true allies and friends, even ersatz parents. At the same time, the institute's instructors provided modified individual therapeutic sessions. These were then also adopted at Goli Otok and turned into regular, compulsory confessional sessions. The instructors might be staff members, police investigators or indeed 're-educated' prisoners who had already climbed the camp's ladder. Just

[8] Petar Kostic, *Psiholoska anatomija Golog Otoka*, Belgrade: Nezavisna izdanja Slobodana Masica, 2012, 72.

[9] Archive of Serbia, Zavod u Smederevskoj Palanci, 3/3-1, 50, 1.

as at Goli Otok, the institute leadership insisted that the inmates produce elaborate narratives about themselves. Along with personal testimonies, they were also required to produce confessional essays on a number of different topics. This coercive form of self-exploration and introspection was regarded as key to the process of re-education.[10]

Despite their radical and liberalising transformations, some of the most progressive members of Yugoslav psychiatry and psychoanalysis could still contribute to the operation of the violent and repressive re-education programme at Goli Otok. Yugoslavia was unique among the socialist countries in providing a medical and political culture in which particular versions of emancipatory psychoanalysis could thrive. But Yugoslav psychoanalysis and progressive psychotherapy could also be involved in violent anti-Stalinist processes, purges and 're-education' projects, and in the subsequent East European psychiatric and pedagogical networks.

In re-thinking the role of psychoanalysis in a Marxist society, Vladislav Klajn proposed and then implemented a curious combination of techniques, which significantly decreased the length of analysis, and sought to give the analyst a more direct and powerful leadership role in the process. It is likely there was an intellectual link between this more authoritarian version of psychoanalysis and the psychological re-education that was implemented in the Goli Otok camp. Klajn argued that, when it was applied to 'primitive', 'undereducated' or 'intellectually less elevated patients', the psychotherapeutic method needed to be more active, more 'authoritative'; in short, the therapist had to lead patients and 'force them to active cooperation'.[11] This was a novel take on the old idea of psychiatrists as teachers and the need for enlightenment. For Klajn, Freud's insights constituted an invaluable contribution to understanding the psyche and mechanisms of mental illness. However, Klajn soon developed into a rather unorthodox 'socialist psychoanalyst', attempting to devise an approach appropriate to Yugoslavia's particular profile. He mostly shunned long-term sessions in favour of shorter, more intense treatments, in which the importance and strength of consciousness and ego were emphasised over the unconscious, and he conceptualised the therapist as akin to a tutor who directed his patients in a firm, disciplined and, if

[10] On the psychoanalytic aspect of the institute's programme, see Antic, *Therapeutic Fascism*.

[11] Vladislav Klajn, 'Problem rehabilitacije – rehabilitacija neuroticara', *Vojno-Sanitetski Pregled*, 1958, 7–8, 531.

necessary, heavy-handed manner, while dispensing 'guidance' much more straightforwardly than an orthodox psychoanalyst would have done.[12] Klajn famously defended psychoanalysis at Party meetings, and claimed that, in his soul, he could combine Freudianism with Marxism, while expressing his admiration for the work of Karen Horney.[13]

Importantly, Klajn was also a high-ranking officer of the Yugoslav state police and a lecturer at the Federal State Police's Polytechnic. Due to his tight connection to police and military structures throughout the 1950s, recent research has related him and another psychiatrist from within the state police, Dr Svetislav Popović, to experiments and developments at Goli Otok.[14] Moreover, Klajn himself worked as the head of the neuro-psychiatric ward at the Belgrade hospital Dragisa Misović, whose director was the senior physician for the Goli Otok prisoners and whose doctors regularly treated the camp's inmates as well as the Yugoslav regime's highest functionaries (in his ward, Klajn introduced and supervised analytic psychotherapy for neurotic patients).[15] But even if Klajn was not directly connected to the Goli Otok experiments—and the exact nature of his involvement remains unclear as the relevant archives have so far been unavailable to researchers—his conceptualisation of 'socialist psychoanalysis' as a more authoritarian version of psychotherapy informed by certain analytic categories probably influenced the formulation of violent 'therapeutic' techniques at the camp, especially since he regularly lectured to state police employees.

The Pedagogy of Self-Management

The Goli Otok camp's psychological outlook was eclectic, complex and contradictory, and characterised by a melange of theoretical and methodological approaches. The leadership insisted on immediately and brutally modifying their inmates' behaviour, through endless repetition,

[12] Petar Klajn, *Razvoj psihoanalize u Srbiji*, Subotica: Pedagoska akademija, 1989, 78–83.

[13] Ibid., 109.

[14] Kostic, *Psiholoska anatomija Golog Otoka*, 41–42.

[15] Ibid.

reinforcement (dispensation of life-saving privileges) and severe punishments.[16] Such insistence reflected the camp's behaviourist approach to re-education, the belief that a structured adjustment of acts—especially public acts—was the precursor to the acquisition of new habits that would transform personality traits and shape choices, most notably political behaviour and convictions.[17] By contrast with the tenets of leading behaviourists, however, the camp authorities did not disregard the relevance of internal mental states. Indeed, its leaders and ideologues were also concerned with uncovering and transforming deeper layers of the psyche. Even behaviourist techniques were often applied with the aim of achieving a deeper—psychoanalytic—transformation of personality, and reworking the subject's personal motivations. This 'therapeutic' ambition bizarrely co-resided, as noted, with techniques of terror and humiliation, an aggressive atmosphere, and the constant possibility of torture. Indeed, 'therapeutic sessions' themselves routinely included a violent component. Introspection and self-analysis played an enormous role in this process, and their application in the violent context of the camp constituted Goli Otok's unique culture of 'therapeutic violence'.

The Goli Otok camp came into operation at approximately the same time as Chinese forces were testing certain 're-education' methods on their American prisoners of war during the Korean War (1950–1953). While there were common features between the Yugoslav and Chinese approaches (most likely stemming from their common Soviet pre-history), the former's re-education experiment introduced the original method of 'self-management' of the inmates, so that the presence of the state, though overwhelming, was not immediately visible in the camp.[18] The Chinese-Korean re-education programme included some elements of the Goli Otok experience: there was a clear prisoner hierarchy, and a particular system of rewards and punishments. The 're-educable' and 'incorrigible' cases were clearly demarcated, so that solidarity within the prisoner community was discouraged and sabotaged. Moreover, the 're-educated' prisoners sometimes surpassed their instructors in their

[16] Ibid., 102.

[17] K. Perucica, *Kako su nas prevaspitavali*, Belgrade: Dereta, 1990, 63.

[18] See A. Bidermann, *March to Calumny: The Story of American POWs in the Korean War*, New York: Macmillan, 1963; R.T. Robin, *The Making of the Cold War Enemy: Culture and Politics in the Military-Intellectual Complex*, Princeton, NJ: Princeton University Press, 2009.

expressions of loyalty to the new cause of communism. They were also soon involved in spying networks inside the camp, and reported on their co-prisoners.[19] Around this time, a wide-ranging and all-pervasive ideological campaign engulfed the entire Chinese society in the early 1950s, aiming at the deep psychological reconstitution of Chinese citizens as well as foreigners living there. This complicated 'thought reform'—as Robert Jay Lifton labelled it—affected prisons, universities and factories. The Yugoslav attempts at re-education, although much more modest and targeted, strikingly involved techniques that similarly focused on participants' intense self-exploration and guided self-analysis.

Since Goli Otok mainly held Communist Party members who had been affiliated with the cause for decades, the system of re-education aimed to convey the message that the imprisoned comrades finally understood the magnitude of their past mistakes and confusions, and led themselves and their colleagues out of the blunder, with the generous help of the CPY. As former inmate Emilijan Milan Kalafatić testified, those who had 'revised' their attitude had to repeat daily at various local political meetings and classes, in front of other prisoners, that 'Yugoslavia was the only socialist country in the world'. They were required to 'celebrate the theory of the withering away of the state, although it was clear to everyone that the state apparatus of violence remained in its entirety, and was even augmented'. This was the cornerstone of Yugoslavia's theory and application of workers' self-management after the 1950s, and it was first formulated and discussed in the violent context of Goli Otok.[20]

Indeed, many former inmates testified that the lower the level of the camp's organisation the less visible became any representatives of state authority (such as policemen). One could get a strong impression that it was in fact the most 'advanced' and 're-educated' prisoners who mostly ran the affairs and conceptualised the camp's programme. As Dragoslav Mihailović remembered, the increasingly porous boundary between the inmates and their keepers (policemen, guards, police investigators) further complicated the situation, making the experience of incarceration even

[19] Peter Watson, *War on the Mind: The Military Uses and Abuses of Psychology*, New York: Basic Books, 1978.

[20] Emilijan Kalafatic, 'Pismo Predsedniku SFR Jugoslavije i Saveza Komunista Jugoslavije Josipu Brozu Titu', in Mihailovic, *Goli Otok*. Belgrade: NIP Politika, 1990, 525–526.

more difficult to handle, since no real community of the imprisoned, no internal moral code of behaviour, could develop.[21]

With its elaborate hierarchical prisoner structure, the camp's unique 'apparatus of compulsion' rested on the core idea that prisoners were constantly to survey and 'read' one another. Furthermore, all inmates were led to believe that 'those ... who saw and understood their own betrayal ask and force the others to do the same'.[22] Each camp within the complex had its own centre for prisoners' self-management (albeit under the watchful eye of police investigators), with their leaders, deputies, foreman and officers in charge of cultural affairs. This pattern was then replicated in the cells and barracks, each of which was organised into a collective (similar to communist front organisations), and within which there were always the 'actives', those who made up the 're-education' vanguard. Barrack heads (room wardens), tasked with ideological leadership roles, were again composed of prisoners who had proved to the police investigators the authenticity of their political 'revision'. What happened in the barracks, the site where all inmates would return each night, determined the prisoners' future.[23]

Finally, each barrack had its own share of 'bandits'—those who still failed to comply, self-criticise and admit their own dangerous past, and who were then subjected to 'boycott'. This included various degrees of physical and psychological torture, and complete isolation from other inmates. Nobody was allowed to communicate to the 'bandits' and they were allocated the hardest, most exhausting and often most meaningless forms of labour. Those who were higher in the ranks—members of the collectives or activists—were tasked with then attending to the 're-education' of the bandits, while ensuring that their time at the camp was kept as miserable and psychologically devastating as possible until their reform. In fact, in order to remain an activist, one had not only to fully 'revise' one's attitudes, demonstrate a complete and accurate understanding of the Yugoslav position in its conflict with the USSR and so on; one also needed to prove one's 'revision' in practice, by using any means available to 'persuade' the bandits to change their orientation and

[21] Mihailovic, Goli Otok, 105.

[22] Milinko Stojanovic, *Goli Otok: Anatomija zlocina*, Belgrade: Strucna knjiga, 1991, 185–186.

[23] Perucica, *Kako su nas prevaspitavali*, 134–144.

join the collective. In reality, this meant that all the activists had to excel in 'chasing up' recalcitrant inmates, in exerting 'psycho-physical methods of compulsion' cursing, yelling at, even hitting the bandits.[24] This was indeed the true test of the validity of their 'rebirth' as honest communists. If they were suspected of faking their pressure on the bandits, activists were likely to be demoted and relieved of previous privileges or even severely punished. In fact, Goli Otok prisoners experienced most of their physical and psychological traumas at the hands of their fellow inmates and often former comrades.

Psychotherapeutic Techniques

In a rare analysis of the psychiatric aspects of Goli Otok 're-education', psychiatrist Todor Baković proposed that psychiatrists and psychoanalysts who advised the state police regarding the organisation of the camp's internal mechanisms drew upon the psychoanalytic concepts of ambivalence and projection. The very nature of the Yugoslav-Soviet split, according to Baković, created conditions for such psychic states and mechanisms. He argued that the passionate ideological and personal loyalty of most Yugoslav communists to Stalin and the Soviet Union, and the uncritical adoration of Stalin in the post-1945 Communist Party of Yugoslavia, meant that the ensuing conflict between Tito and the Soviet leadership came as a dramatic psychological blow. What used to be an idea and an allegiance worth sacrificing one's life for turned into a source of shame, suffering and even imprisonment. People who proved themselves as war heroes were now humiliated, excommunicated and branded as backstabbers. Baković's retrospective interpretation of the techniques applied at the camp, therefore, argued that the notion of ambivalence was deliberately fostered on two levels: first, it was Party members who arrested their own comrades, colleagues, friends, co-warriors and accused them of treason, lack of patriotism, disloyalty; second, within the camp itself, the differentiation of rank occurred among co-prisoners and co-sufferers, with the police keeping their apparent distance: 'the immediate

[24] Miroslav Popovic, *Udri bandu,* Belgrade: Filip Visnjic, 1989, 112–113.

performers of torture were the inmates themselves, and they mostly suffered from each other'.[25]

Baković suggested that psychoanalysts such as Klajn himself, who advised the police on these matters, must have been aware of the powerful defence mechanism of projection, which then inevitably developed from such complex psychological circumstances: if 'revisers' felt any remorse for their humiliating 'revision', if there was any self-contempt or self-recrimination on their part, if they felt the need for self-punishment as a result of their collaboration with the police investigators at the camp, these feelings, he argued, were then probably projected onto the 'bandits', leading to further tendencies of brutalisation: 'They see their punishment of their comrades as a punishment of themselves…. The greater the remorse, the harder the blows. The harder the blows, the greater the relief'.[26] According to Baković, this ensured the spontaneity, the efficiency of the system, as well as its notorious cruelty in requiring the enactment of physical and psychological abuses by one prisoner upon another. Milovan Popovic, a former inmate who had spent most of his incarceration at Goli Otok as a 'bandit', confirmed Baković's points, insisting that the re-educated torturer of his co-prisoners always hated the victim, and this was the result of the complex and painful psychological processes that accompanied his transition to an upper level within the hierarchy: 'a torturer with conscience hated his victim because of the guilty conscience itself'. It was as though, were it not for the victim, there would not have been any guilty conscience either: 'Through his very existence the victim put him in a situation [where he had to] to push and pull him, to scream at him, to treat him, a fellow man, a former comrade, now a co-prisoner, like he never thought anybody would treat [another human being]'.[27] For those reasons, it was suggested here, the conscientious prisoners grew into the worst torturers, and actively strove to sink 'ever deeper in the disgusting earth of evil'. It was this capacity to induce such projections of self-hatred onto the victims, he argued, that kept Goli Otok ticking so successfully. However, although Baković's identification of particular psychoanalytic processes at work at the camp was very revealing, his interpretation of

[25] Teodor Bakovic, 'Psiholoski aspekti golootocke torture i sadistickog mucenja', in *Goli Otok (1949–1956): Radovi sa okruglog stola, Podgorica 27. juna 1995*, Podgorica: CANU, 1998, 212–213.

[26] Ibid., 213.

[27] Popovic, *Udri bandu*.

the Goli Otok mechanisms provides no evidence that psychoanalysis was intentionally applied there. In the rest of the chapter, I will demonstrate that psychoanalytic and psychotherapeutic categories did play a central role in the very organisation and conceptualisation of the camp.

Although this appeared to be a process entirely run from below, almost all Goli Otok convicts agree that the collective's treatment of those making public declarations in their barracks was in fact carefully planned by the police. Yet, as we have noted, the barracks meetings and 'investigations' were set up as though they were collective therapeutic sessions, with inmates obliged to reveal their innermost thoughts, emotions and quandaries, to confess and discuss their life histories, present and criticise their motivations, and dissect their past political and social engagements in front of 'healed' comrades.

Goli Otok, no less than the contemporaneous Chinese re-education experiments, drew considerably upon early Soviet jurisprudence and its conceptualisations of punishment as an opportunity for rebirth and rehabilitation. While the Gulag largely dispensed with the idea of self-managing rehabilitation of prisoners, the 1920s Soviet prisons and labour colonies that had emerged earlier had applied a striking set of measures in order to try and re-educate political offenders, common criminals and juvenile delinquents, as could be seen, for instance, at the Solovetsky labour camp, the Bolshevo camp for juvenile delinquents and at Anton Makarenko's Gorky colony for delinquent, orphaned and/or homeless children in Kharkov. All of these had highlighted—more or less cynically—the goal of re-education and political and moral rehabilitation, and vehemently insisted on the principles of prisoners' self-government inside the camps. Similar to Goli Otok, these early Soviet prisons paid substantial attention to organising cultural, artistic and educational programmes, as well as compulsory political discussion classes. Moreover, self-criticism sessions were regular and compulsory, while prisoners' tribunals were common, and they served to force prisoners publicly to acknowledge their own past mistakes and wrong-doing.[28] However, the Goli Otok

[28] Anne Applebaum, *Gulag: A History of the Soviet Camps*, New York: Doubleday, 2003; Michael David-Fox, *Showcasing the Great Experiment: Cultural Diplomacy and Western Visitors to the Soviet Union, 1921–1941*, New York: Oxford University Press, 2012; D. Tolokontseva, 'Use of Correctional and Labour Measures on the Inmates of the Solovetsky Camp in the 1920s and 1930s', *Arctic Review on Law and Politics*, 2012, 2, 186–199.

camp was exceptional in its heavy emphasis on psychotherapeutic and analytic techniques and concepts, and its attendant and almost exclusive focus on introspection, self-exploration and self-knowledge. It was as though the entire process of investigation, confession writing and interrogation primarily served as a basis for personal, psychological growth, as the following examples show.

In former inmate Rade Panić's book based on his memories of Goli Otok, the room warden utters the following introductory words before the ritual 'declarations of attitude' by a group of prisoners: 'To revise or not to revise, this seems to you as a small difference. It's not. It's everything. It's your life. It's up to you what you will do with it. Until yesterday, I was just like you, a bandit, a stubborn foreign hireling, maybe not personally but certainly objectively speaking an agent of the Comintern. Then I saw the light. This should be your starting point, this realization that you are all bandits and traitors'.[29] Confessions thus did not serve to reveal the truth to the police—the police had already discovered it. Unlike in the Soviet show trials, they also did not have any public, propagandistic or political function, given that the fate of Goli Otok's prisoners was hidden from the eyes of the wider population, and the inmates were never tried or convicted but only received 'administrative sentences'. But the purpose of inmates' public declarations and self-criticism was precisely this self-realisation, guided self-knowledge—that, even though they might not have been conscious of it or purposely engaged in treason and malicious endeavours, every single arrestee was harbouring negative dispositions towards his or her own Party and state, and was in need of a political and ethical 'rebirth'. Goli Otok then served to make each prisoner conscious of these malevolent traits in his or her own personality.

Even though it was a physically brutal labour camp, Goli Otok allotted its inmates more than enough time for such self-reflection. The very living conditions, in a setting of bleak isolation, were supposed to induce introspection. The infamous investigation (*istraga*) never ended here: as there was no trial or conviction, there could be no end to such intimate, soul-searching investigations. On average, every inmate wrote and submitted between 20 and 30 statements in the course of their *istraga*, and the very

[29] Rade Panic, *Titovi Havaji*, Belgrade: Nezavisna izdanja Slobodana Masica, 1997, 41.

process of statement writing and revision was central to the re-education programme.[30]

These life narratives were not focused on particular (real or imagined) crimes; they had to encompass the inmate's entire life, both rational and irrational spheres of his or her personality, and always started in early childhood. Women's camp commander Marija Zelić Popović, whom most remember as an extremely physically brutal figure, would herself later recall how she strove to help the inmates realise and understand their 'true' nature, of which many had not even been aware—that they were traitors and unreliable, that they had harboured negative and pernicious thoughts against their own Party and enmity towards the state—and to assist them to 'unburden' themselves of such orientations and potentials. Although Popovic had no medical, psychiatric or psychoanalytic training, she approached her task of re-structuring the inmates' personalities in explicitly medical terms: 'With each inmate I get her file, just like each patient is accompanied by a medical case history.... Now I see who I am really dealing with'. The files also contained a 'diagnosis', or at least an opinion of the police investigator in the first instance. Zelić Popović then adopted the role of a stern and authoritarian analyst, who pressed the inmates to tell and re-tell, to reconstruct and examine their past decision-making until they realised the underlying source of their betrayal. She suggested how 'they were sometimes not even aware of the path they had started walking down' and related her own traumatisation as a result of this process, because she had to deal with the inmates' 'resistances' to this process of self-realisation.[31] In most cases, this relentless search for 'hidden' treacherous thoughts implied a purely fictional reconstruction of such ideas, which likely never existed but had to be spelled out as unconscious.

It was in order to help this process of 'unearthing' and self-discovery that the camp relied on a set of analytic or quasi-analytic concepts and techniques concerned with intimate self-discovery. During such exercises, the confessing inmate would occupy the centre of the room, while emotionally prodded by the room warden and activists to admit 'what you did, what you used to think, what you are thinking now'. On occasion, encouragement was given to focus on the deepest, most hidden (real

[30] B. Radonjic, *Poruseni ideali*, Belgrade: Interpress, 1995, 76.

[31] Iskaz Marije Zelic, II Programme of Radio Belgrade, 3 May 1990.

or invented) thoughts, dreams and affects. The investigators and camp guards at times confirmed themselves that the perfidious and treacherous thoughts which sometimes existed may not have been entirely known to the inmates themselves, and therefore needed to be 'recovered' and would prove to be a revelation of sorts to the subjects themselves: 'First of all, you will tell your investigator all your ... dirty thoughts. Every single one of your betrayals you will pour out to the investigator, every hostile activity and intention.... All your thoughts. You need to throw up all your filthy thoughts and to re-examine them in the hot light of the sun'.[32]

It is precisely the idea of 'filthy hidden thoughts' which were unknown to the inmates themselves and had to be forcibly dug up and confronted that most resembled—and was most likely inspired by—the Freudian notion of the 'unconscious'. Former inmate Eva Nahiri described in her interview with famous writer Danilo Kis, in 1989, that she was instructed to sit for days and write a report (*zapisnik*), in which she was to reveal 'everything [she] knew and didn't know, everything [she] dreamed about', her entire internal life from the moment she 'sucked in her mother's milk' until the time of incarceration. The investigators would then decide what was relevant, and, even more importantly, whether she was lying or not. Others were asked to write up all of their impressions of the Goli Otok camp and any associations they had in relation to it—if they mentioned anything remotely negative, they were placed back in isolation and 'under boycott'.[33] Soon after his imprisonment, Kosta Perucica was subjected to unspeakable tortures in order to force him into an intimate account of his political development and philosophy: in his report, he was instructed to recount his wartime and postwar doubts about the Party, confusions at certain political developments, to write 'about things that had always been very unclear to me', but also to remember every single letter he drafted, every, even passing, conversation he had had with his colleagues, and the reactions and feelings such conversations elicited in him.[34] Although books, paper and pencils were sorely lacking at other times, the camp provided willing inmates with all the necessary equipment to 'pour their soul and their feelings out in writing'.[35]

[32] Panic, *Titovi Havaji*, 44–45.

[33] Simic and Trifunovic, *Zenski logor na Golom Otoku*, 36–37.

[34] Perucica, *Kako su nas prevaspitavali*, 70–71.

[35] Stojanovic, *Goli Otok*, 231.

Former inmate 'Caca' remembered a particular form of self-criticism (*raskritikovanje*), practised in the female prison camp, in the course of which 'bandits' were required to sit in the centre of a circle made up of other, re-educated inmates, and to discuss the minutiae of their sexual lives, feelings and fantasies, and to describe physical relationships and experiences with husbands, boyfriends, colleagues. In a strongly patriarchal setting, this 'exercise' inevitably served further to humiliate and mortify those considered recalcitrant. Again, there seems to have been a warped application here of the psychoanalytic insistence upon the central role of sexual experiences and drives in the constitution of human personality.

The prisoners had little choice but to engage, therefore, in re-evaluations and re-assessment of their own motives, desires and longings, and to re-interpret their past relationships with their family members and others close to them, in the service of this entwined political and psychopathological model. Even ostensibly trivial inclinations and acts were to be 'poured out' and examined, searched as indicators of particular personality traits. This was meant, so it was claimed, to lead to 'sharpening the criteria, a true transformation, into a man more conscious and more awake than before. Being at Goli Otok creates new people out of us. That new man realizes how naive and blind he was before. Old facts are re-evaluated in a new light. That's why it's normal for the investigation [*istraga*] to be renewed [and open] all time'.[36] The road of self-discovery was supposed to lead ultimately to a more satisfying and self-conscious form of living, and to overcome inner alienation: 'Your entire previous life was one large mistake. You looked around, you saw nothing. You listened superficially, you understood nothing. For some this will be the end, for others real life is only just starting. Life full of clear and sharp views, full of meaning'.[37]

The camp authorities regularly incited—often violently forced—the inmates to 'remember' events from their past lives, communications, relations and encounters with certain people, their impressions, feelings or reactions to particular ideas or news. Partly, the purpose of constantly revisiting these reports and confessions was to achieve this 'remembering' of crucial events that the inmates may have omitted on purpose, forgotten

[36] Panic, *Titovi Havaji*, 44–45.

[37] Mihailovic, *Goli Otok*, 243.

or repressed.[38] Moreover, each new 'remembered' and revealed element indicated a set of relationships and psychological connections which the inmate in question needed to acknowledge and include in a revised self-image: 'Some of you think they had said all they knew. They did not. What looked like everything yesterday, is not sufficient today any more. [Goli] Otok will sharpen your criticism and you will once again speak of all of that from a much sharper point of view'.[39]

In the end, all inmates had to share their new realisation that they had always been 'spineless, cowards, without any memorable merits for the broader community'. As one inmate reportedly declared: 'My greatest disappointment in the conflict between our two parties was not the break between them but a division in my own soul. I believed my entire life that I had been brave... but only after the Resolution was declared did I understand what a coward I have always been'. At Goli Otok he realised that he became a traitor to the Party because he had been afraid of the Red Army's invasion. Moreover, he was stunned to discover yet another hidden motive: 'My next big weakness is my enormous thirst for power. I was hoping to become an editor-in-chief when the Russians arrived'.[40]

According to some of the inmates' testimonies, the ultimate result—and possibly one of the aims—of Goli Otok's measures was not so much re-integration, but in effect the disintegration of the prisoners' personality through self-analysis, 'this perfidious, destructive self-analysis [led to a] demolishing of all life motifs. Convinced of the power of time they have, gradually and patiently they will take [the prisoner] from a rational critical attitude to the self, to pathological contempt for both his own personality and his closest environment'.[41]

A modified, violent and humiliating version of drama therapy, also played a crucial part and was no less perverse in its formulation than the versions of 'psychotherapy' already described. In fact it will already be evident enough how much performance and publicity were required of the inmates anyway in such sessions. But, in addition, the camp's inmates would sometimes have to stage, before audiences of their peers, a largely

[38] Simic and Trifunovic, *Zenski logor na Golom Otoku*, 159–160, inmate 'Jelka'; Stojanovic, *Goli Otok*, 87.

[39] Panic, *Titovi Havaji*, 45.

[40] Panic, *Titovi Havaji*, 60–61.

[41] Mihailovic, *Goli Otok*, 16.

pre-arranged scripted theatrical performance of their political declarations and public repentance for past crimes. The camp's management insisted on the carnivalesque nature of such theatre performances; they pressured inmates to produce plays and collages which ridiculed Stalin, the Soviet Union and the Yugoslav 'bandits', while they celebrated Tito and the Communist Party of Yugoslavia. A frequent theme here was the staged 'burial' of the 1948 Resolution of the Informbureau. These burials were always organised at night, after all prisoners had returned from their physical exertions. A makeshift wooden coffin was prepared, and some of the most stubborn and 'unre-educable' of the inmates forced to carry it throughout the camp, between all the barracks while the rest of the prisoners and guards observed and often laughed. Other 'bandits' were instructed to perform the roles of the dead Resolution's bereaved relatives, to wail and cry, bending their bodies in mock suffering. They were supposed to yell: 'Our Aunt Resolution died, what shall we do without it, poor us without the Resolution', while the activists spurred them on, ridiculing and beating them.[42] In fact, while there was no particular script prepared for this particular elaborate performance, some inmates with professional backgrounds or experience in film or theatre were co-opted to be directors. The burials of the Resolution thus involved all the prisoners at the same time. They were also instituted as further humiliation and punishment for those who refused to participate in 're-education' programmes. With these scorned inmates cast in the ludicrous roles of the Resolution's 'family', such performances served to force them to start re-interpreting their own political orientation in similarly negative terms, as absurd and laughable choices, while they demonstrated to all the others the pathetic and ultimately impotent character of the Soviet attack on the Yugoslav state and of some Yugoslavs' support for the Soviet side. Goli Otok dramas were also quite an efficient way to force such recalcitrant prisoners finally and explicitly to adopt the role that the camp and the police authorities had prepared for them but to which they had difficulties adjusting. In 1953, after the news of Stalin's death was received, a similar procession was organised, in which several prisoners were painted black and dressed in priestly gowns, and led like cattle and with crosses on their necks around the courtyard of the prison.

[42] B. Kosier, *Bezboznici* 2, Sarajevo: Svjetlost, 1991, 388–391.

'Re-education' in Context

In the context of the socialist bloc, the use of such varied 'therapeutic elements' was not confined to the Goli Otok camp. As we already saw, the wartime institute for compulsory 're-education' of young communists took the first steps in the direction of a combined psychoanalytic and behaviourist experimentation, although its applications were mild by comparison. But another socialist country, Romania, adopted similar and equally brutal psychological methods in the infamous Pitesti prison, which mainly incarcerated university students accused of anti-communism and support for the Iron Guard. While there is still, to my knowledge, no evidence regarding potential exchange and transfer of experiences between the Yugoslav and Romanian security police departments, the similarities were striking. The Pitesti experiments in 'depersonalisation', which ran from 1949 until 1952, remain unmatched in the history of Romanian communism, and, like Goli Otok, seem to have drawn on a complex combination of ideas drawn from psychoanalysis, behaviourism, reflexology and Makarenko's pedagogy.[43] It is indeed both fascinating and tragically ironic that very similar torture and brainwashing techniques were applied and developed at roughly the same time on both sides of the Yugoslav–Soviet split in 1948. In the spring of 1950, Veselin Popović, who had since 1949 been head of the first two female prisons for those accused of supporting the Informbureau Resolution in Serbia (many inmates of these prisons soon ended up at the Goli Otok complex), successfully organised his escape to Romania, where he was long held under the surveillance of the Romanian state police and may have shared with them some of the re-education techniques practised in Yugoslavia.[44]

[43] D. Bacu, *The Anti-Humans: Student Re-education in Romanian Prisons*. Englewood, CO: Soldiers of the Cross, 1971. On the Romanian case, see also V. Ierunca, *Fenomenul Pitesti*, Bucharest: Humanitas, 1990; M. Stanescu, *The Re-education Trials in Communist Romania, 1952–1960*, Boulder, CO: East European Monographs, 2010; H.B. Segel, *The Walls Behind the Curtain: East European Prison Literature, 1945–1990*, Pittsburgh: University of Pittsburgh Press, 2012. The Romanian authorities referred to the prison as 'the Centre for Student Re-education', and it also involved elaborate techniques of inmates' 'self-management' and a hierarchical construction of committees run by the most reliable 're-educated' students. The Pitesti inmates were forced to perform humiliating forms of torture upon each other, subjected to long and violent interrogation sessions and 'external and internal unmasking' procedures, in the course of which they had to continuously re-tell and re-write their own life histories.

[44] Mihailovic, *Goli Otok*, 216.

But despite the brutality of the Goli Otok experiment, the concept of democratic self-management was also at the core of Yugoslav psychoanalysts' and psychiatrists' liberal turn in the 1950s, as we have seen in the previous chapter. The very same combination of self-management and psychotherapeutic and psychoanalytic methods developed in 'civilian' psychiatry, where it was applied in pursuit of radically different aims, which centred on individual liberation and self-realisation through self-exploration and discovery.

Yugoslavia thus offered an excellent site for social experimentation in this regard: through the combination of the country's more open version of socialism and Western psychoanalysis, psychotherapists and psychoanalysts hoped to achieve a more humane society, neither capitalist nor Stalinist, a society deeply committed to human emancipation and autonomy that invoked early Marx as its ideological beacon. As we saw in the previous chapter, individual self-realisation was to be achieved only in a self-managing society—in which truly free, authentic, diversely educated workers and citizens took part in making all important decisions regarding their political, social, economic, cultural lives.[45] In other words, Yugoslav psychiatrists and psychoanalysts wanted to create a society devoid of hierarchies, patriarchy and social and political authoritarianism; a combination of psychoanalytic psychotherapy and self-managing socialism was the key, and the experience of psychoanalytic treatment as well as the political conditions of anti-authoritarian self-management were supposed to transform the 'primitive' and dictatorial Yugoslav psyche. Whether it was developed in an authoritarian context, or in the course of discussions regarding anti-Stalinism and liberalisation— self-management shaped Yugoslav psychiatry and psychoanalysis, and fundamentally informed postwar psychiatric theories of the human psyche and its (socialist) transformation.

The continuing importance of self-management within Yugoslav psychiatry indicates another important trait of the profession: its ongoing political involvement with the ideas and practices of reform Communism and its participation in explicitly political discussions. The previous chapter demonstrated that, despite his more authoritarian take on the concept of socialist psychoanalysis, Vladislav Klajn remained an influential figure of Yugoslav mental health sciences throughout the 1960s and

[45] Vojin Matić, *Kada pocinje vaspitanje deteta*, Belgrade, 1955, 61–62.

1970s. He became a head of the neuro-psychiatric ward of Belgrade's elite 'Dragisa Misović' hospital, and his students and mentees availed themselves of the opportunities offered to them by the country's opening up to the West. As one of the very few surviving disciples of Nikola Sugar—the other one was Vojin Matić—he decisively shaped the increasingly liberal field of Yugoslav psychoanalysis and psychotherapy. Even though his early brand of socialist psychoanalysis might appear to be at odds with the subsequent radical liberalisation of the mental health profession, his writings were not particularly exceptional in the context of the widespread debate about the primitivism and backwardness of the Yugoslav population. Klajn's theory was primarily informed by his concerns over the supposed inability of 'primitive' Yugoslav patients to take part in an egalitarian psychoanalytic process. Many Yugoslav 'psy' professionals shared Klajn's worries over whether and how such a mentality could be reformed through psychotherapy and psychoanalysis. In that sense, Klajn was indeed a well-integrated member of the profession, and demonstrated very well its own ambivalence regarding its socialist 'civilising mission'.

Punitive Psychiatry in Yugoslavia

The Goli Otok experiment marked the development of the Yugoslav society and mental health professions at the very beginning of the country's socialist transformation, and demonstrated the authoritarian and repressive potential of some psychiatric and psychotherapeutic concepts and techniques. Decades later, the internationally renowned and politically progressive psychiatric profession in Yugoslavia found itself in the midst of a significantly more public scandal – as it was accused by a group of political dissidents and international human rights organisations of facilitating the government's suppression of political non-conformism and unjustified psychiatric confinements.[46] Such protests and complaints grew increasingly loud throughout the 1980s, and they indicated that Yugoslav psychiatry was ultimately unable to resist the government's political pressures and did not succeed in removing itself sufficiently from the Soviet model. This public discussion about psychiatric abuses implicated

[46] American Psychiatric Association, Letter to Todor Bakovic, President of the Yugoslav Association of Psychiatrists, 1 March 1984; Kosta Cavoski, *Preliminarni izvestaj o zloupotrebi psihijatrije u politicke svrhe*, 1–15, 15 February 1985.

Yugoslavia in human rights abuses and notorious punitive psychiatric practices, which threatened to undermine the country's international status. In the remainder of the chapter, we will explore a rich debate which ensued between the psychiatric profession, dissident advocates and the Yugoslav government itself about the pathology or otherwise of political opposition and dissent.

As we saw in the previous chapter, Soviet ideological approaches quickly lost their influence within the context of Yugoslav psychiatry. However, Yugoslav mental health professionals did eventually resume collaboration with their Soviet and other East European colleagues. As we saw above, even the Goli Otok experiment demonstrated that there were notable similarities between Yugoslavia's approach to the concept of psychological-political re-education and that of other socialist countries, both inside and outside the Soviet bloc. Moreover, there were further parallels between the two 'psy' professional contexts, and, despite its political and medical liberalisation, Yugoslavia did continue to share certain punitive psychiatric practices and conceptual frameworks with the USSR. These were not necessarily related to the lingering importance of the Pavlovian school psychiatry—although discussions about the comparative benefits of organic versus social psychiatric approaches did feature relatively prominently in Yugoslav forensic contexts. But a powerful or dominant position of organic psychiatry was certainly not a precondition for the emergence of repressive practices, and as this chapter has already demonstrated, even the most progressive and potentially emancipatory psychotherapeutic techniques could be used for authoritarian purposes and in punitive contexts.

When it came to psychiatric suppression of political dissenters and non-conformists in Yugoslavia, progressive and liberal psychotherapeutic clinical and theoretical tendencies were combined with abusive practices, sometimes within the same institutions. Yugoslav psychiatrists' involvement in political abuses was first documented in the 1970s on, and it seemed to intensify in the 1980s, decades after the Goli Otok re-education experiment. Such practices were much more conventional and indeed structurally very similar to those in the Soviet Union, and they were less directly shaped by specific ideological or theoretical influences—it was difficult to link them to any particular school of psychiatry. But very tellingly, one of the most important documents evidencing psychiatric manipulations in Yugoslavia was titled *The Psychiatric Goli Otok*—its author, Tomislav Krsmanović, thus implied that these later repressive techniques and strategies were comparable to those implemented in the notorious re-education camp in their brutality and perhaps in their malicious effects on inmates' psychological health and stability.[47] As we will see below, some of the abusive practices and approaches encountered in Yugoslavia's prison psychiatric hospitals could indeed be reminiscent of the above described Goli Otok experiences. However, the core link between these two forms of political suppression was the role that psychiatry, its concepts and institutions played in devising (and implementing) repressive measures for the purposes of the authoritarian political regime. Both at the beginning and towards the end of socialism in Yugoslavia, the non-alignment and intellectual diversity of its 'psy' disciplines had a darker side.

* * *

In 1975, Tomislav Krsmanović, an economist and fledgling human rights activist from Belgrade, was kept in the psychiatric hospital 'Laza Lazarević' for ten days against his will. According to his own testimony, the psychiatrist who treated him made it clear that his medical incarceration was due to his frequent and public complaints of persecution by the authorities: 'you need to get rest and get treatment, you think the government is harassing you, nobody is persecuting you, why would anyone do that, you are not an important person, your difficulties are of your own making, not the authorities'.[48] During his stay in the hospital, Krsmanović was reportedly treated violently and dismissively, diagnosed with 'paranoid reaction' and 'paranoid psychotic episode', and received medications—again against his will—which caused him harm and left long-term organic consequences. This brief incarceration, however, proved to be traumatic not only for Krsmanović: it had very significant negative repercussions for the Yugoslav government. Krsmanović first engaged in a protracted legal battle to disprove the dire label of psychotic illness attached to him during his troubled encounter with the mental health system, drawing in a number of Yugoslavia's high-ranking psychiatric experts and creating a rich personal archive which documented

[47] Archive of Yugoslavia, Tomislav Krsmanović, *Psihijatrijski Goli Otok*, Belgrade: Pokret za zastitu ljudskih prava, 1988.

[48] Krsmanović, *Roman o Briselu*, Sabac: Glas crkve, 2013, 939–951; Krsmanović, *Kaznena psihijatrija, 1975–2004*, Belgrade: Vedes, 2004.

the Yugoslav psychiatric profession's involvement in unethical, politically driven practices.[49] He then founded the Association for the struggle against political abuses of psychiatry and for human rights protection 'Action' (*Akcija*) in April 1981.

Akcija included a number of like-minded Yugoslav intellectuals, who quickly started a relatively successful domestic and international campaign against what they saw as a Soviet-like widespread abuse of psychiatry for political purposes in Yugoslavia. They worked tirelessly throughout the 1980s to collect as many documents as possible to prove that the Yugoslav political authorities used, blackmailed or manipulated psychiatric experts and institutions in order to silence and discredit potentially dangerous political opponents. Krsmanović in particular dedicated his life to shedding light on such psychiatric abuses, offering legal aid and support to the incarcerated and alarming leading international organisations such as Amnesty International, UNESCO and the American Psychiatric Association. It is unclear to what extend the work of *Akcija* and Krsmanović succeeded in damaging Yugoslavia's international standing—which was indeed their ultimate aim so that they could leverage any resulting international pressure to improve the situation in psychiatric hospitals—although all contacted organisations dutifully responded and Amnesty International took particular interest in a number of forcibly incarcerated psychiatric hospital inmates, whom they deemed 'prisoners of conscience'.[50] But one of their most important achievements was the creation of a vast collection of legal, medical and journalistic documents related to practices of punitive psychiatry in Yugoslavia. This was the first time Yugoslavia had been marked as a country responsible for such authoritarian practices, and the international organisations involved regularly expressed their surprise and concern. As we will see below, the Yugoslav authorities attempted damage control through a variety of channels, and always adamantly rejected the suggestion that the individuals in question were anything other than mentally ill people.

Akcija collected more or less detailed dossiers on twenty-four individuals, held in a number of psychiatric hospitals around Yugoslavia, but mostly in psychiatric wards of regular prison hospitals in Belgrade and

[49] Tuzba Tomislava Krsmanovica protiv lekara Zavoda za mentalno zdravlje iz Belgrada, Prvi opstinski sud, Belgrade, 12 May 1981; Resenje, Prvi opstinski sud, 1737/81.

[50] Amnesty International, *Yugoslavia: Prisoners of Conscience*, London: Amnesty International Publications, 1981.

Zagreb. All these people were indicted of politically motivated crimes—the indictments were generally based on their oral and/or written statements critical of the Yugoslav political and social institutions—but in the course of their trials they were declared legally incompetent and unable to understand the significance and implications of their infractions due to severe mental disorders. As a result, according to the Article 63 of the Yugoslav Penal Code, instead of being sent to prisons on political charges, these people were sentenced to indefinite terms in closed psychiatric institutions, supposedly for their own benefit and because they were deemed 'dangerous to society' (*opasni po okolinu*).[51] It was this broad formulation regarding the indictees'/patients' supposed danger (which included not only physical danger and violence but also vaguely defined 'verbal aggression') that elicited angry reactions from the regime's critics, and started a complex discussion over whether a mental ill person might pose any danger to society if they were not physically aggressive.

Moreover, there was a lot of confusion regarding the indictees' legal status: were they to be treated as prisoners, i.e. within the remit of Yugoslavia's criminal law, or as primarily medical patients and thus fully protected by healthcare laws and regulations? As per the Yugoslav Penal Code, those political prisoners deemed legally unaccountable needed to be offered psychiatric treatment as well as 'psychological-pedagogical re-education'.[52] Moreover, in 1977 a by-law was passed by the Yugoslav parliament which aimed to regulate psychiatric confinement of those deemed legally incompetent to stand trial—and it mandated relevant mental health institutions to apply 'modern treatment techniques' and enable regular collaborations between psychiatrists, psychologists and social workers.[53] As we will see later, this legal obligation to offer rounded psychosocial and medical therapy to political indictees was rarely fulfilled—prison hospitals remained brutal custodial institutions—and this

[51] Franjo Bacic and Nikola Srzentic, *Komentar krivicnog zakona*, Belgrade: Savremena administracija, 1978, 269; Archive of the Movement for the protection of human rights (Arhiv pokreta za zastitu ljudskih prava, in the rest of the text: Arhiv Pokreta), Amnesty International, 'Confinement of prisoners of conscience in psychiatric institutions', document 17.

[52] Arhiv Pokreta, Komitet za zastitu ljudskih prava, 'Raport o stanju uslova zivota, medicinske nege i zastite, i opsteg tretmana u zatvorskim psihijatrijskim bolnicama u Jugoslaviji', 17 March 1987, Belgrade, 6–7.

[53] Ibid., 9.

became one of the central complains in Yugoslavia's emerging human rights discourse about psychiatric abuses.

The historiography of East European Communist psychiatry was until recently dominated by accounts of psychiatric misuse for the purposes of suppressing and neutralising political dissent. While Western analyses of East European (primarily Soviet) mental health practices—and innovations—were diverse and often positive in the first decades of the Cold War, the tone changed quite dramatically from the 1970s on, when the framework of political psychiatric abuse became the sole analytical lens through which East European psychiatry was discussed and evaluated in both political and scholarly circles.[54] This lasted until the fall of Communism, when alternative scholarly emphases and questions slowly started emerging.[55] Still, the narrative of Soviet and East European psychiatry as an obedient handmaiden to the authoritarian regimes in the region has maintained significant influence.

Moreover, numerous accounts of such abuses, written by Western observers, Soviet dissidents and psychiatrists, and human rights activists, shed light on a multitude of Soviet psychiatry's problematic clinical practices and conceptual frameworks. Such analyses drew attention to forced hospitalisations and mistreatment mainly of political dissidents, but also of a host of other vulnerable groups in the USSR, such as 'non-political deviants' (e.g. jazz lovers and hippies), nationalists, religious believers etc.[56] Using concepts and diagnoses which were intentionally vague and malleable, Soviet psychiatrists declared large numbers of non-conformists legally unaccountable.

The most notorious of those diagnoses was 'sluggish schizophrenia', a severe disorder which could reportedly at times manifest without any symptoms. While some critics argued that the concept of sluggish schizophrenia was produced within the KGB circles, others pointed out

[54] S. Bloch and P. Reddaway, *Russia's Politica Hospitals: The Abuse of Psychiatry in the Soviet Union*, London: Gollancz, 1977; R. Medvedev and Z. Medvedev, *A Question of Madness*, London: Macmillan Ltd, 1971.

[55] See Marks and Savelli, *Psychiatry in Communist Europe*; Eghigian, 'Was there a Communist Psychiatry?', 364–368; Benjamin Zajicek, *Scientific Psychiatry in Stalin's Soviet Union*.

[56] R. Van Voren, 'Comparing Soviet and Chinese Political Psychiatry', *Journal of the American Academy of Psychiatry and the Law*, 2002, 30:1.

that it was likely a result of Soviet psychiatry's broader conceptualisation of schizophrenia and psychosis.[57] Either way, in relation to political dissidents, the diagnosis proved to be extremely conducive to manipulation—and the clinical symptoms quoted, such as 'reformist ideas' and 'struggle for truth', had distinctly political undertones. Once declared mentally unfit, Soviet psychiatric political prisoners often ended up in 'special hospitals', under the auspices of the Ministry of the Interior, and experienced different forms of additional physical and psychological abuse, such as beatings, physical isolation, involuntary heavy medication, etc.[58] As we will see below, very similar practices were observed in Yugoslavia.

And while Soviet psychiatric abuses were documented exceptionally well, very little is known about comparable abuses in the rest of the Eastern bloc. Scholars have speculated that politically motivated psychiatric malpractice might have been widespread across the Communist world, but little evidence has so far emerged to prove the systematic nature of such manipulations.[59] In the remainder of the chapter, I explore a fragmented but unique archive of documents testifying to the role of Yugoslav socialist psychiatry in political abuses and suppression of political non-conformism.

As will become clear, some of the core questions raised by the Yugoslav experiences were not dissimilar to the Soviet case—questions about the meaning of 'danger to society' and to the state, when that danger was not violent, questions about the motivation of the psychiatric staff involved, as well as questions about the therapeutic versus punitive purposes of political psychiatric confinement. In this sense, Yugoslav and Soviet psychiatry shared a lot, perhaps quite surprisingly, despite the fact that the Yugoslav

[57] Zajicek, 'Soviet Psychiatry and the Origins of the Sluggish Schizophrenia Concept, 1912–1936', *History of the Human Sciences*, 2018, 31:2, 88–105; Helen Lavretsky, 'The Russian Concept of Schizophrenia: A Review of the Literature', *Schizophrenia Bulletin*, 1998, 24:4.

[58] More recently, researchers have explored the history of abuse and violence in communist-era psychiatric hospitals more generally, but still primarily focused on the Soviet Union: Galmarini-Kabala, 'Psychiatry, Violence, and the Soviet Project of Transformation'; Benjamin Zajicek, 'A Soviet System of Professions: Psychiatry, Professional Jurisdiction, and the Soviet Academy of Medical Sciences, 1932–1951', in Susan Grant, ed., *Russian and Soviet Health Care from an International Perspective: Comparing Professions, Practice and Gender, 1880–1960*, Palgrave Macmillan, 2017, 97–117.

[59] See Adler et al., 'Psychiatry Under Tyranny', 3–17.

mental health professions were more internationalised, Westernised and more 'liberal' than their Soviet counterparts. The core difference between the two cases may not have lain in the nature or even brutality of these abuses, but in their extent—while we are aware of several dozen cases in Yugoslavia, such numbers likely reached hundreds, if not thousands, of dissidents in the USSR. But the most striking aspect of psychiatric abuses in Yugoslavia was the involvement of its psychiatric profession—once evidence started coming to light in the 1980s, this certainly surprised major international institutions such as the UN or the American Psychiatric Association, which had known Yugoslav mental health in a decidedly different light.[60]

As we saw in the previous chapters, such a reputation was not unfounded—Yugoslav psychiatry was partly driven by deeply emancipatory and democratic impulses, suffering itself perhaps from 'reformist' ideas and delusions. This clearly did not prevent some of its institutions and professionals from engaging in authoritarian practices and diagnostic exercises. Here, it is important to remember that 'progressive' and 'authoritarian' camps in Yugoslav psychiatry were frequently not clearly separated, and progressive institutions and individuals could engage in, or at least acquiesce to, politically repressive actions. On the other hand, Yugoslav psychiatric prisoners did not reach the international fame of their Soviet counterparts, nor were they particularly important public personalities inside the country. But luckily for historians, the existing archive of Yugoslav psychiatric abuses includes their voices to a surprisingly large extent—through their legal complaints and clarifications, public letters and articles aimed at international and domestic audiences, in which they and their families talked back to the medical and political authorities, and challenged their vague and often problematic definitions of normality and pathology. Through these, we can reconstruct an important three-way conversation between the government, psychiatric authorities and prisoners themselves, which sheds light on some of the most important political as well as psychiatric tensions in 1980s Yugoslavia.

One of Krsmanović's psychiatric evaluation documents demonstrates very well some of the core issues at stake in many of these problematic incarcerations. In 1982, after many years of psychiatric and legal

[60] America Psychiatric Association, Committee on International Abuse of Psychiatry and Psychiatrists, Letter to the Director of the Psychiatric Hospital of the Central Prison, Belgrade, 1 March 1984.

battles in which he was simultaneously disputing his diagnoses and defending himself from political accusations, Krsmanović was ordered by court to undergo yet another assessment by the Belgrade Medical Faculty's forensic psychiatry committee. The committee was made up of leading social psychiatrists—Predrag Kalicanin, Dimitrije Milovanović, Jovan Veljković and Petar Milenković, and headed by renowned professor of neurology Maksim Sternić—and it was tasked with reviewing all of Krsmanović's previous psychiatric documentation as well as with examining Krsmanović himself in order to reach the final diagnosis.[61]

The committee's conclusions could have been read partly as a vindication for Krsmanović: the evaluation did not declare him schizophrenic or psychotic, but stated that Krsmanović had a 'psychopatic personality with a paranoid structure, prone to occasional psychotic episodes'. However, the psychiatrists' explanation of this diagnosis was very indicative of the complex interrelationship between the mental health profession and Yugoslavia's authoritarian political influences. For instance, the psychiatrists noted that Krsmanović suffered from a 'large variety of paranoid (insane) ideas of persecution, and of grandeur', and the main evidence for this 'insanity' was that he 'considered it his duty to fight for the democratisation of our society' and believed he had a right to 'address international organisations, domestic and foreign public opinion, for help'.[62] In other words, Krsmanović's belief in the need for greater democracy in Yugoslavia, and his commitment to participating actively in this process of democratisation, were deemed pathological psychiatric indications, and signs of psychopathy—a borderline personality disorder. When he warned the committee that he would keep informing the relevant international institutions and foreign media of any attempts to abuse psychiatry for political purposes, the doctors described these statements as threats, and quoted Krsmanović's references to human rights breaches as further evidence of mental instability.

Krsmanović's 'ideas of persecution' were particularly worrying for the committee: although he initially left a relatively good impression as a 'sophisticated person', the psychiatrists soon changed their opinion, as 'he was inclined to engage in endless dialogues on everything and anything,

[61] University of Belgrade, Medical Faculty, Sudsko-psihijatrijski odbor, Report number 35/81, 20 April 1982.

[62] Ibid., 5.

and mostly about "his persecutions." On this topics, it was difficult to stop him as he recounted how he had been persecuted and by whom, including by medical doctors'. Moreover, Krsmanović's arguments that he was persecuted by the authorities because of his dissident activities was lightly mocked—the psychiatrists clearly found it laughable that Krsmanović counted himself among some of the most well known critics of the Yugoslav regime such as Djilas, Mihajlo Mihajlov, Franjo Tudjman and others.[63]

As mentioned above, the Medical Faculty's committee also reviewed Krsmanović's previous diagnoses, focusing in particular on the findings of the Military-Medical Academy, whose psychiatrists cleared him of any mental illnesses in October 1977 ('*sine morbo psychico*'), and the Institute of Mental Health's conclusion from June of that year that Krsmanović suffered from schizophrenia.[64] The final meeting of the committee was attended by all the involved psychiatrists from the above institutions, and Krsmanović's psychotherapist at the time, Vladeta Jerotić, was also in contact over the phone—according to the committee's report, Jerotic, too, 'was in full agreement with the committee's opinion'. Therefore, it would appear that some of the most important psychiatric institutions and practitioners in the country were involved in Krsmanović's assessment, and all consented to the medicalisation of his political activities. In particular, as we have already seen, the Institute of Mental Health was one of the most progressive psychiatric organisations in the country, was deeply involved in this case, having offered the most serious diagnosis of 'paranoid schizophrenia'. In fact, Krsmanović had had a long history of communication with and treatment at the Institute of Mental Health, starting before he was forcibly hospitalised, and had always communicated with the Institute's psychiatrist Tomislav Sedmak, who ultimately settled on the schizophrenia diagnosis.

According to Krsmanović's long response to the Medical Faculty committee's report, psychiatrist Tomislav Sedmak always refused to speak about what Krsmanović thought was the main reason behind his insomnia and neurosis: his experience of persistent political discrimination, harrassment and persecution at the hands of the Yugoslav political authorities,

[63] Ibid.

[64] Vojno-Medicinska Akademija, Dr Stevan Petrovic, 'Izvestaj lekara specijaliste', 24 October 1977; Zavod za mentalno zdravlje, file 33800, 6 March 1973.

which targeted him for his public criticism, created obstacles for his professional advancement and even interfered in his private life. In Krsmanović's testimony, Sedmak appeared afraid whenever his patient attempted to discuss the broader political context of his mental health difficulties, and refused to engage in further conversation about this over the phone or in letters whenever Krsmanović contacted him. On the other hand, Krsmanović' version of Jerotic's involvement was significantly different: while the committee noted that Jerotic did not dissent from the collective final opinion, Krsmanović still maintained a high opinion of him, writing that, unlike Sedmak, he was 'very familiar with my life's context'. Jerotic's role was to call the committee and present Krsmanović as an 'innocent exhausted victim' but fully lucid so that he could avoid both prison and psychiatric hospital confinement.[65]

But Krsmanović's response to the report is a unique historical document, not only because it added an alternative narrative to the one put forward in the committee's official report, but because Krsmanović, as a psychiatric patient, used this opportunity to craft a detailed challenge to the dominant psychiatric voice (which, in this case, was further reinforced by the legal and police apparatus, given that Krsmanović was under criminal charges for his political activity). The response is rather long, repetitive at times, and certainly not the most polished piece of writing, but it raised several rather obvious points. In particular, Krsmanović was at his most convincing when questioning those parts of the report which painted him as a paranoid person—if one was exposed to a series of police investigations and criminal charges, and discrimination at work, one's psychological preoccupation with these experiences and their long-term effects could hardly be seen as the 'world of a paranoiac'. In fact, Krsmanović was exceptionally self-reflective in his description of his own behaviour: explaining why he, as the psychiatrists noted, spoke about his persecution all the time, Krsmanović argued that 'violence, as toothache, invades every pore of your personality, it becomes an obsession, the person is only capable of thinking about that one thing', and that 'this was a normal reaction of someone who had no opportunity to protect his rights and to formulate his defence in public'. Krsmanović referred to a recent article by the Croatian trade union association, which warned of increasingly frequent psychological problems caused by workplace

[65] Arhiv Pokreta, Letter to Professor Maksim Sternic, 14 July 1985, document 13.

disputes. Such disputes reportedly had particularly negative effects on those employees who were 'seeking justice' for themselves, to the extent that this was now turning into a serious social and medical problem. Krsmanović (and, as we will see, many other political/psychiatric prisoners) recognised his own predicament in the article's description—he believed that all of his mental health difficulties were 'inauthentic' and caused by his attempts to fight for justice against a much more powerful adversary. He concluded, in line with the dominant psychiatric framework of his time, that his health problems were 'caused by the stresses and violence which lasted for years'.

Regarding the committee's opinion that his belief in his 'duty' to take part in the democratisation of the Yugoslav society was pathological, Krsmanović again offered a radically different interpretation of his own motives and aims—arguing emphatically that his and his colleagues' 'struggle for a better, more humane society' should not be discussed and qualified in terms of psychiatric pathology. In fact, the committee's reference to his 'ideas of grandeur' seems to have preoccupied Krsmanović the most, and he was deeply offended by the implication that his human rights activism was motivated by some pathological self-perception as a saviour or missionary. As he clarified, his activities were first motivated by very personal and 'egotistical reasons' (protection of his own interests and family), and gradually (and naturally) morphed into a broader social project. In other words, Krsmanović's response questioned the very foundations of the concept of psychiatric normality and the solidity of psychiatric diagnostic criteria, pointing out the ease with which a type of behaviour which was celebrated and supported in different socio-political settings (i.e. political struggle for one's rights and better future) could be discredited in a psychiatric context. Why were the interwar Yugoslav Communist Party activists' fierce political activism and opposition to the institutions of the Kingdom of Yugoslavia not deemed signs of lunacy or deranged ideas of grandeur, asked Krsmanović, and by what medical or political criteria was his struggle to protect vulnerable people's human rights categorised differently? Weren't these two struggles—Krsmanović's and the interwar Communist Party's—ultimately motivated by the same desire, to create a better society?

This protracted exchange between Krsmanović and his psychiatrists about the pathology or otherwise of radical political struggle was reminiscent of the famous case of Leonid Plyushch, a brilliant Soviet mathematician turned political dissident, who spent three years in psychiatric confinement for 'anti-Soviet agitation and propaganda' after he publicly criticised the authoritarianism of Soviet political institutions. Due to international pressure, Plyushch was released and allowed to emigrate to Paris, then New York, where he recounted that, in his experience, social maladaptation served as the core clinical criterion of mental illness in the Soviet context. His conversation with Soviet psychiatrists was eerily similar to Krsmanović's responses: when he was told that he was 'abnormal' because he 'couldn't adapt to the situation, [he] risked [his] own and [his] family's life', he, much like Krsmanović did, referred to the political struggle of the pre-revolutionary Bolsheviks and asked if they too were ill. The Moscow psychiatrists then responded that his decision to compare himself with the Bolsheviks indicated his pathological ideas of grandeur—just as Krsmanović's attempts to justify his political activities were dismissed as delusional self-aggrandizement.[66] In both cases, therefore, it was very difficult for the two dissidents to step out of the vicious circle of psychiatric diagnoses—and to disrupt the psychiatric profession's tendency to pathologise critical and non-conformist political attitudes and statements.

In a similar vein, broader discussions which developed around the fate of Yugoslav political psychiatric prisoners focused on the meaning of normality, and on ascertaining the boundary between non-conformist political activity and psychiatric disorder. The cases of these prisoners—the medical and political institutions' categorisations of their crimes, and their own self-narratives—open up an unexpectedly rich window onto the world of political dissatisfaction and critique in socialist Yugoslavia. These people belonged to different walks of life, and their problems with political and psychiatric institutions began because they complained or spoke publicly about a variety of sensitive and controversial issues.[67] Some, like Krsmanović, Milisav Zivanović or Pavle Poljanski, became increasingly loud about their own or their family's political discrimination and about the regime's problematic treatment of dissidents and non-conformists. Some of the complainants pointed out the regime's corruption, abuses, manipulations and non-transparency in legal or industrial institutions, and general political favouritism in public organisations.

[66] John Wing, *Reasoning About Madness*, New York: Transaction Publishers, 1978, 180–187.

[67] Srdjan Cvetkovic, 'Ko je ovde lud? - primeri političke (zlo)upotreba psihijatrije u SFRJ', *Istorija 20. veka*, 2013, 2, 145–163.

Another group of psychiatric prisoners came to the authorities' attention because they criticised the Yugoslav social and political realities from a Marxist rather than liberal democratic positions—people such as Radomir Veljković, possibly the most internationally well-known psychiatric political prisoner in Yugoslavia, and Bajram Ajeti critiqued what they saw as the government's deviations from the correct revolutionary course, and corruption of Yugoslav self-managing socialism. Yet another relatively large group consisted of people, mainly from Croatia, who were accused of espousing and spreading harmful ethnic nationalist views, historical revisionism and even separatist political agenda (Vladimir Perisić, Vladimir Naglić, Vladimir Marković). Therefore, we can see here again that an exploration of psychiatric discussions sheds unique light on the most important political and social cleavages and controversies. Moreover, an analysis of the politicisation of psychiatry, and of the practices and narratives of forensic psychiatry can offer a very significant insight into the Yugoslav society's tensions and the Yugoslav government's core concerns, fears and anxieties.

It is important to note that Yugoslav psychiatrists did not utilise the concept of 'sluggish schizophrenia', but most psychiatric political prisoners were diagnosed with paranoid schizophrenia or psychosis, or a psychotic episode or reaction. The meanings and descriptions of these diagnoses were often not that different from sluggish schizophrenia. As we will see below, those political prisoners diagnosed with schizophrenia or psychosis were often described to exhibit 'ideas of grandeur' or 'delusions of reformism'. In the official clinical description of progressive schizophrenia, used at Snezhnevsky's Institute of Psychiatry in Moscow, such symptoms featured very prominently, and 'delusional ideas of... invention, reformation, grandeur' were indicated as particularly significant symptoms of psychotic illness. When British social psychiatrist John Wing attended a meeting for foreign mental health professionals at Moscow's Serbsky Institute in 1973, he requested clarification regarding precisely this concept of reformist delusion, and a Soviet junior psychiatrist explained that such patients were easily identified because they dealt with 'social problems. The patient thinks it necessary to reform the system of government control in this country. He thinks that he himself is capable of undertaking leadership...'[68] Very similar criteria and descriptions of

[68] Wing, *Reasoning About Madness*, 189.

clinical symptoms were regularly applied to Yugoslav political prisoners and dissenters, and were used to delegitimise and dismiss their critiques of the system and suggestions for political reform.

Furthermore, a majority of Yugoslav psychiatric prisoners had many more than one diagnosis, as they usually underwent a variety of psychiatric assessments and evaluations, as we already saw with Krsmanović, often at their own requests. In order to explain the political aspects of their patients' behaviour, and evaluate them as aberrant, Yugoslav psychiatrists also used a range of parallel or alternative concepts. 'Paranoia querulans' was a relatively frequent one—the diagnosis normally refers to an obsession with litigation and incessant seeking of legal remedies for irrelevant or negligible 'infractions'. In the Yugoslav context, the concept of *paranoia querulans* was a valuable device to describe the behaviour of those indictees who insisted on using the legal system (petitions, legal complaints and pleas) to draw attention to their own experiences of discrimination and harassment. This kind of behaviour was also often referred as 'mania of litigation and justice seeking' ('*manija sudjenja i isterivanja pravde*').[69]

The concept of *paranoia querulans* was, of course, utilised in several cases of Soviet political dissidents, but it was also an internationally recognised diagnosis. In British psychiatry, a person suffering from this affliction was described as touchy, sensitive, egocentric and rigid, and as someone who 'may suffer fancied injustice (or sometimes a real one). He begins to devote his whole energy to trying to put the matter right'.[70] This clinical account depicted quite accurately a number of Yugoslav psychiatric political prisoners, especially since having 'unusual' political ideas seemed to be an accepted feature of this disorder, and patients reportedly often tended to become entirely consumed by their struggle to the point that no other aspect of their life mattered to them. The line between professional clinical practice and political abuse was, therefore, even blurrier in the case of this diagnosis as it certainly was not a peculiar invention of Soviet or communist psychiatry. On the other hand, *paranoia querulans* had a problematic potential to pathologise people's commitment to fighting for their own political or material

[69] Arhiv pokreta, Radomir Veljkovic, 'Protest progresivnom covecanstvu zbog masovnog poludjivanja gradjana u SFRJ', 4 June 1984, document 22.

[70] Wing, *Reasoning About Madness*, 174.

rights, particularly if that struggle occurred in the context of political authoritarianism.

Other psychiatric political prisoners were described as suffering from religious mania (religious insanity), psychopathic personality with extreme suspiciousness, anxiety with a tendency to projection, etc. In all these cases, references to suspicion, projection and pathological paranoid obsession served to send a message that the prisoners' belief that they were indeed targeted and harassed by the political system had no grounding in reality. As prisoner Zoran Stankovic said in passing, when his psychiatrist suggested that nobody was persecuting Zoran and that he was simply self-destructive: 'as if making note of some of this society's injustices were self-destruction'.[71]

Normality, Pathology and the Origins of Mental Illness

The authorities' response was predictable, and when they did feel the need to defend their decisions in public, they attempted to mobilise medical expertise and language in order to prove that the prisoners in question did in fact suffer from grave psychiatric disorders. In response to a petition signed by a number of Yugoslav intellectuals who protested the incarceration of political prisoners in psychiatric institution, Serbian daily *Vecernje Novosti* was, rather shockingly, allowed access to the confidential medical documentation of some prisoners who were mentioned in the petition and held at the Belgrade prison hospital's psychiatric ward. The newspaper then used such information as evidence that the inmates were incontestably abnormal and 'completely incapable of rejoning any social community'. For instance, *Vecernji List* wrote of Radomir Veljković rather mockingly that he spent 'hours, days, months and years "studying" mathematics, quantum physics… and other "high" sciences, from which he [issued] "declarations", "complaints" and other "studies", not caring for rest, walks, TV, socialisation or other normal life activities'.[72]

In some cases, it was difficult to counter such psychiatric charges, as prisoners' behaviour, writing and statements often reflected a tenuous connection with reality, while many of them also had long histories of

[71] Arhiv Pokreta, Letter of Zoran Stankovic, May 1985.

[72] Boro Komad, 'Pucanj u cinjenice', *Vecernje Novosti*, 31 January 1986.

prior psychiatric treatment and even hospitalisation, unrelated to their subsequent politically motivated indictments. In those situations, narratives of human rights organisations such as *Akcija* and of the prisoners themselves applied a common strategy which relied on social psychiatric and psychoanalytic explanations—they admitted that their mental health was indeed undermined, but blamed the regime's actions for the onset of any psychological illnesses.[73] The language of trauma framed such defence narratives: psychological traumatisation was constructed as the main cause of the prisoners' psychological deterioration, as severe psychological traumas were an inevitable result of years, sometimes decades, of oppression and persecution by the Yugoslav government. The case of Radomir Veljković, who eventually spent fifteen years in forced psychiatric confinement, was typical in this sense.

Radomir was a committed communist: a model student of the Military Academy in Belgrade, he was an ambitious and talented officer, as well as a Second World War veteran. His early (involuntary) retirement in 1967, when he was only forty, disappointed him deeply as it cut short his promising career, and he started to complain of a variety of negative trends which he noticed in the Yugoslav society.[74] This culminated in 1969, when Radomir filed a writ against none other than the Yugoslav president Josip Broz Tito, accusing him of political repression and abuse of the state system and services, 'persecution of people', 'participation in joint criminal enterprise', 'undermining of the state's defence and military capabilities', etc. In the early 1970s, Radomir filed further supplements to this writ, in which he accused Tito of strategic and tactical mistakes he supposedly committed as the commander of the resistance army in the Second World War, and of the unnecessary deaths of partisan soldiers which resulted from such mistakes.[75] In March 1973, Radomir was found guilty of 'hostile propaganda' and of 'damaging the reputation of the state', but, since he was diagnosed with a psychotic disorder, he was sentenced to an indefinite term of confinement in the Belgrade prison psychiatric hospital.

[73] Arhiv Pokreta, Dragan Veljkovic, Letter to Vecernje Novosti, 10 February 1982.

[74] Arhiv Pokreta, 'Dokumentacija i informacije o pretrpljenim politickim progonima moga brata Radomira Veljkovica', 197–205.

[75] Optužnica Radomira Veljkovića protiv Josipa Broza Tita pred Okružnim sudom u Beogradu, k. br. 74/69, 14 May1969.

As his brother recounted in one of his complaint letters, Radomir had been 'turned into a robot through years of terror and subversion.[76] He filed a complaint against Tito in an 'inauthentic way, because [his] manipulators wanted that to happen. His ego crumbled under the influence of pent up dissatisfaction and repression'. Radomir Veljković was, moreover, a victim of 'brain washing' by the secret police, so it was no wonder that 'in the recent years, he has had some unusual ideas, which we never noticed before. His psychological state is now bad. But it was not like that before he was placed in this institution'.[77] Veljković himself testified that he had found himself in a state of 'hopelessness and pressure, with weakened nerves (*tankih nerava*), exhausted' by the regime's 'awful Stalinist terror'. Like Krsmanović, Veljković demonstrated an exceptional ability for self-reflection, writing in 1984 that he felt that his 'brain was weakening, [his] memory, health, that [he] was not at all what he used to be'. Veljković firmly believed that such psychological deterioration of inmates was a result of the prison psychiatric hospital authorities' deliberate strategy: 'I see around myself people who were psychologically normal a few years ago, but now they are sinking into madness, alienation', kept indefinitely in an institution he called an Orwellian 'animal farm in the midst of Belgrade, outside the Soviet bloc at the end of the twentieth century'.[78] As his brother once noted, Radomir was 'castrated' and 'diminished' after years of forced confinement, and this was reflected in his behaviour—in the constant, increasingly politically provocative letters and complaints he wrote in the course of his hospital term.[79]

Other psychiatric political prisoners often followed suit. As we saw above, Krsmanović frequently spoke of the deleterious effects of the state persecution on his nervous illness and mental health in general. In his official court complaint, Zoran Stankovic promised to stop critiquing the authorities, because he only did that when he was 'upset, in crisis'. He noted that he 'had fallen seriously ill' as a result of the oppression and the government's 'terror', and his illnesses included a host of psychological problems: 'horrible insomnia, nervous tension, asthenia, depression', in

[76] 'Dokumentacija i informacije o pretrpljenim politickim progonima moga brata Radomira Veljkovica', 202.

[77] Ibid.

[78] Veljkovic, 'Protest progresivnom covecanstvu', 249.

[79] 'Dokumentacija i informacije o pretrpljenim politickim progonima moga brata Radomira Veljkovica'.

addition to a long list of psychosomatic difficulties.[80] Golub Bakic was also a 'traumatised person, dissatisfied with the society's stance towards him and his family'.[81] In the case of Vladimir Perisić's defence, the line between psychological normality and pathology was presented as particularly tenuous, and both *Akcija* and his lawyers emphasised his declining mental health, blaming the obvious deterioration of Perisić's lucidity on the regime's persecutory actions. *Akcija* reported that, after years of 'brutal harassment' and 'traumatisation' by the authorities, he found himself in a 'state of extreme nervous, psychological and physical exhaustion', which led him to act incautiously and commit political provocations.[82] Moreover, Perisić himself reportedly insisted on the 'psychosocial context' of his illness: he confided in Krsmanović that, after spending years in mental hospitals, others saw him as insane and he 'started accepting this as part of my identity'. He was often 'in apathy, confusion, alienation and depression'.[83] On the other hand, the defence narrative occasionally accepted that mental illness was indeed Perisić's reality, and Perisić's lawyer once argued in a complaint that his defendant should not be held accountable due to his long-term diagnosis of paranoid schizophrenia.

But Perisić's case was particularly difficult and this confusion was perhaps understandable. Before his arrest and trial, he spent some time with his family in Germany, where his behaviour was reportedly also disruptive and he had to be briefly confined in a psychiatric hospital. Upon his return to Yugoslavia, he was accused of spreading Croat nationalist 'enemy' propaganda and anti-Yugoslav political attitudes, and of maintaining connections with Croat anti-Yugoslav emigration in Germany. In addition to his diagnosis of paranoid schizophrenia 'expressed in the form of paranoid hallucinations', Perisić was also assessed to suffer from 'religious insanity' by Zagreb psychiatrist Ivan Kosuljendic. After a brief and very traumatising stay in the Zagreb prison hospital's psychiatric ward, he ended up in the Croatian psychiatric hospital 'Ivan Barbot' in Popovaca,

[80] Letter of Zoran Stankovic, 670–673.

[81] Tomislav Krsmanović, *Zloupotreba psihijatrije u politicke svrhe: Slucajevi*, Belgrade, 1988, Golub Bakic, 503–523.

[82] Arhiv Pokreta, Objasnjenje prilozenih dokumenata I informacije o Vladimiru Perisicu, 1.

[83] Ibid., 6–7.

which held prisoners diagnosed with criminal insanity.[84] In Popovaca, even those organisations which spoke on Perisić's behalf and advocated his release had to admit that his behaviour was not always lucid, and that some of his statements gave credence to the official psychiatric assessments of his health. In fact, the Yugoslav authorities used the case of Vladimir Perisic to try and publicly discredit the entire campaign against political abuses of psychiatry, and showcased his behaviour in order to demonstrate that all those prisoners confined to psychiatric institutions for their political statements were indeed mentally ill.

Shortly after Perisić's case caught international attention, a Yugoslav newspaper journalist visited the Popovaca hospital and prepared a feature on its ward for the criminally insane, officially called the 'Institute for treating and keeping mentally abnormal delinquents' (*Zavod za lijecenje i cuvanje dusevno abnormalnih delinkvenata*). To counter *Akcija's* and Amnesty International's increasingly persistent complaints, *Studentski List* presented the Institute and the entire hospital as an example of a therapeutic community, 'in which the staff and patients were equal', and as a model of modern social psychiatry, where patients took active part in the social and cultural life of the institution.[85] Moreover, the hospital's headmaster Jovan Bamburac mounted an impassioned and detailed defence of psychiatry as a discipline, rejecting the claims that psychiatry was being manipulated for repressive political purposes: 'psychiatry is certainly specific within the healthcare system, because it happens that some of our patients… end up in a psychiatric hospital against their will. Then we are always begrudged the fact that we deprived them of freedom…. But nobody remembers to ask why we deprived someone of their freedom'.[86]

In order to demonstrate that psychiatry was not a repressive 'social policeman' and that his patients truly belonged in a hospital for the mentally ill, Bamburac 'randomly' selected one of his patients and talked to him in front of the journalist, who then transcribed the entire conversation. The selected patient happened to be none other than Vladimir

[84] Krsmanović, *Zloupotreba psihijatrije u politicke svrhe*, Vlado Perisic, 11 February 1984, document 20.

[85] 'Put u srediste mozga: Ludilo, delikvencija, institucija', Studentski List, 913/914, 16 January 1986.

[86] Ibid.

Perisić, and his responses indeed served Bamburac's and the newspaper's political purposes very well: he certainly came across as delusional and deeply disturbed, claiming that he was the son of the medieval king Tomislav and had special powers, that he communicated with the dead bishop Stepinac and held 'all the Croats in [his] lymph'. At the end, Bamburac asked triumphantly, 'is this repression what you just saw?', implying, of course, that there was no profession other than psychiatry that could even try to help Perisić (this was also elegantly accentuated by the journalist's withdrawal to the background when they met the patient—he deemed himself incapable of leading that conversation and gave over to Bamburac, the mental health expert, to conduct this part of the interview).[87]

If one was to judge by Perisić's reported words in the article, the psychiatrists were certainly correct in having concluded that he suffered from 'mania of grandeur' or 'reformism', as he spoke of his historical mission to liberate the Croatian people. For Bamburac, Perisic was 'evidently ill', and this was ultimately his message for Amnesty International and similar activist organisations: 'I have no problem if someone believes that he is the conscience of mankind or of the society, but others can be the conscience too. Why would anyone presume *prima faciae* that I or my colleagues… are less conscientious and humane, that we did not share the same vision of freedom as someone who sits in a warm room and writes petitions. When I told one of those people [advocating for a political psychiatric prisoner], well, make friends with him, take him home over the weekend, he responded that [the patient] was not entirely ok in the head'.[88] In his highly colloquial manner, Bamburac thus implied that political activists complaining about psychiatric abuses had no genuine wish or ability to help those patients whom they nominally aimed to protect. On the other hand, psychiatrists were the only ones who truly cared for the wellbeing of such people, who invested time and effort instead of 'sitting in a warm room', but they still got maligned due to the broader society's misunderstanding of the psychiatric profession's mission and difficult tasks.

And while Perisić and his defenders might have claimed that his ruined mental health state was produced by the very system—political and

[87] Ibid.

[88] Ibid.

psychiatric—which Bamburac was trying to protect from criticism, the psychiatrist disagreed. He responded directly to such interpretations of Perisić's behaviour: this man 'could be declared ill for a variety of reasons. As a product of some social climate, some social relations, repression, police... But he is primarily ill because there is a genetic basis—without which there is no real schizophrenia'.[89] It was indeed notable that, despite his early talk of social psychiatry and therapeutic communities—and despite Yugoslav psychiatry's general development away from the biomedical paradigm—Bamburac found the ultimate interpretation of Perisić's illness within the framework of organic psychiatry when faced with accusations of repression and political abuse. This insistence on the organic psychiatric approach went hand in hand with Bamburac's marginalisation of the political aspect of Perisić's statements and behaviour—he argued that Perisic's case only elicited interest and public concern because his organically conditioned illness happened to manifest itself in a way to which 'the society was particularly sensitive, in terms of a symptomatology which smacked of nationalism, chauvinism'. But, in Bamburac's reading, these manifestations, which were indeed socially and culturally shaped, could not possibly be the motivation for Perisić's confinement—the real reason, his 'genetic' schizophrenia, was scientifically incontestable.

Therefore, Bamburac effectively neutralised the meaning of Perisić's political actions and pronouncements by placing them in the context of his supposedly unquestionable organic illness—and by explaining them not as legitimate attitudes of a politically engaged citizen but as products of a diseased, pathological thought process. Of course, there were other ways to frame Perisic's behaviour—and indeed, *Akcija's* report on this case analysed his support for Croatian nationalism in exclusively political terms, emphasising the relatively ordinary and widespread nature of his expressed opinions: 'Vlado often mentions Croatian national history and kings, important personalities, he believes that there is repression, that the people is enslaved (many say this, among them some very reputable individuals, so this in itself could not be seen as a sign of mental illness), that one should fight for national liberation'.[90] In this way, *Akcija* radically reinterpreted Perisić's opposition to the Yugoslav regime, constructing it not as an eccentric liberator's delusion of grandeur but as a legitimate

[89] Ibid.

[90] Objasnjenje prilozenih dokumenata i informacije o Vladimiru Perisicu, 7–8.

belief system of an anti-communist political dissident of nationalist provenance. In this way, a rhetorical battle was being fought between psychiatry and its critics on the very definition of psychological abnormality, and on the relationship between political dissidence and madness. This discussion, of course, simply reiterated in public the main terms and arguments from Krsmanović's psychiatric assessment and his lengthy response—the controversy shed light on the malleability of psychiatric diagnoses, and on the thin line separating socio-political non-conformity from psychiatric pathologisation and confinement.

Bamburac's insistence on organic psychiatry was particularly important here, and as mentioned above, it went directly against his attempts to present the Popovaca hospital as a model therapeutic community. Within the context of Yugoslav psychiatry, moreover, social psychiatric and psychodynamic approaches had by this point been absolutely dominant for nearly forty years, so that even interpretations of schizophrenia in Yugoslav psychiatric literature and in clinical practice were significantly different from Bamburac's analysis. It is telling, therefore, that, when faced with accusations of political psychiatric abuses, even Yugoslav psychiatrists reverted to fairly crude and rigid biomedical explanations, which minimised the importance of socio-cultural political factors, institutions and relations for the onset and development of mental illness. On the other hand, those who advocated against the psychiatric confinement of political prisoners relied very much on psychoanalytic and social psychiatric insights and concepts to frame their narratives and boost their arguments. Here as well, a psychodynamic framework served very well to produce a progressive critique of the social and political system, and to draw attention to potentially deleterious psychological effects of certain social, cultural and political trends and factors. Moreover, such psychoanalytically informed interpretations were used to criticise the functioning of those psychiatric institutions which housed political prisoners, and to analyse harmful relationships which developed between patients and the medical staff, as well as within the patient community.

Anti-Psychiatry in the East

Interestingly, in 1987, in the midst of these increasingly public discussions about the manipulations of Yugoslav psychiatry for political purposes, the leading Serbian daily *Politika* ran an article about the dire situation and plummeting reputation of Soviet psychiatry.[91] While journalist Dusan Pesic omitted to mention the actual proportions of the politicisation of Soviet psychiatry, and its systematic suppression of many prominent political dissidents, the article did problematise the exceedingly broad definition of schizophrenia in the Moscow psychiatric school. Moreover, Pesic emphasised that 'immoderate seeking of justice' could be classed as a symptom of mental pathology, and noted that this could easily be used in bad faith to silence those who had a tendency to criticise the social system as a whole. His example, a diligent employee from Leningrad called Marina, was very illustrative of precisely this tendency—Marina was indeed sentenced to psychiatric confinement as a diagnosed schizophrenic simply because she persistently drew attention to the myriad irregularities and malpractice at her workplace. In the same vein, the article rightly continued, Soviet psychiatry's malleable diagnostic criteria could be abused to neutralise those who took advantage of *glasnost* to air their social and political criticisms and complaints in the USSR.

Even though the article touched upon the issue of punitive political psychiatry, it presented the abuse as instances of individual manipulations by dishonest psychiatrists or local managers and politicians, rather than as a systemic issue. Still, it shed light on the important problem of psychiatric diagnostic criteria, suggesting that there were significant reasons for doubting the legitimacy and scientific solidity of psychiatric concepts and diagnoses (given the existing Soviet criteria, 'it's in fact possible to declare anyone abnormal'). As we will see below, this conclusion certainly resonated with some Yugoslav critiques, which were partly inspired the rich anti-psychiatric literature. The article, however, never made any references to similar tendencies in Yugoslav psychiatry, even though a careful reader would certainly notice some striking similarities.

First of all, *Akcija's* and others' frequent complaints about the brutal treatment of political psychiatric prisoners regularly drew attention to inadequate physical conditions in prison psychiatric wards (especially extremely cold temperatures in winter and broken heating systems), as well as to severe physical violence suffered by inmates—according to Pesic's report, these were exactly the main problems encountered in Soviet psychiatric hospitals, which had recently scandalised the Soviet public. But even more importantly, only three years before the article

[91] Dusan Pesic, 'Lako je postati lud', Politika, 15 November 1987.

was published, Yugoslav citizens were informed of the case of Peter Zemva, Slovene scientist employed at a medical equipment factory, who was forcibly taken to a psychiatric hospital and confined there for a few days because he publicly critiqued the factory's management, their policies and authoritarian decision-making. Luckily, Zemva was quickly released and reinstated in his job, while the factory director resigned amidst public scandal and resentment.[92] But Zemva's shocking psychiatric arrest attracted a lot of journalistic attention, and Serbian, Croatian and Slovene newspapers ran detailed articles about this case. When the article on Soviet psychiatry was published in 1987, it would have been difficult not to notice parallels between Zemva's and Marina's psychiatric confinements.

Overall, Zemva fared significantly better than Marina, who spent longer in the hospital and was then permanently saddled with the diagnosis of schizophrenia—this was perhaps also reflective of the difference in power between the Yugoslav and Soviet psychiatric repressive mechanisms. It remained unclear why Zemva was released so quickly—it was possible that this was partly due to the support he received from his colleagues, as well as to his high social status and education level. The psychiatric hospital where he was briefly kept never explained this in any detail but Jozef Felc, its director, maintained that Zemva had been 'in psychological crisis'[93] and that his treatment at the psychiatric hospital was necessary and medically fully justified. However, several Slovene psychiatric professionals and the Ljubljana Medical Faculty officially protested the critical journalistic coverage of this case, and eminent psychiatrist Joze Lokar defended his profession by noting that 'attacks on psychiatry intensified whenever society was experiencing crisis'.[94]

Zemva's forcible confinement was also unique because it provoked one of the very few critical responses from a psychiatrist. Ljubljana-based alcohologist Janez Rugelj got involved in this public discussion in no uncertain terms: his article in Slovene newspaper *Temeks* not only took a clear stance against this particular instance of psychiatric abuse,

[92] Krsmanović, *Zloupotreba psihijatrije u politicke svrhe*, Petar Zemva, 601; 'Istraga nad besprekornim novinarom', *Duga*, 274, 25 August 1984.

[93] Miodrag Govedarica, 'Sa posla na posmatranje', *Vecernje Novosti*, 15 August 1984.

[94] Janez Rugelj, 'Psihijatrija bi rada "zatusala" protizakonito "psihiatricno arestacijo" dr Petra Zemve', *Temeks*, 45/84, 8 November 1984.

but also made damning statements about the general state of psychiatry in Yugoslavia.[95] Rugelj was the first Yugoslav psychiatrist who, in response to Lokar's observation, spelled it out that 'psychiatry was only attacked in times of crisis if it became a force of repression'. Writing from personal experience, Rugelj concluded that Yugoslav psychiatry was 'dangerously obedient' to the political repressive structures (primarily, he argued, because of its traditionalism and backwardness) and that Zemva's case was certainly not unique: 'in our society psychiatry is not a medical science but – entirely in line with Szasz's definition – a social service for controlling non-criminal transgressions'. But Rugelj's article was additionally important because it was not limited to socialist psychiatry—he placed his critique in a much broader context, drawing on some of the leading thinkers and practitioners in antipsychiatry and radical psychiatry – Basaglia, Szasz, Goffman, Laing, Bierer. In that sense, his intervention shed light on the relationship between the public criticism of political abuses of psychiatry in Yugoslavia and the anti-psychiatry movement, which primarily developed in the West. While the other advocates for the rights of psychiatric political prisoners in Yugoslavia rarely quoted such anti-psychiatric literature, they did engage, as we have seen above, in lengthy discussions of the scientific value of psychiatric diagnostic criteria, and of the malleable and socially/politically conditioned meaning of the concept of psychiatric normality. In that sense, the broader discussion about repressive psychiatry in Yugoslavia possibly constituted an important anti-psychiatric moment in the history of East European mental health sciences.

Quoting none other than the legendary Yugoslav alcohologist and psychiatrist Vladimir Hudolin, Rugelj reminded his readers of psychiatry's time-honoured social role—to 'lock up people with inappropriate behaviour in psychiatric hospitals, in order to protect the society from the "danger" of mental health patients'. Moreover, he emphasised the predominant importance of social, cultural and political environments for the emergence and development of mental illness, arguing that traditional psychiatry in general avoided to tackle the broader pathology of family and society—which caused and conditioned mental suffering—choosing instead to 'sacrifice the affected individual' in order to safeguard

95 Ibid., 14–15.

the existing social order. In Rugelj's thoughtful critique, the authoritarian character of socialist political regimes could not on its own explain the existence of psychiatric abuses—the reason was in the very nature of psychiatry as a medical discipline and clinical practice, in its historical commitment to conforming to dominant social norms and values, and defending social relations and hierarchies. The notion of psychiatric normality and health remained, consequently, a matter of social agreement and not a scientific issue. Furthermore, rather than helping resolve people's mental difficulties and aiding their social integration, psychiatry produced pathology: 'with the diagnosis of schizophrenia, psychiatrists created millions of life-long psychiatric patients, whom psychiatry needs in order to justify its own continued existence'.[96]

It was clear from Rugelj's discussion, however, that his views were less radical than those of Szasz or Laing; for him, the solution to the problem of psychiatry's harmful and abusive politicisation, which happened both in the East and in the West, was in the development of progressive and emancipatory social psychiatry. This 'alternative psychiatry', as he called it, was sorely needed in Yugoslavia, and its main aim would be 'to gradually activate people suffering from psychological distress and build their capacity for life struggles', as well as to 'enable them for full social participation'.[97] Rugelj believed that these aims were sabotaged by the existing repressive psychiatric practices in Yugoslavia, but he also argued that a progressive socialist society was certainly capable of revolutionising traditional institutional psychiatry. In other words, in Rugelj's narrative, socialism did not automatically go hand in hand with psychiatric abuses; in many ways, socialism was psychiatry's only hope, the only system which could 'fully socialise' mental health professions. Thus revolutionised, psychiatry and psychotherapy would not aim to tutor, control or confine people with psychological distress but instead work to strengthen their independence and social abilities (of course, as we already saw in the previous chapter, these were precisely the theoretical and clinical goals of many socialist psychiatrists and psychotherapists in Yugoslavia, and their emancipatory practice existed in parallel with the political psychiatric abuses to which Rugelj was responding). Here again, social psychiatry was pitted against 'traditional' approaches which tended

[96] Ibid.

[97] Ibid.

to disregard broader socio-political factors and repressive structures, and social psychiatric and psychotherapeutic frameworks were constructed as the only ones capable of overcoming psychiatry's inherent authoritarian inclinations. Bamburac's observations about the predominantly organic origins of schizophrenia thus confirmed this division between social and 'traditional' biological psychiatry, and also marked the latter as a more likely ally of politically repressive tendencies.

Conditions and Therapy in Psychiatric Prison Hospitals

In March 1987, the Yugoslav Committee for human right protection published a lengthy report on the state of psychiatric wards in the country's two prison hospitals in Belgrade and Zagreb, where most political inmates were held.[98] Writing about the hospitals' excessively brutal practices, the authors of the report argued that such measures served to 'break passive resistance, re-educate inmates, and create obedient, terrified, broken and submissive citizens, who will not in any way obstruct the normal functioning of the society'. The report was primarily based on the prisoners' own testimonies, and their accounts of the physical and psychological brutalities suffered at the two psychiatric wards, and their intended outcomes, were indeed very reminiscent of the re-education strategies practised several decades earlier in the Goli Otok camp. In fact, the parents of one inmate, Janos Vibok, reported the words of a male nurse from the Belgrade ward, which could have easily been uttered in the context of Goli Otok: the personality of 'political enemies needs to be completely annihilated, humiliated, only when they are truly humiliated are they also defeated, in the prison we aim to break resistance in people, to demean them, make them terrified and submissive, or if that's not possible—to destroy them'.[99] This was the most effective way to 'incapacitate the prisoner as a person who might formulate a critique of social injustices', and act in unconventional or non-conformist ways.[100]

[98] Komitet za zastitu ljudskih prava, 'Raport o stanju uslova zivota', 1–35.

[99] Lujza Vibok, Letter to Mr Nigel Rodley, Amnesty International, 26 March 1985; Gradski sekretarijat za unutrasnje poslove, II Odeljenje UZSK, Krivicna prijava, 23268/79, Belgrade, 12 December 1979.

[100] 'Raport o stanju uslova zivota', 22–23.

The report made it clear over and over again that these hospital psychiatric wards applied none of the recommended therapeutic strategies and practices, and that, furthermore, the psychiatrists employed at these institutions invested no efforts in developing productive and therapeutic relationships with their patients/inmates. Following a mandatory mental health exam at admission, inmates were scheduled no further regular meetings with their psychiatrists, and when psychiatrists did see them for check-ups or assessments, their demeanour was 'curt, dry, formal', and there was no genuine communication. Instead, the staff developed and employed what the report deemed to be a 'subversive sophisticated psychiatric technique' in order to disrupt and neutralise any remnants of the prisoners' disobedience and political insubordination. The report utilised an explicitly psychoanalytic language to critique the conduct of the psychiatric staff, who were 'more akin to prison administrators than medical doctors dedicated to these people's health': because the psychiatrists in question demonstrated very little empathy towards their patients, 'so-called negative transfer emerged', while 'negative counter-transfers' were inevitable, and many patients experienced emotional and verbal abuse at the hands of their doctors and nurses. It was therefore impossible to create a necessary atmosphere of confidence and 'positive transfer situations' in these institutions, which had a disastrous effects on the inmates' overall psychological and emotional state.[101]

The psychiatric staff were described in damning terms: reportedly held in low esteem by their colleagues in other mental health institutions around Yugoslavia, prison ward psychiatrists were 'cold and formal', emotionally ambivalent towards the patients and profoundly disinterested in exploring the patients' inner world or listening to their 'doubts, fears, uncertainties'. Furthermore, the report evaluated the psychiatrists' own psyche, concluding, rather expectedly, that they were 'unable to imagine themselves in their patients' shoes, to feel their traumas and suffering, and to assess them realistically'. They were ideologically indoctrinated (they believed that political prisoners posed an 'even greater danger to society than murderers', as they threatened the entire social fabric with their subversive political activities and propaganda), and also keen to preserve their material and political benefits and privileges.[102] Between the lines,

[101] Ibid., 29.

[102] Ibid., 30–32.

the authors of the report argued that the prison psychiatrists were unable to feel empathy, and were therefore themselves psychologically damaged. This rhetorical manoeuvre in fact turned the tables on the psychiatrists and the prison authorities—constructing *them* as psychologically pathological, and it was quite common in political and literary narratives about political abuses of psychiatry in socialist Eastern Europe.

Reasons for marking the psychiatric staff as pathological—'paranoid' and 'sadistic' in different critical narratives—were, of course, more than merely rhetorical. In this regard, Yugoslav psychiatric political prisoners' experiences were strikingly similar to those of their counterparts in the USSR's notorious 'special hospitals'. According to the report, the inmates of the two prison psychiatric hospitals were not only denied standard therapeutic care; they were also exposed to policies, treatments and experiences which were explicitly intended to undermine their mental health, such as frequent and severe physical beatings for any sign of noncompliance, or for criticising any aspect of the hospitals' functioning and heavy pharmacological therapy, while the patients rarely if ever had an opportunity to meet with psychologists or social workers.[103] Complaints and non-conformist or even vaguely defiant statements could easily land one in an isolation unit for long periods of time. For instance, prisoner Vladimir Marković testified that an Albanian inmate was sent to isolation merely for saying that, if he died, he did not wish to be buried in Serbia but in Kosovo.[104] In the Zagreb hospital, electro-convulsive therapy was also used regularly, primarily as a punishment for non-conformist behaviour—for example, Vladimir Perisić was reportedly treated with ECT systematically after he asked for the Bible and to see a priest.[105]

[103] Ibid., 10–28. It is important to note here that such treatment and conditions were not necessarily dissimilar to those experienced by non-political patients in regular psychiatric hospitals, especially outside the largest cities and research centres. As Ivan Simic and other researchers have documented, patients in Yugoslav psychiatric hospitals such as Donja Toponica regularly endured brutality and violence at the hands of auxiliary staff and guards in the early postwar decades, while these underfunded and understaffed institutions offered virtually no psychotherapy nor psychological counselling, and witnessed a breakdown of patient-psychiatrist relationships. While the situation in mental healthcare institutions certainly improved over the following decades, prison psychiatric hospitals might have simply been kept in an unreformed state, partly intentionally and partly out of inertia. See Simic, 'The curious case of Aleksandar Milivojevic', 1350–1362.

[104] 'Raport o stanju uslova zivota', 23.

[105] Ibid., 26.

Finally, all psychiatric political prisoners at all institutions regularly complained that their relationships with the external world were disrupted very efficiently; most importantly, their family visits were obstructed in different ways, family members were threatened and discouraged from visiting and maintaining contact, and letters and packages were rarely delivered. This in spite of the fact that, as the authors of the report rightly noted, the dominant psychiatric approaches in Yugoslavia (and the world) emphasised the therapeutic importance and benefits of involving family in all aspects of mental health treatment and healing.[106] Some family members, furthermore, reportedly experienced exceptional levels of harassment, psychological coercion, blackmail as well as physical and sexual violence at the hands of hospital staff—the case of Janos Vibok's family is particularly instructive here. A male nurse from the Belgrade prison hospital targeted his parents for years, extorting money and material gifts from them while threatening to 'drive their son insane' if they did not comply with his wishes. Finally, the male nurse raped Janos's mother and threatened her into silence. Janos's situation, unfortunately, never improved.[107]

* * *

As we saw throughout this chapter, the history of Yugoslav psychiatry's involvement in repressive and authoritarian practices is complex and thought-provoking. It demonstrates the multifaceted and often contradictory character of the Yugoslav 'psy' disciplines, but it also sheds light on the political functioning and aims of the Yugoslav regime. In fact, the contradiction at the heart of this story—that progressive and emancipatory psychotherapeutic concepts, techniques, institutions and individuals could be engaged in some of the most violent practices aimed at political dissenters—reveals a vital trait of the Yugoslav government and society. Lauded as the most liberal and Westernised of all the East European socialist countries, the experimental homeland of workers' self-management and humanist Marxism was also a site of violent political repression throughout the postwar period. The analysis of psychiatric and psychoanalytic participation in such practices offers a unique insight into the aims and mechanisms of the regime's authoritarian political

[106] Ibid., 16–20.

[107] Ibid., 20–21.

control. Punitive psychiatry in Yugoslavia still contained some unique characteristics. The Goli Otok experiment in political re-education relied precisely on those principles of self-management, radical democracy and revolutionary personal transformation that fundamentally marked the subsequent liberalisation of Yugoslavia's 'psy' professions. On the other hand, the 1970s and 1980s saw a more conventional form of punitive psychiatry develop in Yugoslavia, although these practices also seemed to implicate some of the country's flagship progressive psychiatric and psychotherapeutic institutions. Still, Yugoslavia's more relaxed political atmosphere affected the practices of punitive psychiatry to an important extent, and a rather elaborate public and legal discussion ensued, which allowed many psychiatric victims and survivors to tell their own story, and involved a variety of international and local organisations. For those reasons, this chapter has attempted to write the history of political manipulations of Yugoslav psychiatry as an (unequal) conversation between a variety of voices and participants. Overall, the instances of political psychiatric abuses in Yugoslavia remind us that, despite its rather unwilling departure from the Cominform in 1948, the country had significant socio-political and medical similarities with the other states in the socialist bloc. Yugoslavia's Westernisation was complicated by the persistence of both political and psychiatric authoritarianisms, and even the Goli Otok experiment, directly provoked by the very break from the Soviet Union, brought Yugoslavia closer to the Soviet bloc's authoritarian practices. In that sense, the history of Yugoslav psychiatry yet again opens an unexpected window onto the country's multiple and often mutually contradictory internationalisations, and demonstrates Yugoslavia's continuing links to the community and experiences of East European socialism.

CHAPTER 5

Global Imaginations and Non-alignment: Waging War Against Backwardness

As some of the most prominent Yugoslav psychiatrists and psychoanalysts increasingly joined their Western colleagues in transnational exchanges, professional organisations and intellectual debates, the Western 'psy' disciplines were undergoing their own process of soul-searching and radical transformation in the aftermath the Second World War and in the midst of violent decolonisation. This was both an exciting and a rather disruptive time to develop close and intense links with West European mental health professions. On the one hand, this was the 'great psychiatric moment' of the twentieth century. Following the end of the Second World War, many relied on psychiatry, psychotherapy and psychoanalysis to offer crucial insights into social pathologies, sources of violence, psychological roots of fascism and fascistic leanings.[1] According to many observers in the 1940s and 1950s, the world was on the brink of a disaster, and it was only those who had deep knowledge of all the intricacies of the human psyche who could work to prevent further aggression and effect a major transformation in temperaments and mentalities.[2] Psychiatrists were called

[1] Ian Dowbiggin, *The Quest for Mental Health: A Tale of Science, Medicine, Scandal, Sorrow, and Mass Society*, Cambridge: Cambridge University Press, 2011.

[2] Brock Chisholm, 'The Psychiatry of Enduring Peace and Social Progress (The William Alanson White Memorial Lecture)', *Psychiatry*, 1946, 9, 3–20.

A. Antić, *Non-Aligned Psychiatry in the Cold War*, Mental Health in Historical Perspective, https://doi.org/10.1007/978-3-030-89449-8_5

to contribute to warding off the core challenges to the post-WWII peace: they were sought to ensure success in a variety of very important political endeavours, such as eradicating fascism in Europe or dealing with the challenges of economic reconstruction, modernisation and social development throughout the world.[3] To these global anxieties, the 1950s and 1960s added what Europeans perceived as the extreme dangers of decolonisation: not only the anti-colonial movements and their challenge to the colonial order, but also the radical social, political and cultural transformations brought about by the withdrawal of the colonial powers and independence of their former non-European territories. In many ways, the new post-WWII global system seemingly could not even be conceived without a fundamental input of those specialising in the human psyche. Socialist psychiatrists had a lot to contribute in that regard, even though their attempts to engage with broader social, cultural and political issues have so far been largely neglected in scholarly literature.

In the mid-twentieth century, any belief in the possibility of long-term peaceful and harmonious cross-cultural communication was fragile, and the 'psy' sciences and anthropology contributed significantly to debates around psychological preconditions for and limitations of cross-cultural understanding in a rapidly globalising decolonised world. But Western psychiatry had many skeletons in its own closet: the profession as a whole in large part served to support and legitimise oppressive and violent regimes and explicitly racist hierarchies, both in the colonies and in Europe. If Western psychiatry was to have any meaningful social and political role in the turbulent postwar world, it needed to rethink its own core assumptions and involvements. The emerging discipline of transcultural psychiatry aimed to serve this precise purpose, as its proponents attempted to leave behind the profession's racist and colonial legacies, and lay the foundation for a more inclusive union between Western and non-Western concepts of mental illness and healing.[4] From the 1950s on, cross-cultural research became one of the most important and fast-growing fields in global psychiatry. And while historical accounts of this period are scant and focus almost exclusively on West European

[3] Daniel Pick, *The Pursuit of the Nazi Mind: Hitler, Hess and the Analysts*, Oxford: Oxford University Press, 2012.

[4] Alice Bullard, 'Imperial Networks and Postcolonial Independence: The Transition from Colonial to Transcultural Psychiatry', in Sloan Malone and Megan Vaughan, eds, *Psychiatry and Empire*, Basingstoke: Palgrave Macmillan, 2007.

contributions and former imperial connections, the main aim of this chapter is to analyse for the first time the role of socialist East European (Yugoslav) mental health practitioners in the emergence and development of post-colonial cross-cultural psychiatry.[5]

As part of their intense internationalisation in the aftermath of the 1948 Tito–Stalin split, Yugoslav psychiatrists embarked on lengthy educational and advisory trips to the non-aligned world which allowed them to conduct sociological, medical, psychiatric and anthropological research in the non-Western territories. Some of them were keen to join the budding discipline of cross-cultural psychiatry as they considered themselves well placed to explore the transcultural sociological and political aspects of mental illness and to contribute to comparative global studies on psychiatric normativity, epidemiology and universal diagnostic techniques. As professionals coming from 'in-between' different cultural, ideological and political spaces, they thought themselves particularly capable of combining a variety of theoretical and clinical approaches in order to develop culturally sensitive but globally applicable norms for diagnosing mental illness and for defining its social, cultural and anthropological elements, causes and consequences. Moreover, as East Europeans, they believed that they had a much less complex relationship to colonial histories and legacies than their West European colleagues, and their socialist background gave them further anti-colonial credentials. It is indeed debatable to what extent transcultural psychiatry succeeded in removing itself from erstwhile intellectual and clinical colonial frameworks in the aftermath of the Second World War, and, as we will see below, East European contributions to the field were far from unproblematic in this regard. Still, intellectuals and professionals traveling to the global South from the Balkans (and Yugoslavia) could claim that their own 'whiteness' and Europeanness were conditional, and that their own cultural and geographical background placed them in a position from which they could better understand those oppressed by European colonial powers. Their liminal civilisational position indeed bred some of their most interesting psychiatric and anthropological contributions, which will be the core themes of this chapter.

[5] Mahone and Vaughan, *Psychiatry and Empire*; Heaton, *Black Skin, White Coats*; Jock McCulloch, *Colonial Psychiatry and the 'African Mind'*, Cambridge: Cambridge University Press, 1995; Katie Kilroy-Marac, 'Nostalgic for Modernity: Reflecting on the Early Years of the Fann Psychiatric Clinic in Dakar, Senegal', *African Identities*, 2013, 11:4, 367–380.

Not only socialism but also the practices and discourses of non-alignment at times appeared to take Yugoslavia outside of Europe altogether. Even though the Balkan region might have seen itself as politically, geographically and civilisationally European (even under socialism), its historical legacy was one of imperial subjects rather than imperial rulers, and the attachment to a 'European identity' was accompanied by narratives of cultural inferiority and experiences of rejection by Europe.[6] In that sense, non-aligned Yugoslavia's geopolitical and civilisational status was permanently unstable, and a close analysis of Yugoslav psychiatric discussions of socialist, Western and non-European psyche will demonstrate how this instability shaped these professionals' clinical contributions to transcultural psychiatry as well as their political engagement with decolonisation and the notions of race, modernity and primitivism.

This chapter traces such transnational and interdisciplinary engagements as they peaked in the 1960s, and as they took a different turn with the onset of 'new cross-cultural psychiatry' in the 1980s. It focuses on two distinguished Belgrade psychiatrists and psychoanalysts Vladimir Jakovljević (1925–1968) and Časlav Hadzi-Nikolić (1942), who undertook clinical and anthropological research in the global South (Africa, India and South and Central America), and intervened in a unique and original manner in Western-dominated global transcultural psychiatry.

The chapter begins by considering Jakovljević's work in Guinea, the former French colony in West Africa, where he spent over thirty months (1961–1963) as a clinical and research psychiatrist and a member of the technical aid mission financed by Yugoslavia's Federal Bureau for international scientific, educational-cultural and technical cooperation.[7] Jakovljević was the most prominent Yugoslav psychiatrist to participate in any professional or clinical exchange with the decolonising world, as well as the most prolific one, publishing numerous reports, books and journal articles on his involvement in Guinea and its implications for the field of transcultural psychiatry. He was the pioneer of Yugoslavia's (and Eastern Europe's) transcultural psychiatric research, and quickly became the leading figure in that field in the regional context.[8] On

[6] Baker, *Race and the Yugoslav Region*.

[7] Archive of Yugoslavia, Savezni zavod za medjunarodnu naucnu, prosvetno-kulturnu i tehnicku saradnju, F-465 box 545, 'Opsti dosije'; box 1645, 'Naucno-tehnicka saradnja SFRJ-Gvineja'.

[8] Klajn, *Razvoj Psihoanalize u Srbiji*.

the other hand, Hadzi-Nikolic belonged to a later generation of cross-cultural researchers, who grew increasingly critical of their intellectual predecessors in the field of transcultural psychiatry, viewing them as deeply influenced by Eurocentric, even colonial frameworks and unable or unwilling to understand non-Western concepts of mental illness and healing on their own terms. Hadzi-Nikolic was a particularly outspoken representative of the much more anthropologically minded 'new cross-cultural psychiatry', and, to my knowledge, its only East European exponent. He spent the 1980s working in a series of South American states such as Peru, Ecuador and Bolivia as a chief medical officer of 'Energoprojekt', Yugoslavia's flagship construction company which pursued contracts and investment throughout the world and particularly focused on collaboration with developing countries.[9]

By tracing Yugoslav psychiatrists' efforts to establish links and communication models between Western, Eastern and (global) Southern epistemological systems and networks, this chapter aims to inscribe the region of Eastern Europe into the broader history of global medical and psychiatric knowledge production.[10] It is particularly important to explore socialist East European contributions to the field of transcultural psychiatry. The topic of colonial rule, decolonisation and the pernicious legacies of imperialism became increasingly important for the political regimes in Eastern Europe as they sought to get involved with the global South through a variety of economic, cultural and political schemes, and offer an alternative to the failed Western project.

It was perhaps not accidental that the only East European transcultural psychiatrists came from Yugoslavia: the ideological influence of

[9] Časlav Hadzi-Nikolić, *Kad se vidi ono sto se ne vidi: Samani i halucinogeni*, Belgrade: Itaka, 2004 (reprinted).

[10] The literature on Cold War encounters between the socialist bloc and the 'Third World' is growing, and it largely focuses on networks of experts and university student exchanges, while the history of medical collaboration remains neglected for the most part. See Maxim Matusevich, 'Revisiting the Soviet Moment in Sub-Saharan Africa', *History Compass*, 2009, 10, 1–10; Matusevich, 'Probing the Limits of Internationalism: African Students Confront Soviet Ritual', *Anthropology of East Europe Review*, 2009, 27:2, 19–39; Benjamin Tromly, 'Brother or Other? East European Students in Soviet Higher Education Establishments, 1948–1956', *European History Quarterly*, 2014, 44:1, 80–102; Lukasz Stanek, 'Architects from Socialist Countries in Ghana (1957–1967): Modern Architecture and Mondialisation', *Journal of the Society of Architectural Historians*, 2015, 74:4, 416–442; Stanek, 'Mobilities of Architecture in the Late Cold War: From Socialist Poland to Kuwait, and Back', *International Journal of Islamic Architecture*, 2015, 4:2, 365–398.

non-alignment should not be underestimated in this field. Postwar global transcultural psychiatry attempted to grapple with the legacies and afterlives of colonial power structures, and to transform the professional relationships and models of communication between the decolonising world and the former colonial powers. Yugoslavia was well prepared to join this global discussion: non-alignment built the identification with global anti-colonial struggle into the very narrative of Yugoslav identity, and the intense contacts with the global South through the framework of non-aligned solidarity and collaboration certainly affected the development of socialist transcultural psychiatry in the country. As Oskar Davico claimed in his well-known travelogue 'Black on white', Yugoslavs were 'slaves for centuries themselves'[11] (according to writer Nikola Vitorović, they were 'different white people'),[12] and hence more capable of solidarity with the non-European world. At the same time, both Yugoslav politicians and psychiatrists relied on the universalist language of 'civilisation' vs the 'uncivilised world' which permeated social, cultural and medical discourses. Yugoslav (and any other East European) socialism ultimately adopted Eurocentric narratives of linear progress and modernity, while symbols of 'backwardness' and 'primitivism' were regularly associated with Asian and African nations. In such a contradictory political and professional context, how did Yugoslav socialist psychiatrists affect the global field of transcultural psychiatry, and how did socialism and/or non-alignment shape their legacies?

East European Pioneers in Transcultural Psychiatry

Jakovljević—a Marxist psychiatrist educated in France and deeply interested in French and British psychoanalysis and psychotherapy—personifies the in-between position inhabited by Yugoslav researchers and clinicians; this chapter traces how such political, ideological and geographical-cultural displacement moulded his and his Yugoslav colleagues' interventions in the field of transcultural psychiatry. Jakovljević's 'in-betweenness' was multidimensional. Geographically and culturally they were caught between Western Europe (the home of transcultural psychiatry) and a

[11] Oskar Davico, *Crno na belo*, Belgrade: Prosveta, 1962, 20.

[12] Nikola Vitorovic, *Crne Suze Konga*, Belgrade: Biblioteka Marko Polo, 1961.

small Balkan country, whose own developmental stage was questionable and uncertain. Ideologically, even though he declared himself a committed communist, Jakovljević's affiliation was to a non-Soviet, non-aligned form of socialism, which meant that his approach to social and mental health problems in the 'Third World' was a combination of Marxist (even Soviet) psychiatric concerns, West European theoretical frameworks and ideas of workers' self-management and non-aligned solidarity. Finally, as a socialist Eastern European psychiatrist, Jakovljević was extremely critical of the legacies of Western colonialism, but as a prominent transcultural psychiatrist he never managed to completely break out of the profession's lingering colonial paradigm: as he grappled with the concepts of primitivism, backwardness and decolonisation, Jakovljević combined colonial and anti-colonial discourses to try to define the global position and developmental possibilities of the decolonising world.

One crucial consequence of Jakovljević's complex background was his complicated and constantly changing relationship to his Guinean area of study: he was a white European researcher but emphatically not Western in a crucial political/ideological sense, and a representative of a state which consciously strove to offer a communist alternative to the Western colonial project.[13] Jakovljević's global engagements were ultimately driven by his domestic concerns—his implicit perception of the fundamental similarity between Guinea and Yugoslavia as two 'backward' and rapidly modernising societies. While he never explicitly drew parallels between Yugoslavia and any African country, this chapter close reads Jakovljević's texts in order to reveal the similarity of his analyses of and conclusions about the two regions, and to interrogate Jakovljević's uncertainty regarding the cultural-geographic and civilisational position of socialist Yugoslavia.

In this chapter I also aim to demonstrate that such transcultural involvements exposed some of the core ideological and conceptual inconsistencies within Marxist psychiatry in Eastern Europe.[14] Jakovljević's

[13] For a recent discussion of the role of psychiatry and psychiatric concepts in the Western colonial project in the twentieth century, see Erik Linstrum, *Ruling Minds: Psychology in the British Empire*, Cambridge: Harvard University Press, 2016.

[14] On the history and intellectual frameworks of Marxist and Communist psychiatry in Eastern Europe, see Ari Kiev, *Psychiatry in the Communist World*, New York: Science House, 1968; Marks and Savelli, *Psychiatry in Communist Europe*.

contradictory relationship to colonial legacies was not simply a function of his education in (Western European) transcultural psychiatry; it should also be placed in the context of Marxism's (and Marxist psychiatry's) own 'civilising mission'. One of the core debates in Yugoslavia's socialist psychiatry revolved around the problem of 'primitive' patients, and the psychiatrists' role in modernising those 'archaic' and 'uncultured' sections of the population. Because of the multiple meanings of 'primitivism in the Yugoslav psychiatric context, Jakovljević applied the same language of backwardness and civilisation to his Macedonian and Guinean patients, and, consequently, there were no fundamental differences in his descriptions of the developmental stages of the two regions.

Jakovljević belonged to one of the first post-World War II generations of Yugoslav psychiatrists. Graduating from the Medical Faculty in Zagreb in 1951, he completed specialisations in neuropsychiatry at several clinics in Yugoslavia as well as a one-year postgraduate psychoanalytic training in Paris (1956–1957). Before settling in Belgrade he spent three years as a psychiatric clinician, researcher and teacher in Skopje, Macedonia, Yugoslavia's southernmost republic and one of its most underdeveloped territories, which became very important for his subsequent contributions to comparative and transcultural psychiatry. Jakovljević belonged to a powerful psychoanalytically oriented psychiatric and psychotherapeutic group gathered around Vladislav Klajn at the 'Dragiša Mišović' hospital, where Jakovljević himself was briefly employed. Throughout his varied career he was committed to reconciling modern psychoanalysis with humanist Marxism, Marxist anthropology and the core tenets of workers' self-management, a synthesis which remained the principal mission of Yugoslavia's postwar psychiatry.

The development of Marxist and socialist psychiatry in post-1945 Yugoslavia saw a radical departure from the previously dominant biological and organicist models, which interpreted mental illness as exclusively understood in the context of hereditary, constitutional and physiological deficiencies. As Marxist mental health professionals argued, these earlier paradigms conveniently ignored the pervasive pathological influences of socio-economic factors and contexts in capitalist societies and medicalised social conflicts and economic inequalities. In that sense, Yugoslav socialist psychiatry became increasingly interested in the social, psychological and environmental aspects of patients' experiences.[15] As Jakovljević wrote in his 1959 article on the sociopsychology of neuroses in Macedonia, the development of the concept of psychogenesis of mental illness in cultural psychiatry had enabled clinicians and researchers to 'disprove fatalist interpretations regarding the supposedly exclusively hereditary nature of a variety of [mental] disorders, including neuroses'.[16] In addition, as the political experiment with workers' self-management was underway, a growing number of both psychiatrists and social scientists began to explore the relationship between humanist Marxism, personal emancipation and psychoanalysis, and suggested that psychoanalytic techniques such as self-reflection and self-exploration might be central to achieving individual liberation and self-realisation in a self-managing context.[17] Jakovljević remained keenly interested in different psychoanalytic approaches as tools for personal liberation and development but still maintained a critical voice towards classical psychoanalysis and its tendency to eschew sociological analysis and focus predominantly on internal psychological conflicts and processes. Like Klajn he represented a sociologically oriented and materialist school of thought within psychoanalytic circles inspired by Karen Horney, Erich Fromm and Igor Caruso in particular.[18] Jakovljević was also something of an outsider to the profession because his sociological and anthropological interests led him, in 1963, to a professorship at the Faculty of Philosophy, rather than of medicine, at the University of Belgrade.[19]

Jakovljević's Marxist orientation inspired his interest in the socioeconomic and contextual determinants of mental pathology and his efforts to bridge disciplinary boundaries between psychiatry and social sciences. 'All internal (intra-psychic) conflicts', he opined, 'are, in the final

[15] See Antic, *Therapeutic Fascism*, esp. chapter 2.

[16] Jakovljević, 'Prilog Proucavanju Sociopsihogeneze Neurotickih Poremecaja Licnosti', *Sociologija*, 2 (1959), 55.

[17] On the relationship between Yugoslav psychoanalysis and the theory of workers' self-management, especially as it was discussed within the Praxis school, see Antic, 'The Pedagogy of Workers' Self-management: Terror, Therapy, and Reform Communism in Yugoslavia After the Tito-Stalin Split', *Journal of Social History*, 2016, 50:1, 179–203.

[18] Jakovljević, 'Predgovor', in Igor Caruso, ed., *Socijalni Aspekti Psihoanalize*, Belgrade: Kultura, 1969.

[19] Zagorka Pesic-Golubovic, 'Vladimir Jakovljević (1925–1958)', 6–7. There, he maintained fruitful, if informal, professional relations with some of the leading members of the Praxis school of critical Marxist philosophy.

analysis, merely intimate sediments of broader social conflicts, expressed to a greater or lesser extent in an individual personality [Such mental disturbances] were conditioned by major imbalances within the core social institutions (family, class, social group), which were then reflected in the mental structure of an individual'.[20] His proclaimed aim was not only to draw more attention to the socio-cultural aspects of mental health and abnormality but to 'bring together as much as possible medical and sociological research activities'.[21] Jakovljević's core contribution to the humanities was his comprehensive examination of the concept of social pathology, in the course of which he combined psychiatric insights with anthropological, philosophical and sociological methodologies, aiming to explore alienation, mental distress and pathological maladjustment by identifying and addressing their social, economic and cultural roots and causes.[22] Therefore, when discussing psychiatric illnesses he remained primarily interested in social relations, societal norms and cultural institutions predominant in the patient's social environment, and aimed to develop generalised definitions regarding the relationship between individual psychological malfunctioning and broader socio-economic and cultural conditions.[23] His transcultural explorations served the same purpose and constituted an essential part of his life-long research into socio-economic and cultural determinants of mental illness and health.[24]

In addition, as we will see below, Jakovljević's Marxist orientation shaped his reading of Guinea's rapid modernisation and socio-economic development. While he agreed with most transcultural psychiatrists of his time that the forces of modernisation produced mental pathology in the decolonising world, his experiences of social revolution in Yugoslavia made him more optimistic regarding the Guinean population's ability to overcome psychological breakdowns, adapt to radical changes and achieve

[20] Jakovljević, 'Prilog Proucavanju Neurotickih Poremecaja', 76.

[21] Ibid., 59.

[22] Jakovljević, moreover, often published in non-medical anthropological, ethnographic and sociological journals, and relied on psychoanalytic and psychiatric insights to discuss mentalities, cultural habits and folk customs. See, for instance, Jakovljević, 'Preziveli Oblici Orgijastickog Vidaarhaicnih Rusaliskih Obreda - Homoljske Rusalje, Padalice', *Etnoloski pregled*, 1960, 2, 7–23.

[23] Pesic-Golubovic, 'Vladimir Jakovljević (1925–1958)', 6–7.

[24] On the development and institutionalisation of Yugoslav psychiatry in the 1940s and 1950s, see Antic, *Therapeutic Fascism*.

a more 'progressive' stage of development.[25] As a researcher from a fellow socialist country, Jakovljević remained more sensitive to Guinea's potentials for development and radical social change.

Jakovljević first travelled to Guinea in March 1961, where he worked to establish the psychiatric services in a country which had previously had no mental health facilities other than one neurological department and one psychiatric centre in the main hospitals in the capital city, Conakry (as a rule, psychiatric patients in Guinea had been treated in general hospitals). He was thus engaged in organising the work of Guinea's fledgling mental health departments and in educating various types of psychiatric hospital staff. In addition to his work with psychiatric patients in the Donka and Baley hospitals in Conakry, Jakovljević treated and interacted with mental health patients in prisons and asylums, as well as regularly visiting a variety of hospitals and private homes in the interior of the country. As a result, he obtained access to a diverse population of psychiatric patients, engaging with Guineans from various social, ethnic and cultural backgrounds as he travelled across the country. Alongside what appears to have been a very hectic schedule of clinical and organisational work, Jakovljević remained interested in anthropological psychiatric research and collected epidemiological, sociological and ethnographic data, aiming to produce conclusive work in the fields of comparative and transcultural psychiatry.[26]

In the postwar era, Jakovljević was among the very few Eastern Europeans to join the budding field of transcultural psychiatry, which was spearheaded by the Western psychiatric community and fundamentally tied to the process of decolonisation. For Yugoslavs, as well as for their Western colleagues, the rapidly decolonising African continent presented an unprecedented opportunity for exploration and experimentation, a research laboratory of sorts where the new, post-colonial international psychiatry might begin to be forged.[27]

[25] Jakovljević, *Kulturna sredina i psihički poremećaji ličnosti: transkulturno-psihijatrijsko proučavanje u Afričkoj Gvineji*, PhD dissertation, University of Zagreb, 1967.

[26] Jakovljević, 'Transkulturno-psihijatrijska Proucavanja u Gvineji: Preliminarno Saopstenje', *Neuropsihijatrija*, 1963, 11:1, 24–25.

[27] Jakovljević, 'Social Science in Medicine (review)', *Sociologija*, 1959, 2, 178–180.

Transcultural Psychiatry: The Birth of a New Field

In itself, transcultural (or cultural) psychiatry proved to be a complicated, contradictory discipline, which intersected in multiple and controversial ways with colonial mindsets, post-colonial realities and post-Second World War universalism and humanitarianism. Even though scholars have recently shed more light on the history of the discipline, its links to colonial psychiatry remain difficult to fully understand. Alice Bullard defined transcultural psychiatry as one of the multiple sets of practices into which colonial psychiatry transformed itself in the mid-twentieth century: with the slow and agonising death of the West European colonial project, Western psychiatrists searched for more productive ways of thinking about traditional non-Western concepts of mental health and healing strategies and sought to integrate non-European ideas of psychological abnormality and therapy into the dominant psychiatric science[28] On the one hand, as Emmanuel Delille has argued, the emergence and professionalisation of transcultural psychiatry as an academic discipline signified a period of radical transition, driven by the uncertainties and reassessments of the decolonisation period.[29] At the same time, however, the discredited colonial background was difficult to shed: some of the continuities between colonial and transcultural psychiatry are striking, while several champions of late-colonial psychiatry became part of post-Second World War transcultural psychiatric circles.[30] Early transcultural psychiatric scholarship tended to perceive the cultures of former colonies as self-contained, static entities and described them as exotic and archaic, reifying their forms of communication and core traits. In the 1960s and 1970s transcultural psychiatrists still understood 'cultures' as 'out there', residing entirely with the other, while professionals were assumed to base their work on a universal system of knowledge grounded in science that was viewed as

[28] Bullard, 'Imperial Networks and Postcolonial Independence'.

[29] Emmanuel Delille, 'On the History of Cultural Psychiatry: Georges Devereux, Henri Ellenberger, and the Psychological Treatment of Native Americans in the 1950s', *Transcultural Psychiatry*, 2016, 53:3, 393.

[30] For particularly critical assessments of ethnopsychiatry in France, see Didier Fassin, 'Ethnopsychiatry and the Postcolonial Encounter: A French Psychopolitics of Otherness', in Warwick Anderson, Deborah Jenson, and Richard Keller, eds, *Unconscious Dominions: Psychoanalysis, Colonial Trauma, and Global Sovereignties*, Duke University Press, 2011.

acultural'.[31] As a result, as Arthur Kleinman has pointed out, transcultural psychiatry tended to pay lip service to ethnographic and anthropological research, assuming that cultures merely determined the 'camouflage' of disease and at best shaped their symptoms and superficial expressions.[32] Such medical universalism reinforced Eurocentric classification and treatment systems, disregarding a careful analysis of local cultural, social and economic contexts and working with simplified notions of non-European societies and values.

Jakovljević aligned himself with international currents of transcultural psychiatric research, initially through studies comparing Macedonia and France, and later in explorations of the former French colony of Guinea in Western Africa. As France was one of the homelands of post-Second World War transcultural psychiatry, Jakovljević's exposure to transcultural psychiatry during his studies in Paris had shaped his already existing interest in the socio-cultural determinants of mental illness and guided him towards the bourgeoning field of international post-colonial psychiatric research. Initially Jakovljević took part in the WHO's initiatives in postwar international psychiatry as well as in the ambitious research projects emerging around the Canadian journal *Transcultural Psychiatry*, which was based at the McGill University's increasingly influential Division of Social and Transcultural Psychiatry. Such projects largely focused on gathering information regarding the frequency and symptoms of a variety of psychiatric disorders from around the world.[33]

In his thirty months of clinical and research work in Guinea Jakovljević aimed to address some of the core questions and problems of transcultural psychiatry. Are there cultures in which mental disorders do not exist or are extremely rare? Are there epidemiological differences between cultures when it comes to mental illness?[34] But beyond these questions typical of post-Second World War cultural psychiatry, Jakovljević was also influenced

[31] Laurence J. Kirmayer, '50 Years of *Transcultural Psychiatry*', *Transcultural Psychiatry*, 2013, 50:1, 3–5.

[32] Arthur Kleinman, 'Depression, Somatization and the "New Cross-cultural Psychiatry"', *Social Science and Medicine*, 1977, 11.

[33] See, for instance, H.B.M. Murphy et al., 'Crosscultural Inquiry Into the Symptomatology of Depression: A Preliminary Report', *Transcultural Psychiatry*, 1964, 1, 5–18; Ibid., 'A Crosscultural Survey of Schizophrenic Symptomatology', *International Journal of Social Psychiatry*, 1963, 9:4, 237–249.

[34] Jakovljević, 'Kulturna sredina i neuroze', *Medicinski Glasnik*, 1959, 50: 2–2a.

by a long line of psychiatric and psychotherapeutic forays into anthropological and ethnographic research, which questioned whether a universal psychological (or psychoanalytic) self could be assumed and sought to ascertain to what extent it was bound by socio-cultural determinants.[35]

This then was an ambitious and comprehensive project of exploring the role of socio-cultural factors in the onset and understanding of mental illness. In it Jakovljević relied on a variety of scientific and political influences to which he was exposed in order to move beyond the simplistic binaries of complete relativism, on the one hand, and (what he termed) Western 'ethnocentric' universalism, on the other, in evaluating mental normality. This position stood in implicit contrast to psychoanalytic anthropological research such as Geza Roheim's famous interwar explorations of Australian Aborigines, which argued for a universal, global concept of the unconscious.[36] Jakovljević opined that socio-anthropological research in psychiatry should encourage the profession to revise all those theories of pathogenesis which assume 'a universally identical psychogenic content'.[37] Such 'idealist speculation' divorced from careful engagement with social and historical conditions clashed with Jakovljević's Marxist approach, which led him to focus much more carefully and systematically than most of his fellow transcultural psychiatrists on the role of socio-economic and cultural factors in shaping the psychological world of his patients.

As an alternative to relativism or universalism Jakovljević proposed what he termed 'cultural-integrationism', or 'integrationist universalism'. Rather than descending into extreme cultural relativism or Western-centric universalism, Jakovljević proposed that 'it [was] necessary, on the contrary, to study common principles, by synthetically generalising their specific expressions in a particular socio-cultural environment'.[38]

[35] See Sadowsky, *Imperial Bedlam*; Ashis Nandy, *Savage Freud and Other Essays*, Princeton: Princeton University Press, 1995; Stephen Frosh, *For and Against Psychoanalysis*, Abingdon: Routledge, 2006; Roland Littlewood and Maurice Lipsedge, *Aliens and Alienists: Ethnic Minorities and Psychiatry*, Abingdon: Routledge, 1997; Ranjana Khanna, *Dark Continents: Psychoanalysis and Colonialism*, Durham: Duke University Press, 2003.

[36] Joy Damousi, 'Geza Roheim and the Australian Aborigine: Psychoanalytic Anthropology During the Inter-War Years', in Anderson et al., eds, *Unconscious Dominions*, 75–95.

[37] Jakovljević, 'Kulturna Sredina i Neuroze', 50–53.

[38] Jakovljević, 'Transkulturno-psihijatrijska Proucavanja u Gvineji', in *Prilozi za Socijalnu Patologiju*, Belgrade: Sloboda, 1984, 134.

Such common principles should then be built into the foundations of the new field of international psychiatry. This approach recognised the overwhelming importance of specific socio-cultural factors in causing psychiatric disorders in a given social setting. It required a careful assessment of both patients' and therapists' socio-cultural backgrounds and relied on comparative epidemiological and phenomenological analyses to identify those notions in mental pathology, therapy and prophylaxis which might be shared among cultures and civilisations.[39] It was globe-trotting researchers such as Jakovljević himself who offered to resolve the existing tension between 'ethnocentrism and relativism in psychiatric diagnostics'.[40]

In his clinical applications of the cultural-integrationist approach, Jakovljević relied on interpreters to communicate with most of his native patients. Recruited from among local auxiliary medical staff as well as those studying to become psychiatric social workers, these interpreters also helped Jakovljević develop what he called the 'socio-psychiatric' component of patient reports—a detailed exploration of every patient's sociological and environmental surroundings developed through specific questionnaires as well as lengthy interviews with family members and carers. According to Jakovljević's descriptions, the translators were able to provide a more comprehensive socio-cultural interpretation of patients' behaviour and attitudes in addition to the basic linguistic translation of patients' statements. Helpfully, Jakovljević's medically trained interpreters could situate patients' reactions and symptoms in a broader Guinean context and evaluate whether those reactions truly deviated from the Guinean 'norm'. This reflected Jakovljević's insistence on relativistic socio-cultural criteria of normality and abnormality: by consulting his translators in this way, for example, he claimed that he 'avoided any possibility of Euro-American centralism, as well as anarchical relativism'.[41]

Still, in his concern to move away from such 'anarchical relativism', Jakovljević consistently applied the American Psychiatric Association's classification of illnesses and ultimately translated all psychiatric disorders which he encountered in Guinea into 'universal' medical diagnoses developed in the United States—for all his interest in detailed anthropological

[39] Ibid., 170.

[40] Jakovljević, 'Kulturna Sredina i Neuroze', 52.

[41] Jakovljević, *Prilozi za Socijalnu Patologiju*, 130–133.

research and socio-cultural particularities, his Guinean patients, just like his Yugoslav and French patients, were diagnosed with schizophrenia, mania, different forms of neurosis, reactive psychosis and a variety of psychosomatic and sociopathic disorders.[42] According to Jakovljević, 'there existed certain specific manifestation of individual mental disorders, which could be classified within the traditional schemes [only] with some difficulty'. Nonetheless, he concluded that such specificities did not warrant the creation of novel diagnostic categories, as 'in essence [they] belonged to the already existing nosological groups'.[43] Therefore, Jakovljević's own conclusions about mental illness patterns in Guinea had important universalist aspects, and his Marxism did not lead him to question Eurocentric nosologies. But, as we will see below, his universalism was further informed by a sense of socialist solidarity between Eastern Europe and the global South, and by his belief that all societies can be evaluated as progressive or otherwise according to the universal Marxist standards of historical development.[44] This set him apart from most of his Western European colleagues.

Eastern Europe and Guinea

In 1958 Guinea was the only French territory to opt for immediate independence in the September constitutional referendum. All the other parts decided to remain junior partners in a newly formed French Community, defined in the Fifth Republic's recently passed constitution, and accepted the continuation of French tutelage for an indefinite period of time. On the other hand, the Guineans were urged by their national branch of the African Democratic Assembly (*Rassemblement Démocratique Africain*; RDA), an inter-territorial association of political parties in French West Africa and one of the most powerful political forces in the region, to choose a more radical and disruptive path of fully independent

[42] Ibid., 124.

[43] Ibid., 134.

[44] This was perhaps more akin to the early universalist trends in African transcultural psychiatry, such as the school of thought championed by Nigeria's Thomas A. Lambo, who promoted the notion of the 'unity of mankind' when it came to patterns of mental health and disease because he believed that such a platform would help fight racism in European psychiatry (Heaton, *Black Skin, White Coats*).

statehood and socialist transformation.[45] The reasons behind this were many and mainly had to do with the unusually successful national mobilisation strategies of the country's dominant political party and its close links with the broadest sections of its membership. The national RDA, which was to rule Guinea in the coming four decades, was an organisation openly styled after the Communist Party of France, and by 1958 it grew to be largely shaped by its grassroots militant left-wing factions—trade unionists, radical students and youth and women's associations.[46] These resolutely pushed the political leadership towards the left in the months leading up to the 1958 referendum and radicalised the RDA's vision of post-colonial revolutionary politics. This was a startling and potentially promising beginning to Guinea's decolonisation, and the country soon embarked on an exceptionally ambitious programme of modern nation-building and social, cultural and political transformation, allying itself with Soviet, then Chinese communism.

But this auspicious start was ultimately not indicative of the overall success of the national revolution. Guinea's decisive bid for socialism entailed not only a distancing from the French colonial education and ideological value systems but also an assault on what the leadership termed 'primitive' cultural and religious traditions, the controversial 'demystification campaign'. In their attempt to culturally and socially 'rehabilitate' the nation, the Guinean post-colonial leadership aimed to counter 'the intellectual elitism and Eurocentrism bred by colonial schooling' and raise a new generation of nationalist youth by thoroughly transforming their 'historical consciousness, cultural sensibilities, and future aspirations'.[47] This far-reaching concept of reform, modernisation and revolutionisation of mentalities understandably 'triggered multiple, multifaceted disruptions

[45] Elizabeth Schmidt, 'Anticolonial Nationalism in French West Africa: What Made Guinea Unique?', *African Studies Review*, 2009, 52:2, 1–34.

[46] Schmidt, 'Cold War in Guinea: The RDA and the Struggle Over Communism, 1950–1958', *Journal of African History*, 2007, 48:1, 95–121; see also Schmidt, *Mobilizing the Masses: Gender, Ethnicity and Class in the Nationalist Movement in Guinea, 1939–1958*, New Hampshire: Heinemann, 2005, and Schmidt, *Cold War and Decolonization in Guinea, 1946–1958*, Athens: Ohio University Press, 2007; Claude Riviere, *Guinea: The Mobilization of a People*, New York: Ithaca, 1977; Tony Chafer, *The End of Empire in French West Africa: France's Successful Decolonization?*, London: Bloomsbury, 2002.

[47] Straker, Jay, *Youth, Nationalism and the Guinean Revolution*, Bloomington and Indianapolis: Indiana University Press, 2009, 11.

of local life everywhere in Guinea'.[48] Moreover, the enormous disruption was soon accompanied by growing authoritarianism of an increasingly brutal and intolerant RDA regime, whose charismatic leader Ahmed Sékou Touré clamped down on his opponents from the early 1960s on, declaring the beginning of a 'Socialist Cultural Revolution' in 1968 and remaining the uncontested leader of the country until his death in 1984.

For many commentators Guinea's attempted revolution was a prime example of a failed decolonisation, the democratic potential of the late 1950s apparently squandered in the subsequent decades of dictatorship, violence and political and ethnic strife.[49] On the other hand, the radical reforms of the 1960s and 1970s thoroughly transformed the face of Guinean society, and this sweeping change made the country seem like a dynamic laboratory for revolutionary policies and designs. Guinea's experiences of modernisation, urbanisation and dismantling of the old socio-cultural structures might well have resonated with those of experts arriving from Eastern Europe's newly socialist republics. Guinea itself was also attracted to the promise of East European socialist revolutions and developed extensive educational and technical exchanges with the Eastern Bloc in the 1960s. As Mike McGovern has argued, socialist states in Africa often 'had more concrete political and economic links to the socialist countries of Europe and Asia than to some of their neighbours on the African continent'.[50] Yugoslavia's path of non-alignment proved additionally attractive to newly sovereign African states, which hoped to avoid falling under the hegemony of either side in the Cold War. Signifying the importance of Yugoslavia in particular, the face of Josip Broz Tito featured on Guinea's 10,000 silly note.[51]

From Jakovljević's Eastern European perspective, the decolonising world was of notable interest as well. The rapid socio-economic, political and cultural changes involved in both the socialist revolution and post-colonial modern state-building featured very importantly as pathogenic

[48] Ibid., 12.

[49] David Rieff, 'In Defense of Afro-pessimism', *World Policy Journal*, 1998–1999, 15:4, 10–22; Patrick Chabal and Jean-Pascal Daloz, *Africa Works: Disorder as Political Instrument*, Oxford and Bloomington: James Currey and Indiana University Press, 1999; Manthia Diawara, *In Search of Africa*, Cambridge: Harvard University Press, 1998.

[50] Mike McGovern, *Unmasking the State: Making Guinea Modern*, Chicago: University of Chicago Press, 2012, 160.

[51] Ibid., 161.

factors in his interpretations. Even though Jakovljević never explicitly equated Yugoslavia and Guinea, his descriptions of Macedonia's 'primitiveness' corresponded very closely to his analyses of Guinea's core social problems. In that sense, Jakovljević's texts (unintentionally) indicated that, despite its 'Europeanness', Yugoslavia might be eminently comparable to the decolonising world. It is this unspoken similarity between Eastern Europe and Guinea—which leaps off the pages of Jakovljević's writings—that I am now going to explore.

Before his long-standing engagement with Guinea Jakovljević conducted psychiatric epidemiological and sociological research in Macedonia and made comparisons with the mental health situation in Paris. Aiming to apply ethno-psychiatric methodology and theoretical frameworks to the study of the pathogenesis of neuroses, Jakovljević used the research material he collected during his employment in Macedonia: in 1953–1954 alone, for instance, he interviewed over 1,500 neurotic patients at the Skopje neuropsychiatric hospital, and compared the results and statistical information with those he compiled in psychiatric clinics and consulting rooms in Paris in 1956 and 1957.[52]

In his writings on Macedonia Jakovljević regularly set it up against 'civilised countries', noting that the rate of neurotic disorders was much lower in Macedonia—a standard trope of colonial psychiatry which insisted that psychological disease such as neurosis or schizophrenia was a unique characteristic of highly industrialised, urbanised and cultured regions of the world. But Macedonia was also undergoing dramatic transformations, which meant that its rate of psychiatric morbidity was alarmingly on the rise. Focusing on the 'primitive' and 'underdeveloped' regions of Yugoslavia, Jakovljević delineated the core socio-psychological characteristics of this 'primitive mentality:' 'totemistic beliefs and appropriate rituals all the way to exorcism;... extreme patriarchy in families; open aggression in the form of blood vengeance; buying of women who are evaluated as merchandise', and a 'marked submissiveness of women', etc. Moreover, Macedonia was reportedly characterised by 'extremely archaic' social structures, which exhibited 'exceptional forms of socio-psychological backwardness;'[53] this resulted in an 'exceptionally levelled

[52] Jakovljević, 'Doprinos Proucavanju Uloge Psiholoskih Uticaja Sociokulturne Sredine u Patogenezi Neuroza', *Neuropsihijatrija*, 1959, 7:1–2, 41–42.

[53] Jakovljević, 'Prilog Proucavanju Neurotickih Poremecaja', 62–63.

collective psyche' that defied and precluded the process individuation or the formation of richer forms of internal life.[54] Especially among the Muslim population, psychiatric research identified further symptoms of severe underdevelopment: 'extreme fatalism and even more developed primitive beliefs', 'propensity to sexual deviations', a 'great rigidity of personalities', as well as a tendency to assign mystical causality to a long list of life events and to resort to magic acts, protective amulets or 'bizarre medications of archaic or religious origin'.[55]

Jakovljević's descriptions of cultural, ethnographic and anthropological aspects of post-colonial Guinean society relied on the same set of terms and concepts: in the African country's primary and secondary social institutions, Jakovljević identified a similar combination of 'primitivism', 'hierarchy', 'patriarchy' and 'archaic' relations, and he particularly emphasised the remarkably unequal position of women and youth in traditional settings. Just as in the south of the Balkans, he wrote, most Guineans' 'life is still full of magical rituals, with an almost universal application of magic for the purposes of attack and defence'. Moreover, in Guinea 'one believes that the world constitutes a certain vitalistic unity, inhabited by a variety of supernatural and natural creatures'; the 'fatalistic actions' of these beings explain the course of all events and history.[56] For these reasons, prayers, sacrificial rituals, amulets and invocations of magical powers appeared to be the core strategies for surviving life's calamities.

However, the largest number of socially conditioned psychological disorders stemmed from a 'dynamic process of abrupt changes of one social environment'—a condition equally applicable, as it transpired, to Macedonia/Yugoslavia and Guinea/the decolonising world. In the more developed parts of Macedonia, a 'patriarchal-oriental' lifestyle and mentality gradually became entangled with more modern, Western European influences, and this profoundly reshaped the collective psyche of the region. The process of change which triggered the largest proportion of psychiatric disorders had to do with industrialisation, modernisation and urbanisation, as well as the implementation of some of the core

[54] Jakovljević, 'Doprinos Proucavanju Uloge Psiholoskih Uticaja Socio-kulturne Sredine u Patogenezi Neuroza', 42.

[55] Jakovljević, 'Utjecaj Kulturno-socijalne Sredine na Psihopatiku Sizofrenih Stanja', *Neuropsihijatrija*, 1957, 5:2, 143.

[56] Jakovljević, 'Transkulturno-psihijatrijska Proucavanja u Gvineji: Preliminarno Saopstenje', *Neuropsihijatrija*, 1963, 11:1, 24.

principles of the socialist revolution, such as workers' rights and gender equality. In all these respects Macedonia emerged as surprisingly akin to Guinea and other sub-Saharan African countries, despite their dramatically different historical, political and cultural contexts. In the Macedonian case, this process denoted 'a change of lifestyle from simple and primitive ... to complex and cultured; ... a change of belief system from a mystic-causal to a rational-causal type', as well as a move towards more abstract thinking and linguistic structures and radical transformations of large, 'backward' and highly hierarchical families.[57] In 1960s Guinea, similarly, the dramatic transformations of the post-colonial era were primarily marked by 'a completely serious cultural emancipation, which is implemented both through education and through political propaganda', as well as by 'mechanisation, industrialisation and socialisation [implementation of certain socialist organisational principles], which results in the sudden migration to cities and change in occupations and lifestyles'.[58] The 'rural exodus' plagued the collective mental health of Guineans, but it was a price that needed to be paid for social, cultural, economic and political progress. In the African context the most common social conflicts reportedly concerned gender and age divisions, as 'women and youth were in the process of obtaining an increasing list of legal rights, which men and the elders did not want to grant them without resistance'.[59]

Moreover, by far the harshest and most universal forms of interpersonal conflict Jakovljević observed were between those 'faithful to the traditional norms and those willing to abandon them'. But the very process of 'civilisation' was troubled and uneven, so that 'the new was permanently pregnant with the old', and those who started undergoing modernisation or 'Westernisation' were often quite torn between different aspects of their personality: a civilised person would be rather polarised in all their activities—'superficially Westernised but intimately traditional, superficially rational but intimately irrational, superficially controlled but fundamentally impulsive'.[60] According to Jakovljević, 'new layers of

[57] Ibid., 75.

[58] Jakovljević, *Prilozi za Socijalnu Patologiju*, 106.

[59] Ibid., 121.

[60] Ibid., 176. Interestingly, Ksenija Kondic used almost identical language to talk about Yugoslav socialist families caught up in the broader dynamics of social transformations and modernisation: 'Both parents, both spouses carry within themselves from their primary (mostly patriarchal) families a lot of old, patriarchal [traits and beliefs], which have been

Western culture [were] successfully grafted onto these primitive layers, so that in the cities they usually co-exist[ed] or [were] indeed deeply interrelated, and only [got] separated in illness'.[61] Such polarisation led to a large number of psychological breakdowns whose roots were in this bifurcated 'pseudo-European' and African existence, the result of forcing ancient systems into novel, modernised conditions. In fact, in his recent anthropological study of the Demystification programme, McGovern has argued, along similar lines, that the most violent aspects of the Guinean state's assault on polytheistic religious traditions signalled a pervasive 'modernist anxiety' and the modernisers' deep-seated psychological need to 'purge' the lingering backwardness and primitivism from themselves. This fundamental uncertainty about the nation's ability to become and remain modern, according to McGovern, drove Sékou Touré's brutal campaign to 'eradicate the embarrassing residue of pre-modern backwardness from the body politic'.[62] Jakovljević could, of course, recognise such problems and complications in his own rapidly modernising home country.

However, such comparisons or parallels were never stated in an explicit manner. But the language which Jakovljević used to describe the cultural and psychiatric situation in both Macedonia and Guinea/African countries in general was extremely similar and betrayed a set of assumptions which Jakovljević might have been hard pressed to fully support openly. Throughout his comparative studies, he tended to reiterate that 'European cultures'—including Yugoslavia and France as his clinical case studies—presented a very different 'configuration/layout of structure of specific mental disorders'; moreover, Yugoslavia in particular had a much higher frequency of mental disorders than Guinea or Africa as a whole, which placed her firmly in the camp of developed, Western countries

woven into their personalities in their formative years, but which is often incompatible with the contemporary, new, modern norms' (Kondic, *Povezanost decjih neuroticnih smetnji sa strukturom licnosti odnosno patologijom roditelja*, 12). This example further demonstrates how the dominant socialist psychiatric discourse in Yugoslavia placed East European and African societies, as well as the challenges they faced in the course of modernisation and revolutionary changes, within the same analytic framework, even when parallels were not drawn directly nor explicitly.

[61] Ibid., 24–25.

[62] McGovern, *Unmasking the State*, 20.

(such as, for instance, the United States or United Kingdom).[63] As he claimed in his comparative study of neuroses, both Macedonia and France 'originated from the same archaic family' and had experienced similar historical events and influences, which explained a basic similarity and comparability of certain formative social institutions. At the same time, however, even though Yugoslavia was not an 'archaic' society such as, say, Guinea, its specific historical development still set it radically apart from the French case, producing very dissimilar forms of cultural identity and secondary social institutions.[64] This constantly shifting political and cultural image of the author's home country was in fact quite telling of the complex position Yugoslavia inhabited on the international scene: its political alliances were as complex as its (apparent) psychiatric identity, and it was at different times comparable to a variety of very different states and cultures, from Africa, to Central and Western Europe.

Colonial Psychiatry and Its Legacies

This confusing state of affairs was further complicated by Jakovljević's tendency to quote and ally himself with both Western colonial psychiatrists such as John Colin Carothers and prominent anti-colonial and post-colonial psychiatric experts such as Lambo. This was in large measure a product of the complex and intellectual incoherent nature of transcultural psychiatry as a field: these internal tensions marked the development of post-Second World War global psychiatric clinical and research practice, and they are of central importance to understanding Jakovljević's own contradictory conclusions and intellectual legacies. In that sense, Jakovljević's perception of Guinea's position on the international scale of civilisations was extremely ambiguous: while he emphasised the relevance of African research for understanding the effects of dramatic social shifts in Eastern Europe, he also accepted, relatively uncritically, an openly colonial binary of civilised Europe versus primitive Africa. In this latter constellation, the Yugoslav lands, despite their socialist reorientation, belonged firmly to the European family of nations and cultures, which

[63] Ibid., 177.

[64] Jakovljević, 'Doprinos Proucavanju Uloge Psiholoskih Uticaja Socio-kulturne Sredine u Patogenezi Neuroza', 51.

was reportedly characterised by a significantly different structure and phenomenology of mental illness.

This was a longstanding phenomenon: from well before the Second World War, Yugoslav psychiatrists for the most part adopted the terminology of Western colonial psychiatry in the domestic context and regularly referred to local mental health patients as 'primitive' and 'uncivilised'. The growing literature on the history of colonial psychiatry thus might be useful for illuminating the nature of the relationship between psychiatrists and their patients of very different social and educational backgrounds in the Yugoslav context. The historiography of colonial psychiatry described the complex and potentially explosive encounters between the West European psychiatric elite, with their modernising and 'civilising' agendas, and local patients, who challenged the tropes and classificatory systems of European medicine and brought with them a set of traditional beliefs and explanations. Such a clash of paradigms turned clinics into sites of fierce contestation: 'psychiatrists and patients engaged in a protracted argument about incompatible approaches to illness'.[65] According to Richard Keller's description of the French Algiers school of psychiatry, the psychiatrists were regularly baffled by patients who presented 'diffuse complaints' and were 'unable to translate their experience of illness into a comprehensible symptomatology'.[66] This description is reminiscent of the attitudes and diagnostic behaviour of Yugoslav psychiatrists, who, while sharing a cultural and ethnic background as well as a native language with their patients, were prone to pathologise ineloquence and unfamiliarity with medical paradigms. Moreover, colonial patients often understood their own mental anguish in the context of traditional and magic beliefs, while their psychiatrists tended to treat the allegiance to such notions as a symptom of pathological mental deterioration; in a similar vein, the lack of education, literacy or Western hygienic habits tended to mark entire societies as more likely to develop forms of insanity in the European psychiatrists' worldview.

In this sense, commonalities with the Yugoslav case are striking and instructive, and they might be explained by reference to a civilising mission of sorts which the Western-educated Yugoslav psychiatrists shared with their colonial counterparts in the first half of the twentieth century.

[65] Keller, *Colonial Madness*, 87.

[66] Ibid., 110.

Working in a slowly (and painfully) modernising yet predominantly agricultural country, interwar Yugoslav mental health professionals entertained glorious ideas of their important social and political role. Keller's note that, in their own minds, 'colonial psychiatrists occupied the front lines in a struggle between Western biomedicine and what they considered to be superstitious tradition',[67] could be applied to the Yugoslav psychiatric profession with very little qualification. In fact, Yugoslav medical practitioners as a whole seemed to wage an all-out war against the rural population's conceptions of health, illness and hygiene.[68] Yugoslav psychiatrists, trained in Western Europe and deeply involved in broader European professional networks, thus likely had more in common with French or German doctors than with their illiterate peasant patients.[69]

Some of that intellectual affiliation certainly survived the revolution of 1945, and the literature produced by West European colonial psychiatrists formed a very important part of Jakovljević's own bibliography. Within the context of Yugoslavia's own project of socialist modernisation and urbanisation, there was no dramatic change in psychiatrists' conceptions of their 'civilising mission' in a largely under-educated and rural country. In fact, under socialism the task of turning the existing population into a collective of much more progressive, modernised, forward-looking Marxist citizens was more pressing than ever, and Jakovljević and his colleagues constantly referred to the prominent role of psychiatrists in

[67] Ibid., 119.

[68] In the countryside as well as in recently urbanized areas, moreover, fortune-tellers emerged as the psychiatric profession's rivals of sorts for popular attention and trust. They offered alternative, supernatural interpretations of psychological malaise, provided specific advice for resolving mental problems and even served as a particular kind of psychotherapists, in the context in which no psychotherapy was practiced in hospitals. Consequently, since the late nineteenth century, the state attempted to eliminate or at least restrict and control their practice, but those efforts proved largely unsuccessful.

[69] Foreign visitors to Yugoslavia and Belgrade in the 1920s and 1930s regularly noted particularly strong conflicts and contradictions between traditional and modern (Western) forms of life, the extreme conservatism and poverty of the countryside which clashed with internationalist currents and Westernized mass culture of large cities, so that "East and West created a specific mix, and one felt with certainty the existence of a gap...There is nothing that could bridge it, and one is constantly afraid of suddenly falling into a hole" (Marie-Janine Calic, *Sozialgeschichte Serbiens 1815 – 1941: Der Aufhaltsame Fortschritt wahrend der Industrialisierung*, Munich: R. Oldenbourg Verlag, 1994, 120). Psychiatric hospitals well represented the nature and implications of this "unbridgeable" gap.

effecting these major social, cultural and psychological changes. As Jakovljević noted in relation to the rapid socialist transformation of Yugoslav families, the transition from 'primitive', more diffuse type of families to much narrower, nuclear families characteristic of 'civilised societies' was at the core of the social changes of the postwar period, and the psychiatric profession had a foremost duty to alleviate the psychological toll of this dramatic move.[70] In that sense, Yugoslav psychiatrists could be both colonial-minded and extremely critical of colonial legacies, and this became particularly pronounced when they actually travelled to and engaged with the former colonies.

In the context of socialist societies in Eastern Europe, moreover, the idea of modernising and civilising backward cultures and peoples was not uncommon. As Bruce Grant noted in connection with the Soviet political attitude towards the indigenous populations of Siberia, the political project of building communism and communist consciousness in the entire country inevitably entailed the speeding up of the cultural development of those peoples who were not advanced enough on the Marxist historical scale. For the Soviet authorities and ideologies this meant that the core goal of socialist development was to quickly move these people and areas from 'tradition' to 'modernity', to accomplish a 'heroic leap from primitive-communal society to socialism'.[71] At the same time, however, Grant argues, the dominant perception of the Siberian peoples in Russian consciousness remained largely unchanged: they were primitive, 'untamed' and wild, unintegrated in the broader Soviet society despite the state's monumental effort. In the final analysis, the socialist state's extreme paternalism likely aided the persistence of that image of backwardness and primitivism. In the African context as well, 'scientific socialism... insisted upon a single path to modernity. Although socialism identified problems of exploitation within European modernity, it did not hesitate to treat non-European societies with Eurocentric disdain'.[72] In fact, socialist Yugoslav intellectuals, political commentators and Party functionaries often wrote very affirmatively about the

[70] Jakovljević, *Neuravnotezena porodica*, Belgrade: Centar za obavestavanje roditelja, 1961, 4.

[71] Bruce Grant, 'Siberia Hot and Cold: Reconstructing the Image of Siberian Indigenous Peoples', in Galya Diment and Yuri Slezkine, eds, *Between Heaven and Hell: The Myth of Siberia in Russian Culture*, New York: St. Martin's Press, 1992, 227–228.

[72] Mcgovern, *Unmasking the State*, 19.

progress of socialism in Africa (singling out Ghana and Guinea as particularly successful examples), but their analyses regularly focused on the 'insufficient maturity' of particular African societies to fully adopt and implement socialist ideas and institutions. This reported immaturity, a concept integral to linear models of social and political development, was characterised by a variety of marks of economic and political underdevelopment and lagging behind, including an 'unusually low' level of culture and civilisation.[73] As curator of Belgrade's Museum of African Art Dejan Sretenović noted in his analysis of images of Africa and NAM in Yugoslavia, African partners were seen as a 'younger brother' who needed to be helped and led 'on his path of socialism', having changed from 'leopard skins [to] worker overalls'.[74] The Marxist and Western colonial ideas of the 'primitive' thus coexisted and overlapped in the socialist world. East European medical doctors' perception of their own domestic patient populations as primitive or unmodern shaped their understanding of both the decolonising world and Western colonial medical/psychiatric discourses.

The Problem of a 'Primitive' Patient

As we saw in the Chapter 2, there was a significant linguistic confusion in the dominant psychiatric discourse regarding the exact connotation of the concept of 'primitivism'. Yugoslav socialist psychiatrists, and practitioners such as Jakovljević in particular, tended to conflate different meanings of the word, and rarely reflected on the fact that the same notion could be used to refer to both 'uncultured' Europeans (and Yugoslavs) and 'pre-modern' African tribes. In that sense, Jakovljević's clinical and anthropological observations about Guinea were directly relevant to his Yugoslav colleagues' everyday practice. Many psychiatrists' stance towards the majority of their patients in Yugoslavia tended to be rather ambivalent, as their 'primitivism' and 'backwardness' apparently complicated the application and ultimate success of analytic interpretive therapeutic frameworks. At the same time, the psychiatric profession considered its 'civilisational' struggle against 'backwardness' to be its most

[73] Branimir Banovic, 'Crna Afrika i socijalizam', *Nase Teme*, September 1964, 8:9, 1461–1481.

[74] Dejan Sretenovic, *Crno telo, bele maske*, Belgrade: Museum of African Art, 2004, 26.

important ambition, and a vital aspect of its contribution to raising a new generation of revolutionary citizens. As we saw in Chapter 3, the question of whether and under what circumstances such primitivism could be overcome informed the majority of postwar professional debates in Yugoslavia.[75]

The issue of social and cultural 'primitivism', and its effects on psychiatric practice, thus loomed large in the minds of Jakovljević and his colleagues, and this domestic concern crucially affected Jakovljević's own explorations of a different (but not too different) kind of 'backwardness' in Guinea. Still, in Jakovljević's own worldview, the terms did get redefined to a significant extent. Unlike in the prewar psychiatric jargon, the concept of primitivism employed by postwar socialist psychiatry was imbued with expectations of progress and the overcoming of backwardness. At the same time, Paris—Jakovljević's symbol for civilisation and cultural sophistication—demonstrated clear signs of degeneration and decay, so that the very terms 'primitivism' and 'civilisation' assumed somewhat altered meanings. As Jakovljević concluded, Macedonia constituted a simpler environment 'which was radically advancing' and which had a predominantly negative attitude towards complex neurosis. On the other hand, France, an incomparably more complex social and cultural setting 'which was in the process of destructuring', tended to have a peculiar appreciation for neuroticism, so that a patient 'could easily achieve a certain provisory, abnormal balance, not attacked by his social milieu'.[76]

As discussed above, while modernisation necessarily carried with it a sharp increase in psychological suffering and disorder, it was not a failed mission: even 'primitive' African inhabitants could adapt to a more technically and culturally advanced surrounding. The pessimism and biological determinism of the pre-socialist years were gone, and the new trends and assumptions in Jakovljević's rendering of transcultural psychiatry predicted ultimately positive outcomes of the momentous social and political transformations of both sub-Saharan Africa and the socialist bloc. Writing of Guinea's ever fluctuating social makeup, he observed that 'it became clear that inherited phylogenetic cultural models do not necessarily repeat themselves in the course of development, but are always

[75] Vladislav Klajn, 'Problem Rehabilitacije – Rehabilitacija Neuroticara', *VSP*, 1958, 7:8, 529–531; Klajn, *Razvoj Psihoanalize u Srbiji*, 78–83.

[76] Jakovljević, 'Prilog Proucavanju Neurotickih Poremecaja', 80–81.

learnt and, in the course of that learning, can always be changed'.[77] This clearly boded well for the Yugoslav socialist development too, and perhaps even echoed Yugoslav psychiatrists' experiences with 'partisan hysteria', when 'primitive' peasant soldiers underwent temporary bouts of neurosis following the end of the war but were then successfully integrated in a modernising socialist society.[78]

Since cultural patterns and dispositions were so malleable and dependent on socio-cultural environment and political and economic structures, Jakovljević could not draw a straightforward line between 'primitive' civilisations and the 'childhood stage of humanity'—a common trope not only in twentieth-century Western psychiatry, but also in more progressive psychoanalytic and anthropological discourses, which saw the 'savages' of the non-white world as fascinating snapshots of humanity as it was before the onset of 'civilisation'. As Freud's close associate and biographer Ernest Jones noted, 'it is possible that the conscious thinking of savages is more directly and extensively influenced by unconscious factors than is that of civilised people, just as is so with the child'.[79] In contrast, Jakovljević criticised the 'infantilism thesis'. Even though he admitted that 'primitive adults' of Guinea shared certain mental traits with children from the civilised world, differences were equally if not more important.[80] As we saw in Chapter 2, Marxist psychiatry and psychoanalysis—although they assumed that progress was unidirectional and that Guinea had to 'catch up'—could hardly view African civilisations in a static manner within the evolutionary context, but instead argued that cultures and societies could, under propitious circumstances, make revolutionary leaps in their own development and progress: 'our experiences have clearly demonstrated that a primitive personality, who is young and capable enough, can successfully integrate in a technically and culturally developed environment, even though that integration might be accompanied by temporary mental disorders'.[81] In that sense, despite being heavily influenced by Western European psychoanalytic thinking, Jakovljević distanced himself

[77] Jakovljević, *Prilozi za Socijalnu Patologiju*, 167.

[78] See Antic, 'Heroes and Hysterics: "Partisan Hysteria" and Communist State-Building in Yugoslavia After 1945', *Social History of Medicine*, 2014, 27:2, 349–371.

[79] Quoted in Damousi, 'Geza Roheim', 75–95.

[80] Jakovljević, *Prilozi za Socijalnu Patologiju*, 142.

[81] Ibid., 167.

from those transcultural psychoanalytic and psychiatric discourses which saw the 'contemporary "primitive" as a version of the early stages of human society' who could consequently have no history.[82]

Outside psychiatric discussions, socialist Yugoslavia saw similar contestations of the thesis that African cultures were static, inferior and incapable of development. In 1961, for instance, reporting from the first congress of black writers and artists in 1956 Paris, renowned Yugoslav linguist Petar Guberina objected vehemently to some 'European researchers of Africa', who viewed it as a 'civilisation of a lower type', a 'static phenomenon of eternal traditions and exoticism', and a 'museum exhibit.' He drew attention to Western ethnographers' common mistake of seeing African cultures solely 'horizontally, at the moment when colonialism destroyed their creative development'. Guberina, on the other hand, wrote of African cultural production as a 'great human civilisation' in the pre-colonial times, and as dynamic and exceptionally adaptable, managing to thrive even in the most oppressive circumstances of slavery, colonisation and broader societal oppression. In discussing the work and performances of Guinea's national dance company *Compagnie des Ballets Africains* at the Paris congress, he emphasised their extraordinary capacity to combine modern and traditional elements, and thereby to express the rapid development and progress of the Guinean society. African societies were, therefore, not static, underdeveloped and trapped in a lower stage of civilisational progress, but were comparable to any other cultures in their ability to give and receive, modernise and develop while remaining authentic.[83] In other domains as well, African societies tended to be portrayed as eminently capable of modernity and modernisation, and perfectly adept at organising their own political, economic and social life, and administering its own populations.[84]

In the same vein, Jakovljević complicated the standard narrative regarding psychiatric epidemiologies in the non-Western world. On the one hand, he subscribed to the thesis that the overall frequency of

[82] Khanna, *Dark Continents*, 6.

[83] Petar Guberina, 'Tragom africke crnacke kulture', *Nase Teme*, 'Suvremena Afrika', July 1961, 5:7, 985–1019.

[84] See Radina Vucetic, 'We Shall Win: Yugoslav Film Cooperation with FRELIMO', *Revista de Ciencias Sociais*, 2019, 118, 131–150.

mental disorders was lower in Guinea than in the 'civilised' world—Jakovljević's statistics on Guinea's psychiatric morbidity broadly corresponded to the figures Carothers identified in Kenya.[85] However, he still insisted that 'even underdeveloped countries could see relatively high numbers of mental disturbances' and that 'there existed highly complex psychopathologies even among the most backward sections of the [Guinean] population'.[86] British imperial psychiatrists and psychoanalysts often assumed that lower rates of mental illness meant that 'Africans and Asians were incapable of examining their feelings' or did not have 'a distinct personality', but instead '[shared] a communal mind attuned to the elementary collective consciousness of his tribe'.[87] However, Jakovljević concluded that it was not the assumed inherent and unchangeable simplicity of the mind that predetermined the status of mental health or illness in the African world; it was a complex web of social, political and cultural circumstances.[88] In fact, 'the complexity or otherwise of abnormal mental structures depended primarily on the nature and composition of the corresponding social institutions, and not on the level of civilisation, as it is commonly assumed', and Jakovljević argued that even 'primitive' cultures could often develop highly intricate sets of social relations.[89]

This was not merely an ideological distancing from the core tenets of Western European colonial psychiatry and colonially minded transcultural psychiatric concepts but also an attempt to reinterpret the long-standing and rather influential Freudian tradition of '[transposing] the racial assumptions of the cultural evolutionary scale onto the modern psyche'.[90] Jakovljević's attempt at a Marxist re-interpretation of the West African subjectivity was thus crucially informed by his consideration of the position and developmental potential of socialist Eastern Europe on the global civilisational scale, and we can speculate that it was this cultural, geographical and ideological displacement of Jakovljević himself

85 See Carothers, 'A Study of Mental Derangement in Africans', 142–166.

86 Jakovljević, *Prilozi za Socijalnu Patologiju*, 162.

87 Littlewood and Lipsedge, *Aliens and Alienists*, 66–67.

88 Jakovljević., *Prilozi za Socijalnu Patologiju*, 168.

89 Ibid., 166.

90 Celia Brickman, *Aboriginal Populations in the Mind: Race and Primitivity in Psychoanalysis*, New York: Columbia University Press, 2003.

as a Yugoslav psychiatrist in the 1960s that determined his distinctive take on the concept of primitivism in the context of post-Second World War international psychiatry.

'Revolutionary Personality'

Jakovljević's distancing from some important aspects of Freudian psychoanalysis spread to other areas of his work as well. In his discussions of the definition of pathology and normality in different cultural contexts, Jakovljević criticised exclusively psychological interpretations of mental disorders, which he thought disregarded the revolutionary potential of conflicts between individuals and their social environment: 'socially caused conflicts might constitute a progressive factor in the development of a society' and lead to revolutionary resistance against the social organisation or structure.[91] This was a new platform for Marxist psychiatry and psychoanalysis, and it radically redefined the role of social conflict in causing mental illness. While a discord or conflict between an individual and her social environment (which traditional psychoanalysis tended to see as the core origins of neurotic disorders) might lead to mental pathology and personality deviation, pathological or pathogenic sociocultural factors did not necessarily cause psychological disorders, if a robust individual in an 'abnormal' society found ways to overcome or affect the existing circumstances. Quite to the contrary, a 'conformist adaptation of an individual to an abnormal social environment might lead to an even more fundamental form of [psychological] abnormality'. In that sense, what Jakovljević defined as a 'non-conformist' personality was a phenomenon critically different from a mentally ill individual, although it did emerge from a similar structural setting. In fact, the natural conclusion of such reasoning was that the 'non-conformist personality' was the healthiest type of individual in any reactionary or 'anachronistic' society. Jakovljević articulated his theory of revolutionary personality following his work in Guinea but based it on his research findings in both Africa and Yugoslavia. This is where universalism came to inform Jakovljević's conception of comparative psychiatry: in order to evaluate the existence and intensity of mental disorder in a particular culture or society, it was not enough to consider conflicts between individuals and broader

[91] Jakovljević, 'Prilog Proucavanju Neurotickih Poremecaja', 76.

structures; those very structures, environments and socio-political values needed to be assessed against a set of universal, 'objective' standards, which would mark them as progressive or otherwise.

Mental pathology developed if individuals clashed with the norms of a progressive society, but if a similar conflict occurred in a reactionary setting, it was not necessarily a sign of an abnormal personality. If the person in question could not adapt to the anachronistic or 'decadent' demands of a non-progressive social environment, they could be seen as abnormal only if such conflicts were destructive, rather than constructive or progressive in a revolutionary sense. In fact, such intra-psychic conflicts need not lead to mental illness at all, and might even result in the 'growth of personality and society, which happens precisely as a consequence of ever more complex internal conflicts and new solutions built into that society by the personality [in question]'. At the same time, 'absolute social adaptation to anachronistic and obsolete forms of sociability would necessarily impoverish and alienate the individual', and possibly push them into difficult neurotic disorders.[92]

It was in this context of non-conformist and revolutionary personalities that Jakovljević implicitly recognised one of the strongest connections between Eastern European and Guinean/African experiences of dramatic social change. While revolutionary activity in wartime and postwar Yugoslavia established the foundations of the new state and was celebrated at every political, social and cultural level, Guinea had undergone comparable political experiences, primarily in the course of its recent decolonisation struggle which produced different forms of anti-colonial cultural and political expressions. According to Jakovljević, this clearly demonstrated that 'pathogenic' social and political situations were not necessarily destructive because not all individuals would be broken by such potentially psychologically destabilising circumstances. To the contrary, certain personalities might be 'stimulated [by such illness-inducing settings] to develop creatively new forms of reacting (such as the creation of novel political forms in the context of fighting colonialism instead of conformist subordination)'.[93] The creative potential embedded in social and political conflicts in certain types of societies, therefore, allowed both Yugoslavia and Guinea to turn possible psychological disorders into productive and

[92] Jakovljević, 'Prilog Proucavanju Neurotickih Poremecaja', 76–77.

[93] Jakovljević, *Prilozi za Socijalnu Patologiju*, 163.

progressive political behaviour, which fundamentally marked the profiles of both countries regardless of their dramatically different circumstances. It was in this theory of revolutionary personality and its complex relationship to mental illness that the original contribution of Yugoslavia's postwar Marxist psychiatry lay, and the comparative anthropological, ethnographic and psychiatric research conducted by Jakovljević and his associates in Guinea and Europe played a crucial role in the development of this thesis. The experience of Guinean decolonisation confirmed Jakovljević's conclusions drawn from Yugoslavia's and Eastern Europe's recent socialist revolutionary past. Moreover, it allowed the Yugoslav psychiatrist to generalise his Marxist-informed tenets regarding the role of social conflict in causing mental illness and to combine his transcultural research goals with politically salient explorations of the psychological impact of revolutionary environment or activity.

'New Cross-Cultural Psychiatry' in the Socialist World

In 1977, Arthur Kleinman famously critiqued what he saw as the universalising and Eurocentric trends in transcultural psychiatry, which threatened to consign to marginality and irrelevance any local cultural differences in how mental distress was experienced and understood around the world. As new global psychiatric nosologies were being developed, based largely on Western categories and definitions, Kleinman called for the creation of a new cross-cultural psychiatry: he pointed out that there were many conceptual problems and inconsistencies in what he referred to as 'old transcultural psychiatry', which 'involved a breathless search through large amounts of data from different societies looking for "universals."'[94] Kleinman argued for a much larger role for anthropology in cross-cultural research of mental illness, insisting that 'culture' was not merely a force that shaped how a universal psychiatric disease was expressed but that cultural contexts were absolutely central to understanding how any idea of mental illness was even conceived. As a result, Kleinman and his followers warned against transcultural psychiatry's employment of Western-developed and -influenced cultural

[94] Arthur Kleinman, 'Depression, Somatization and the New Cross-Cultural Psychiatry', *Social Science and Medicine*, 1977, 11:1, 1977, 3–10.

models of illness to the exclusion of anthropological and phenomenological accounts, urging their colleagues in transcultural psychiatry to try and understand mental illnesses in the terms of their patients' culture instead of focusing on supposedly universally applicable 'disease entities'.[95]

It was these disease entities which came under heavy scrutiny following Kleinman's programmatic article. 'Old transcultural psychiatry' assumed that Western psychiatric categories were culture-free rather than products of a highly culturally specific West European epistemology, and acknowledged local cultural contexts and meanings solely in order to ascertain to what extent they fit with these categories or departed from them. On the other hand, this new generation of researchers 'advocated a radical "process of changing theoretical and methodological paradigms" in order to develop an approach which would take into account the local meanings of any pattern together with a wide range of related behaviours before attempting any comparisons across societies'.[96] The theoretical and methodological frameworks of the 'new cross-cultural psychiatry certainly challenged some of Jakovljević's own universalising and Eurocentric assumptions, despite his own critical departures from many tenets of mainstream global transcultural psychiatry. Two decades after Jakovljević's Guinean pursuits, Eastern Europe saw another Yugoslav psychiatrist who responded to the changing international trends in transcultural psychiatry, and aimed to integrate Kleinman's and others' core principles in his own research in the global South territories. In the process, he departed from some of Jakovljević's important assumptions, but also intervened in global debates from an original scholarly and cultural position.

Throughout the 1980s, Časlav Hadzi-Nikolić visited a number of indigenous communities in the Andes and in the Amazon rainforest in order to attempt to explore their concepts and experiences of shamanism, their shaman-led rituals (used for therapeutic purposes), and their notions of the relationship between humans, nature and the universe. Unlike Jakovljević the objective clinical researcher, Hadzi-Nikolic sought to attain full membership of these groups in order to be able to experience and understand their symbolic and cultural universes 'from the inside':

[95] Jatinder Bains, 'Race, Culture and Psychiatry: A History of Transcultural Psychiatry', *Transcultural Psychiatry*, 2005, 16:2, 139–154.

[96] Roland Littlewood, 'From Categories to Contexts: A Decade of the "New Cross-Cultural Psychiatry"', *British Journal of Psychiatry*, 1990, 156, 308–327.

he joined rather than observed the shamanistic ceremonies, used hallucinogenic substances as any other participant, and reportedly experienced feelings of deep solidarity and understanding with the communities he was researching. According to his own testimony, what he encountered amounted to a 'highly refined therapeutic system whose importance and dimensions we could only begin to understand'. Moreover, this system held truths and realisations which 'the West was only now discovering, while these peoples have known them for thousands of years'. Because of that—and in contradistinction to Jakovljević, who still functioned within the parameters of 'primitivism' and civilisation—Hadzi-Nikolic concluded that both "primitive peoples" and "primitive cultures" were Western constructions created out of ignorance or malice'.[97] Hadzi Nikolić's writings were thus part of the explicitly anthropological and relativist turn in global cross-cultural psychiatry—proponents of this new approach aimed not to translate different conceptualisations of mental illness and healing in exclusively Western psychiatric terms—but he went farther than most of his colleagues in his critique of the role of Western systems of knowledge. His criticism also led him to rather disturbing conclusions regarding the prospects and benefits of cross-cultural contact and mutual understanding.

Even though Jakovljević adopted a linear model of progress and modernisation, in many ways, as we already saw, his was an optimistic cross-cultural psychiatry. Although he emphasised the psychopathological potentials of modernisation, social transformation and Westernisation, his concept of revolutionary personality and his focus on sociological rather than exclusively cultural explanations of mental distress enabled him to conclude that rapid social change did not need to be disastrously disruptive, and that even 'primitive' personalities could adjust and advance rather quickly and successfully in a revolutionary situation. Jakovljević's take, therefore, on the possibility and limitations of constructive cross-cultural exchange and communication was overall positive—as he observed in both Yugoslavia and Guinea, such cross-cultural contacts could lead to productive situations and social and political progress. But by the 1980s, such optimistic beliefs in the power of progress and social change were seriously shaken globally as well as within the socialist

[97] Hadzi-Nikolic, *Kad se vidi ono sto se ne vidi*, 7.

world. Hadzi-Nikolic professed his utmost admiration for the sophisticated cultural and therapeutic principles of the Andean and Amazonian peoples, but he also concluded that their cultures were incompatible with 'ours'—and that any contact with the materially (but not spiritually) superior Western civilisation only impoverished these indigenous systems of knowledge and beliefs. Ironically, then, a deeper anthropological and phenomenological understanding of non-Western cultures within the context of 'new cross-cultural psychiatry' led to a much more pessimistic view of the possibility of transcultural contact and communication.[98]

Hadzi-Nikolic thus addressed directly the issue of transculturation and deculturation of native peoples across the non-European world—one of the most important themes in both colonial and post-colonial psychiatry[99]—and even though his geographical area of research was not part of the same wave of decolonisation as Africa and Asia, it was clear that he viewed the Westernisation of South American territories in the same context of aggressive European colonisation and imperial rule, and compared their experiences explicitly with those of other parts of the decolonising world such as India or Nigeria. For Hadzi-Nikolic, an 'encounter between members of a native culture with another, more efficient, more equipped and more armed civilisation represented in fact a demise of their own culture'. The purpose of native shaman rituals changed radically in the context of Westernisation. While, before the encounter with European religious traditions, shamanistic therapeutic rituals served to find 'an individual's place in a larger cosmic scheme, and to establish a connection between individuals and their theogonic and cosmogonic principle', following the Westernising influences and the introduction of a different God, 'the possibility of synthesis with divine powers was lost'. Now, the purpose of therapeutic rituals was not to realise a harmonious integration with the Universe, but simply to aid suffering acculturated individuals in resolving specific conflicts which

[98] It remained unclear whether Hadzi-Nikolic meant to say that cultural interpenetration would be harmful in itself and under any circumstances, but it is likely that his theory focused on the destructive and detrimental effect of the West in particular.

[99] In particular, cross-cultural encounters remained one of post-colonial transcultural psychiatry's core concerns and pre-occupations, as well as a central aspect of its mission to facilitate global understanding and communication. See, for instance, Ari Kiev, *Transcultural Psychiatry*, New York: Free Press, 1972.

emerged from a 'clash between two cultures'.[100] In other words, South American indigenous cultures were incompatible with the Western one—it was not only that their therapeutic concepts and systems could not be translated into and understood by Western observers, but the very contact between the two led to catastrophic consequences.

Cross-cultural communication, therefore, amounted to a cultural clash, which undermined the most important and refined elements of indigenous therapeutic cultures. Hadzi-Nikolic used explicitly militaristic language to describe the inter-civilisational encounter. The dominant Western civilisation was spreading through 'authoritarianism and indoctrination', but 'old divinities defended themselves fiercely and that resistance persists until present day'. Moreover, these traditional gods never 'surrendered' but 'continued their battle underground'.[101] Hadzi-Nikolic's pessimistic take on cross-cultural encounters undermined one of the most important political and professional goals of post-colonial transcultural psychiatry: with its strong universalist component, the discipline was conceived as both a facilitator of inter-cultural exchanges and a field which dealt with potentially disruptive consequences of cross-cultural encounters and clashes. European colonial psychiatrists argued in the early twentieth century that exposing non-Western natives to Westernising influences such as education or urbanisation would have dangerously negative psychological consequences, and that 'primitive' non-Europeans were racially, culturally and biologically unsuited to such alien cultural endeavours.[102] In response to that, post-colonial transcultural psychiatry sought to radically reconsider the nature, necessity and possible consequences of intense transcultural connections, and to offer a framework for understanding cross-cultural communication and experiences. The very concept of universal humanity served to smooth the progress of inter-cultural understanding, dialogue and tolerance.

In that sense, Hadzi-Nikolic's insistence on the notions of cultural incompatibility might have been surprising, but his reasoning was fundamentally different from that employed by colonial psychiatrists. While the latter warned against intensive cross-cultural interpenetration because they

[100] Hadzi-Nikolic, *Kad se vidi ono sto se ne vidi*, 191–192.

[101] Ibid., 49–50.

[102] Carothers, 'A Study of Mental Derangement in Africans', 197–219.

saw non-Western peoples as too underdeveloped to withstand it, Hadzi-Nikolic objected to the Western influences precisely because he tended to view the South American shamanist therapeutic systems of knowledge as intellectually superior to those of the West—the Western culture, as his argument went, was more powerful only in a narrow political and military sense. Even though he argued that indigenous cultural and therapeutic concepts were unique, incomparable and untranslatable, he still at times referred to the Andean and Amazonian shamanistic rituals in psychoanalytic terms—proposing that they were so ahead of supposedly more sophisticated Western theories that, thousands of years before the West, their rituals had perfected working with the unconscious and used hallucinogenic substances and group séances to project and interpret its most disturbing elements in culturally acceptable terms.

Despite such occasional celebrations of shamanistic rituals as superior, overall Hadzi-Nikolic proclaimed himself agnostic with regard to different therapeutic systems—indigenous rituals and shamanism, psychoanalysis and psychodynamic psychiatry, biological psychiatry. Speaking of a psychoanalytically inflected interpretation of Mexican indigenous rituals by one of the leading US transcultural psychiatrists Ari Kiev, Hadzi Nikolic noted that 'we should approach Kiev's explanation with as much enthusiasm as we would that of the *curanderos* [shamans] themselves'.[103] These different epistemological systems existed on parallel planes, without any hierarchical relationship between them. Here, Hadzi-Nikolic achieved what few of his colleagues ever did, even in the context of the new cross-cultural psychiatry—he set up Western psychiatric models as merely another version of ethno-psychiatry instead of seeing them as the yardstick against which to measure the effectiveness of all other therapeutic cultures.

Just like Jakovljević's, Hadzi-Nikolic's relationship with the 'Western culture' was ambiguous and unclear. He did at times refer to the Western therapeutic concepts and traditions as 'ours', perhaps because he himself had been trained in psychodynamic and psychoanalytic psychiatry both in Yugoslavia and in Western Europe. At the same time, in his anthropological analysis he assumed the position of an outsider—someone who bore no political or cultural responsibility for colonial aggression and injustice, and who could easily step outside European and Western educational

[103] Hadzi-Nikolic, *Kad se vidi ono sto se ne vidi*, 166.

traditions precisely because he occupied a position in between different therapeutic and civilisational models. His socialist or Marxist leanings never factored in his writings and interpretation in any open or explicit manner, however—this might have been a symptom of the decreasing significance of socialist and Marxist ideology in Yugoslav psychiatric practice and theory in the 1980s—and his solidarity with his research subjects seemed to stem from a much broader sense of shared humanity.

As we saw above, Jakovljević's universalism was complex and at times contradictory: despite his careful sociological and socio-cultural analyses, he used Western psychiatric nosological categories unproblematically to diagnose his Guinean patients, and his implicit comparisons between the Balkans and West Africa fed into his universalist frameworks for evaluating social progress and backwardness. Hadzi-Nikolic, on the other hand, viewed psychiatric universalism particularly negatively—the core problem with it, he opined, was the West's 'unpreparedness to see another culture in its uniqueness and inimitability, and our persistent and misleading ambition to understand the life of other cultures applying exclusively our categories'. But Hadzi-Nikolic's cultural relativism was ultimately tempered by his musings about possibly universal human characteristics, and those elements of human nature which supposedly crossed geographical, racial and civilisational boundaries. We might say that his universalism was primarily philosophical and spiritual, as it concerned states of existential fear and anxiety, which he thought marked the human condition regardless of historical or cultural background. Hadzi-Nikolic viewed Andean and Amazonian shamanism as expressions of a broader human search for answers to what he considered the core questions: 'who am I? where do I come from and where am I headed? who do I belong to? what is my place in the Universe?' It was in the course of rituals and shamans' interventions that individuals were integrated with the 'absolute' cosmic and divine powers. The need to realise such an integration and find answers as to the purpose of human existence in this world was universal, according to Hadzi-Nikolic, and he compared the structure and aims of shamanistic rituals to the questions raised by Russian religious philosopher Nikolai Berdyaev, who hoped to 'discover the secret of his own personality, to reveal who he was, where he came from', as well as the 'secret of the world with which he was connected in ways that defy rational comprehension.'[104] Hadzi-Nikolic concluded that such inquiries were pursued by both the most refined European academics *and* 'primitive' shamans and their followers, and therefore stemmed from an 'insuperable human yearning for protection and anchor', expressing universal existential fears and sense of powerlessness.[105]

* * *

As we have seen throughout this chapter, discussing Africa and the developing world often meant discussing Eastern European developmental concerns: similarities and comparisons abounded, and it remained unclear whether, in Jakovljević's mental universe and clinical conclusions, Yugoslavia had more in common with Africa or Western Europe. This shaped Jakovljević's understanding of concepts such as 'primitivism' and civilisation, and even though he tacitly accepted the cultural and medical assumptions of the colonial psychiatric framework, he subscribed to a much more dynamic view of non-Western societies and cultural traditions. In this way, he revised the traditional psychiatric, psychoanalytic and anthropological interpretations of non-European civilisations as inhabiting the childhood stage of the history of humankind, and insisted on Guinea's remarkable possibilities for progress and development. In this regard, Jakovljević echoed broader cultural and political discourses in Yugoslavia: in 1963, for instance, Bozo Milačić, a distinguished journalist and author, wrote in his travelogue about Libya that, even though some Western authors depicted it as 'a crate of sand, a child ... Libya is not a child who is learning to walk, it is a grown up, stronger and richer every day'.[106] Perhaps precisely because Yugoslav psychiatry remained preoccupied with the purported primitivism of its own peasant and working-class population, Jakovljević strove to make inferences regarding the cultural and psychological consequences of Guinea's extremely disruptive social(ist) transformation, and attempted to frame his conclusions in a way that would be relevant for the far-reaching transformations affecting the Yugoslav society. For understandable reasons, Jakovljević was crucially interested in the psychological repercussions of radical social changes; his experiences in Guinea, where the period of decolonisation and quest for

[104] Ibid., 181.

[105] Ibid., 185.

[106] Bozo Milacic, *Suncana putovanja i bijele noci*, Zagreb: Stvarnost, 1963, 45.

a local version of socialism was accompanied by seismic societal shifts, helped him develop a nuanced theory of revolutionary personalities and their roles in times of social and political disruption and uncertainty. In the context of Marxist psychiatry, Jakovljević's concept of revolutionary personality radically redefined the relationship between social conflict and mental illness, as he relied on anthropological, ethnographic and clinical evidence from both Yugoslavia and Guinea.

Jakovljević's work and special position within the emerging discipline of transcultural psychiatry were thus marked by both his (and his home country's) political and ideological background, and the position of Yugoslavia on the cultural and political periphery of Europe. His involvement in transcultural psychiatry demonstrated the inherent contradiction of Eastern European Marxist psychiatry: its dubiously colonial 'civilising mission' towards the subalterns in its own populations, and its progressive, emancipatory agenda. Jakovljević's use of Africa as a testing ground for the relative significance of cultural and civilisational factors in the development of mental illness ultimately turned into an unprecedented opportunity to shed light on and attempt to resolve some glaring internal inconsistencies from Yugoslavia's own socio-political context.

Jakovljević was a representative of the first generation of transcultural psychiatry, one marred by complex and contradictory legacies of colonial psychiatry, and deeply anxious about the pathological effects of massive social and cultural changes brought on by decolonisation. Moreover, Jakovljević's interventions revealed Yugoslav socialism's ambiguities with regard to race, anti-colonialism and non-aligned solidarities: despite his pronounced anti-imperialist politics, Jakovljević's classification systems and diagnostic procedures were predominantly Eurocentric, and he associated backwardness and primitivism exclusively with the African continent and cultural traditions. Jakovljević's socialist solidarities with his Guinean patients could not undo his straightforward acceptance of a variety of colonial frameworks and medical nosologies, and his loyalty to a linear model of progress and development whose parameters were decided by white European men. It was not until the 1980s and the emergence of a large number of critical voices in global anthropology and cross-cultural psychiatry that some of these assumptions began to be challenged in the socialist world.

Hadzi-Nikolic, Eastern Europe's sole representative of this new trend in cross-cultural psychiatric research, dismissed 'primitivism' as a concept that held any analytic usefulness for understanding Andean and Amazonian indigenous cultures, and the possibility of cross-cultural understanding and exchange. Even after Kleinman's critique, global postcolonial psychiatry struggled to overcome its tendency to view Western psychiatric models as the most valuable interpretive frameworks for understanding and healing mental distress. Hadzi-Nikolic was one of the very few psychiatrists who aimed to undermine such hierarchical assumptions, and placed Western and indigenous systems of knowledge and belief on the same level—as incomparable and largely untranslatable but equal in their sophistication and cultural effectiveness. Hadzi-Nikolic's interventions were not framed as explicitly socialist or Marxist, but they were enabled by his position of epistemological 'in-betweenness' which he shared with Jakovljević, and which made it possible for him to engage critically with a variety of cultural and psychiatric educational traditions (in this sense, both Jakovljević and Hadzi-Nikolic belonged to a long succession of Yugoslav socialist intellectuals who claimed, more or less explicitly, that they could understand the non-Western world better than West European authors). Still, his cultural relativism was not unlimited: his writings suggested that he did believe in the existence of universally shared human characteristics. Unlike Jakovljević's universalism, which was largely informed by his sense of socialist solidarity, Hadzi-Nikolic's was broader and primarily driven by humanist and ethical concerns. It signalled that the need for transcultural psychiatry to broaden and reframe the boundaries of humanity, and to include the indigenous people of South America in a global human community as members equally deserving of respect and transcultural empathy as white Europeans—and not as primitives and second-class citizens who ought to catch up and modernise.

CHAPTER 6

'Psy' Sciences Beyond the Consulting Room

As we saw in the previous chapters, from the late 1950s on and especially throughout the 1960s and 1970s, Yugoslavia was an exception in the socialist world. Its unique 'path to socialism' was explicitly based on Marxist humanist ideas of freedom and personal liberation, and the country strove to distinguish itself from Soviet-dominated state socialist model by insisting on political decentralisation and the doctrine of the gradual 'withering away of the state'. Even though such circumstances were still significantly different from institutionalised political pluralism and liberal democracy, a greater sense of freedom and political independence was nevertheless felt in a variety of professional and artistic fields, as well as in the public sphere more generally, and the 'psy' professions in particular certainly benefited from Yugoslavia's unique ideology and geopolitical position. Even more importantly, in different spheres of public life, a significant number of influential critical voices emerged both from the arts and from academic circles, who aimed to analyse and condemn the origins of what they saw as a betrayal of the socialist ideals in Yugoslavia, and the failure of a full liberation of the socialist consciousness. In the 1960s and 1970s, politically engaged writers, film directors, political theorists and philosophers defined important aspects and institutions of the Yugoslav Communist state as elitist, bureaucratised and ossified, and entirely out of sync with the fundamental principles

A. Antić, *Non-Aligned Psychiatry in the Cold War*,
Mental Health in Historical Perspective,
https://doi.org/10.1007/978-3-030-89449-8_6

of the theory of workers' self-management. This critique emphasised that, despite years of institutional and legislative reforms, and despite the Yugoslav leadership's official condemnation of Soviet-style dictatorships, the Yugoslav system remained almost instinctively repressive, ideologically dogmatic, and based on discipline, political conformity and psychological manipulation.

But these intellectuals, artists and dissident activists were generally not anti-Communists: they themselves came from the left, and insisted not on the subversion of Marxist ideals but on their full-fledged implementation, attempting to hold the Yugoslav state responsible for its own unfulfilled promises. In other words, they demanded a return to early Marxist humanism and the creation of a genuinely free socialist society, fundamentally based on ideas of workers' self-management, where all citizens would take active part in economic and political decision-making, and be allowed to lead full and authentic lives. For such a political community to be viable, they rightly noted, a very different form of education and political practice was urgently needed, as well as a radically changed model of citizenship.

These wide-ranging critiques of the Yugoslav system's shortcomings and unfulfilled promises regularly engaged with different models of the human psyche, and the artists and intellectuals in question often phrased their political interventions in psychiatric, psychotherapeutic or psychoanalytic terms. Moreover, they frequently relied on the 'psy' disciplines and their core concepts and theories to discuss some of the country's most pressing political and social concerns. The chapter will explore these peculiar interrelationships between artistic, academic, political and psychiatric discourses, and trace the role of the 'psy' sciences outside psychiatric hospitals and consulting rooms. It will also demonstrate that psychiatry was hardly a marginal and unknown discipline in the Balkans. These political discussions often constructed the psychiatric profession and institutions as particularly instructive examples of a punitive custodial system—a microcosm of political dictatorship: psychiatry and its long tradition of compulsory commitments and forced, frequently violent treatment served as an excellent metaphor for the broader social community and its experience of political suppression and helplessness. At the same time, however, many dissident intellectuals and artists coached their calls for freedom and authenticity in psychoanalytic and psychotherapeutic terms, presenting the conceptual apparatus of the 'psy' disciplines as a valuable means of achieving personal emancipation and resisting dictatorial demands. This demonstrated once again that there existed an exceptionally close relationship between political revolutions and different conceptualisations of the human psyche.

Yugoslav Cinematography and the 'Psy' Sciences

Far from being a marginalised, socially irrelevant discipline, which operated far from most Yugoslav citizens' interest and awareness, psychiatry and related 'psy' sciences became very important to the cultural critique of Yugoslavia's political realities, and served as a powerful inspiration for such critical artistic discourses. What does political authoritarianism do to the human mind? How are individuals pacified and turned from creative beings with humanist motivations into obedient Party apparatchiks, enforcers of the Party dogma, and vice versa? These were some of the core concerns of Yugoslav socialist cinematography, which often aimed to undertake psychological studies of individuals in constraining social and political contexts in order to demonstrate the societal and state institutions' responsibility for undermining the goals of humanist Marxism. In fact, Yugoslav film authors struggled with the fundamental contradiction at the heart of the country's political system: between the government's aspirations to achieve genuine Marxist democracy through workers' self-management, decentralisation of power and grassroots participation on the one hand, and its lingering repressive institutional practice and expectations on the other.[1] This conflict marred Yugoslavia's ideological experiment from the very beginning, and, importantly for this study, some of the most significant films of the socialist era addressed it by relying on psychiatric and psychoanalytic metaphors, synecdoches and concepts. In other words, Yugoslavia's difficulties with implementing the innovative system of workers' self-management in the context of one-party authoritarianism were often retold as narratives of psychological experimentation and/or manipulation, with a focus on how such incoherence might affect the psyche of citizens and their ability to develop into autonomous and free personalities.

Yugoslav cinema addressed some of the most important political and social issues of the socialist era; from the late 1950s on in particular,

[1] Daniel Goulding, *Liberated Cinema: The Yugoslav Experience, 1945–1991*, Bloomington: Indiana University Press, 2002; Pavle Levi, *Disintegration in Frames: Aesthetics and Ideology in the Yugoslav and Post-Yugoslav Cinema*, Stanford University Press, 2007.

artistic and so-called 'black wave' films focused on exploring the concepts of human freedom, creativity and responsibility in authoritarian regimes, and examined the fate of personal fulfilment, liberty and happiness in the context of socialism and its utopian promises.[2] These films were, of course, highly critical, but this critique often came from within Marxist ideology, and held out the hope for improvement and for the fulfilment of the Communist promise. At the centre of these debates was the relationship between the human psyche and authoritarian political systems, and primarily for this reason, Yugoslav cinema relied on a variety of psychiatric and psychoanalytic concepts in order to tackle its broader social and political concerns. The socialist political project involved a complex and ambitious psychological restructuring in pursuit of a new socialist man and woman. As world-renowned Yugoslav director Dušan Makavejev asked in his 1966 film 'Love affair or the case of a missing switchboard operator' (discussed below), 'Will man be remodelled? Will the future man retain certain old organs?' Answering such questions about the influence of political utopias on human mind required some basic psychoanalytic and psychotherapeutic conceptual apparatus. Such restructuring and remodelling was unlikely to be discussed without reference to the 'psy' disciplines and their potential for political manipulation and/or liberation. Yugoslav cinema, as well as literature, explored complex relationships between the 'psy' sciences and politics, whether psychiatrists and psychotherapists were portrayed as hypocritical, sometimes sadistic abusers of political power, or as harbingers of personal freedom and emancipation.

In the East European literary and film tradition, the notions of psychiatric hospital and psychiatric treatment have held a significant amount of symbolic power, and have long been used to raise broader social, cultural and political issues, or to offer sharp criticism of socio-political problems. In particular, the psychiatric hospital ('madhouse' or 'psychushka) became a common chronotope in Russian and Soviet literature, and was often used to 'to consider the Soviet experience and the Soviet hero'.[3] Within this tradition, the trope of the psychiatric hospital could serve a number of different purposes, and acquired a variety of meanings: as a site of violent

[2] Radina Vucetic, *Koka-kola socijalizam*, Belgrade: Sluzbeni Glasnik, 2016, 144–162; Bogdan Tirnanic, *Crni talas*, Belgrade: Filmski Centar Srbije, 2011.

[3] Rebecca Reich, 'Over the Cuckoo's Nest: Russian Variations on a Psychiatric Theme', in Marks and Savelli, eds, *Psychiatry in Communist Europe*, 196–215.

repression, torture and restriction (or complete annulment) of citizens' human rights, or as a refuge, where an independent and free-thinking individual can continue to exercise his or her unrestrained creativity beyond the reach of an oppressive civil society. Moreover, the theme of 'madmen' as the only free and creative individuals in an authoritarian society proved to be an extraordinarily significant and lasting one. Those who were diagnosed as psychologically deviant and in need of psychiatric treatment were often cast in the roles of the regime's conscious or unconscious opponents: whether they meant it or not, they came to resist the authorities' rigidity and onslaught on their citizens' creative minds. As Angela Brintlinger has argued in relation to contemporary Russian literature, the 'madness [of the psychiatric patient] then, lies precisely in his lack of respect for authority' and in his commitment to independent thinking.[4] In a similar vein, Rebecca Reich has noted that one of the most important tropes in East European anti-psychiatric dissident literature was that of mental health patients who challenged their psychiatric diagnoses, and removed diagnostic authority from the (compromised) psychiatric profession.[5]

In Yugoslav cinematography, such themes and metaphors played a very important role. In fact, one of Yugoslavia's most successful, internationally acclaimed and domestically popular films was entirely focused on a psychiatrist—alcohologist—and his troubled therapeutic community of semi-recovered alcoholic patients. Goran Paskaljević's *Poseban tretman (Special treatment)* premiered only a few short months after the death of Yugoslavia's President Tito, and despite offering what could be read as an exceptionally harsh critique of his rule, it was well received by Yugoslav film critics and scored unprecedented successes at both domestic international film festivals (including three awards at Yugoslavia's flagship Pula Film Festival, a nomination for the Golden Globe awards, and a prestigious prize at the Cannes Festival for Milena Dravić, one of its brilliant

[4] Angela Brintlinger, 'The Hero in the Madhouse: The Post-Soviet Novel Confronts the Soviet Past', *Slavic Review*, 2004, 63:1, 43–65.

[5] Rebecca Reich, *State of Madness: Psychiatry, Literature, and Dissent after Stalin*, De Kalb, IL: Northern Illinois University Press, 2018.

supporting actresses).[6] It was also the Yugoslav film of the year in 1980.[7] The director and two screenwriters, Filip David and Dušan Kovačević, used the intriguing figure of Dr Ilić and his unusual therapeutic methods to comment on the nature of 'benign totalitarianism' and its broader societal effects in Yugoslavia. In fact, Paskaljević indicated that the character of Dr Ilić was structured and developed in such a way as to convey criticism not only of dictatorial personalities in general, but also of the Yugoslav model of soft authoritarianism, where people were led to believe that their liberties and freedom of choice were curtailed for their own benefit while their limited participation was still solicited.[8] The Yugoslav political society was imagined as a psychiatric community, while psychiatric relations emerged as the most appropriate framework for depicting and critiquing socialist authoritarianism.

Paskaljević's film certainly relied on those constructions of 'madmen' explored and discussed by Reich and Brintlinger: in it, psychiatric patients emerged as symbols of freethinking, healthy hedonism and independence—in addition, they diagnosed the psychiatrist himself in a memorable reversal of roles. At the same time, however, *Special treatment* diagnosed the entire Yugoslav society as pathological, which destabilised and complicated the image of mental patients as courageous free thinkers and representatives of sanity (in opposition to the state's repressive insanity).

The plot of the film revolves around the final test which the renowned alcohologist prepares for his patient group—they are to demonstrate their sobriety and strength of character by performing a morality tale in a small brewery. Dr Ilić, an ambitious and committed psychiatrist, is bent on proving that his methods for engaging alcoholic patients and instilling in them self-discipline and a rational desire to recover can be effective even in the most challenging of circumstances. However, the core problem undermining his therapeutic project is that he runs a clinic for compulsory treatment of alcoholics, and while some of his patients seem internally driven to overcome their addiction, it becomes increasingly obvious throughout the film that Dr Ilić's is an experiment in forced

6 *Poseban tretman*, 1980, dir. Goran Paskaljević; Nino Milenkovic, 'Posebno tretirani tretman', *TV Novosti*, May 1980.

7 Jasmina Sopova, 'Serbian Film-Maker Goran Paskaljević', *UNESCO Courier*, February 2000, 53:2.

8 *The Cinema of Goran Paskaljević*, Belgrade: Stubovi Kulture, 2010, 62–69.

healing, in the course of which participation and compliance are secured through rather repressive measures.

It is particularly intriguing that one of the most prominent signs of Ilic's authoritarianism is his rigid commitment to 'civilising' his patients. Throughout the film, his general dissatisfaction with the patients' level of cultural awareness and understanding comes across strongly, and belies his declarations of equality within their therapeutic community. Despite his proffered beliefs in his patients' capacities and responsibility, he clearly views them as less sophisticated than himself, and considers their cultural advancement to be essential to their psychological recovery. In one of the film's most memorable scenes, Ilić irritably interrupts the patients singing a folk song which they evidently enjoyed ('enough with that tavern music', he chastises, 'the landscape around us deserves something more beautiful'), and plays them Wagner's 'Ride of the Valkyries' instead, which dampens the mood significantly, and fails to elicit any honest participation. In fact, the legendary melody becomes the film's core soundtrack—an apt symbol of the top-down nature of Ilic's re-education strategy. By banning the patients' authentic celebrations of life and joy through folk music, Ilić effectively cuts them out of his therapeutic/political project of re-education, and aims to found their happiness and success on a platform which is profoundly alien to them. There are many other ways in which Ilić strives to change his patients' values and personalities from 'primitive' to 'advanced': by introducing a variety of 'hygienic' measures such as a regular physical exercise regime or 'healthy' eating habits (in another important scene, the patients longingly gaze at—but the psychiatrist scorns—a group of men enjoying pork roast and beer; instead, the patients are distributed apples as snacks). The film zooms in on the undemocratic, exclusionary potentials of the psychiatric civilising mission, and links it to the broader socialist political experiment in Yugoslavia.

Whether consciously or by accident, Paskaljević's film tapped into one of the most important themes in Yugoslav psychiatric discussions of alcoholism: the strong link which Yugoslav psychiatry established between high levels of alcohol consumption and Yugoslav folklore/traditional behaviour. Almost all of the leading alcohologists in Yugoslavia commented on—and lamented—the exceptionally tolerant attitude that traditional and 'backward' peasant communities had towards the use of alcohol. According to prominent Serbian alcohologist Borislav Djukanović, alcohol played a central role in the social life of Yugoslavia's traditional peasant communities: its socio-psychological functions were multiple, and included enabling social participation and increasing group cohesion. Alcohol drinking was also vital to a number of traditional (mainly religious) rituals, some of which had already lost their traditional form and meaning but not the drinking component: 'at one funeral, people could drink over one hundred litres of alcohol'. Finally, alcohol had a foremost utilitarian purpose in traditional communities, and helped people achieve a variety of personal, social and economic goals. In that sense, Yugoslav psychiatrists-turned-ethnographers believed they were facing an exceptionally formidable enemy, as alcohol, even excessive drinking, was such an important factor in facilitating social contacts, relieving social and psychological tensions and establishing and reinforcing social bonds that a large number of common social situations were simply unimaginable without it. To make matters worse, 'the orthodox church had relatively early taken a liberal stance towards using wine and... rakia' in the context of religious ceremonies, which then resulted in further persistent increase in hedonistic drinking once the societal influence of the church deteriorated.[9]

In other words, traditional peasant communities associated excessive alcohol consumption with positive personality traits and good social standing ('families [who do not take part in traditional rituals of offering and consuming alcohol in relevant social situations] lose face in the social life of their village and are likely to experience a decline in their participatory capacity in collective activities'). Moreover, it was precisely those communities which faced the most severe social, cultural and economic dislocation in the midst of socialist Yugoslavia's rapid industrialisation and urbanisation: they migrated in large numbers from villages to urban environments, where they experienced poverty, a housing crisis as well as, according to alcohologists, cultural conflicts and a breakdown of their primary social contacts. In such challenging circumstances, alcohol consumption reportedly skyrocketed, while alcohol fulfilled an important psychological function and alleviated severe psychological disturbances. As Djukanović concluded, 'a tavern [*kafana*] became the most important bond between urban and rural environments', so that it was not at all surprising that Yugoslavia had more taverns than primary schools. This was then the core aspect of Yugoslav psychiatrists' understanding of the

[9] Borislav Djukanović, 'Drustveni stavovi prema picu i obicaji', *Socijalna psihijatrija*, 1974, 2, 345–354.

problem of alcoholism: it was tightly and inextricably related to the backward, rural and traditional nature of the fledgling socialist society, the final and most tenacious remnant of its 'primitive' past which was slowly and painfully disappearing in the course of modernisation. Alcoholism was a price that 'one generation had to pay for being wrenched from their rural social context'.[10]

The film's Ilić undoubtedly agreed with this interpretation, and objected aggressively to his patients' attachment to various 'folkloric' elements, such as traditional music or tavern food and atmosphere (his patients mostly came from the margins of Yugoslavia's cities and towns, demonstrating the failures of the country's urbanisation and development). For Djukanović as well, the psychiatric profession had a historic responsibility to offer different—more civilised and 'rational'—ways of assuaging the loneliness and internal cultural tensions of this migrant, in-between class of Yugoslavs, and to show them alternative avenues for fulfilling and developing their 'humane needs'.[11] This was the most important task of socialist psychiatry's civilising mission.[12] Here again, despite their socially and politically progressive outlook, Yugoslav socialist 'psy' disciplines appropriated one of the core tropes of Western colonial psychiatry, its 'acculturation' thesis—the argument that 'primitive' groups were particularly vulnerable to mental pathology when faced with large-scale social and cultural changes and modernisation (in the form of industrialisation and urbanisation).[13] As we saw in the preceding chapters, the concept of 'acculturation' was used by West European psychiatrists to theorise the colonised world's responses to rapid modernisation both before and after decolonisation, and to pathologise non-European societies by depicting them as incapable of handling the challenges of modernity.[14] In the Yugoslav (and East European) case, very similar ideas informed the psychiatric profession's thinking about alcoholism: exposing the Yugoslav peasant population to the vagaries of socialist development

[10] Ibid., 352–353.

[11] Ibid., 353.

[12] For further discussion of Yugoslav socialist psychiatry's engagement with alcoholism, see Savelli, 'Diseased, Depraved or Just Drunk? The Psychiatric Panic Over Alcoholism in Communist Yugoslavia', *Social History of Medicine*, 2012, 25:2, 462–480.

[13] Carothers, 'A Study of Mental Derangement in Africans', 197–219.

[14] Megan Vaughan, *Curing Their Ills: Colonial Power and African Illness*, Stanford: Stanford University Press, 1991.

led to grave psychological consequences, as such 'primitive' social groups were bound to struggle with adapting to more advanced forms of life, to which they were culturally (if not racially) unsuited.

It is not accidental that Ilić is a specialist for treating alcoholism: this particular social illness caused major concern among Yugoslavia's leading psychiatrists and political decision-makers. In psychiatric publications, experts on alcoholism engaged in raising a veritable moral panic as the number of diagnosed and treated alcoholics rose. As Djukanović noted with alarm in 1979, post-WWII psychiatric research and questionnaires indicated that even children in primary and secondary schools were not spared the deleterious effects of excessive drinking.[15] Moreover, as many as 14% of children from a Croatian town in a wine-making region were found to be chronic alcoholics, while over a half of pre-university students and pupils in the whole of Yugoslavia reportedly drank alcohol occasionally or regularly.[16]

The persistence, let alone the exacerbation, of the illness was difficult to understand in ideological and political terms: given that Yugoslavia's socialist (and social) psychiatrists believed that alcoholism was rooted in social and economic problems, and caused by damaged and unhealthy interpersonal relations, it should have long been extinguished in a developed and accomplished socialist society such as Yugoslavia. In fact, as Croatian psychiatrist Ivan Hercog noted in 1950, capitalism, with its exploitative social relations, could never tackle alcoholism in the same way that socialism could: alcoholism was a product of 'the systematic exploitation of man against man that could be found under capitalism' but that was bound to disappear in the socialist world.[17] Two decades later, however, according to Yugoslav psychiatric epidemiologists, alcoholism was far from eradicated, and its rates were rising twice as fast as those of any other mental illness despite the enormous efforts of the socialist public health system, while it disproportionately affected the working-class population and undermined its ability to contribute to the country's development. Matthew Savelli rightly noted that Yugoslav socialist psychiatrists spoke of alcoholism in apocalyptic terms: alcoholism was marked as

[15] Djukanović, *Alkoholizam i porodica*, Belgrade: Privredna stampa, 1979.

[16] Josip Dojc, 'Alkoholizam kao posledica uticaja drustva I okoline', *Higijena*, 1957: 2–3.

[17] Ivan Hercog, 'Borba protiv alkoholizma u socijalistickoj drzavi', *Lijecnicki Vjesnik*, 1950, 72, 261–262.

'the number one national problem', a comprehensive social, health and political threat to the nation's survival (while it was also described as one of the world's most serious and intractable problems).[18] The very severity of the affliction among the Yugoslav population served as an indictment of the system as a whole, and of socialism's failure to deliver its utopian promise. In the context of such psychiatric debates, it is not difficult to see why Paskaljević and the screenwriters might have chosen their focus in the film: alcoholics were perceived as almost akin to social rebels and critics—they were also an enormous social and political threat—and Ilić's obsession with eradicating alcoholism mirrors the political regime's commitment to transforming and revolutionising the Yugoslav society.

The film's script was based on a short theatre play, authored by Dušan Kovačević, who subsequently adapted it for the screen. The play, titled *What is it in the human being that forces him to drink* (also the film's subtitle), was written in 1976 and performed in a provincial theatre in Serbia, but its narrative structure was substantially different from the film's—although several core themes persisted, and Dr Ilić remained the main character.[19] The play's Ilić is much more laughable, in the tradition of theatre of the absurd, than the grave and increasingly psychopathological figure of the psychiatrist in the film. However, the former character dedicates much more time to catastrophising statements about the dangers of alcoholism, and seems to parrot the above-mentioned pronouncements from psychiatric journals. In the play, they sound increasingly absurd and mocking: '[alcoholism] is no longer an "individual disease", it's a national tragedy', as well as a 'great civilisational illness', which is 'immeasurably' more lethal than cancer. This Ilić also (half-jokingly) develops an image of alcoholics as politically threatening and rivals to the Communist Party: 'alcoholics are the oldest and most vital party organisation. Their membership is fanatical…'[20] In other words, because their loyalties lay elsewhere, their political unreliability was only to be expected (and feared)—or, as another Yugoslav expert in

[18] Savelli, 'Diseased, Depraved or Just Drunk?', 465.

[19] Dusan Kovacevic, *Sta je to u ljudskom bicu sto ga vodi prema picu*, Belgrade: Laguna, 2018 (reprinted).

[20] Ibid.

alcohology concluded, 'there is no self-managing socialism among drunk people'.[21]

It was in the field of alcoholism studies that Yugoslav psychiatry bred one of its most important and internationally renowned figures. Dr Vladimir Hudolin made a lasting impact on global social psychiatry and its struggle with curing alcoholism; his clubs of treated alcoholics—famous 'Hudolin clubs'—mushroomed across the world and his methods of treatment were adopted and lauded globally.[22] While Hudolin's personality was never criticised in any professional publications, his therapeutic philosophy was strikingly similar to Ilić's 'special treatment', and it is possible that the film's main character was developed as a parody of Hudolin's socialist approach to re-educating alcoholics.

Hudolin never hid the fact that, in his therapeutic communities, he was after altering his patients' personalities: his entire professional career was 'an attempt at re-educating the adult man, re-educating the personality'.[23] However, like Ilić, he did not think this could be achieved without his patients' full participation, and he wanted to see patients as equal contributors to the process: 're-education of the personality cannot be completely successful if the patient is only the object of such treatment, so that social psychiatry requires that the patient should present himself as an equal subject in the therapeutic process'.[24] For that reason, Hudolin and his collaborators developed an original programme of comprehensive health education, which was vital to alcoholics' successful recovery: alcoholic patients were to undergo regular therapeutic and rehabilitative treatments, but, in addition to that, they were required to attend lectures and seminars and learn in great detail about the core theoretical, medical, legal and sociological aspects of their illness, as well as to receive 'general health education'. Moreover, just like with Ilic's patients, Hudolin's programme of re-education also involved 'achieving a general hygienic minimum' as well as improving 'the general education of the

[21] Vladimir Hudolin, *Klubovi lijecenih alkoholicara*, Zagreb: Jumena, 1982, 119–120.

[22] See Dusko Wolfl, ed., *Vladimir Hudolin and his work*, Rijeka: Regional Centre for Alcoholism, 2007; Vladimir Hudolin, S. Stojiljkovic, and R. Percinkovski, 'Socijalno-medicinski aspekti alkoholizma u SFRJ', *Zbornik radova jugoslovenske konferencije o alkoholizmu*, Belgrade, 1967.

[23] Hudolin, 'Health Education of Patients in the Field of Social Psychiatry, Notably Alcoholics', *International Journal of Social Psychiatry*, 1972, 18:3, 1–9.

[24] Ibid., 2–3.

patient' (in the sense of raising their cultural levels and engaging them in various artistic pursuits, such as music and song).[25] In the course of the programme, the 'civilising mission' was thus allowed to run its full course, while the most successful patients were then given an opportunity to attend a 'postgraduate course' in alcoholism studies, for which Hudolin developed an ambitious and detailed syllabus filled with specialist lectures and seminars. Having once achieved this postgraduate level, former alcoholics would ideally stand shoulder to shoulder with psychiatrists, nurses and social workers, and would engage as equal partners—often as fully paid employees—in the treatment of other alcoholics.[26]

In other words, even though Hudolin devised a decidedly top-down project of social engineering, his aim was ultimately to bridge the gap between 'experts' and 'ordinary' patients, and to create a truly radical therapeutic community. He directly related his experimental treatment to the socialist ideology by referring to his groups as 'self-managing therapeutic communities'.[27] In that sense, Hudolin's project was profoundly contradictory in its aims and motivations—both quite authoritarian and radically egalitarian—and as such could serve as a perfect model for Ilić's fictional therapeutic experiment. *Special treatment* focused on socialist psychiatric approaches and experiments to critique what its authors saw as the paradoxical nature of Yugoslav socialism as a whole—a system which purported to create free, emancipated, self-managing and 'equal' citizens through coercive and dictatorial measures. The project of socialist revolution and transformation was inseparable from (authoritarian) psychiatric re-education.[28]

This irresolvable contradiction is central to all relationships and character development in the film. The patients in Ilić's clinic all look like prisoners in their identical striped pyjamas, and the therapeutic community is clearly presented as more akin to a prison than any other egalitarian or

[25] Hudolin, *Klubovi lijecenih alkoholicara*, 123–126.

[26] Hudolin, 'Health Education of Patients', 7–8.

[27] Hudolin, 'Alcoholism in Croatia', *International Journal of Social Psychiatry*, 1969, 15:2, 85–91.

[28] With Ilic set up as the undisputed leader of the group, the film also plays on the idea of political leaders as psychiatrists, which effectively eliminates the population as a collective of citizens; instead, they are all constructed as less than fully rational human beings—either children or mental health patients in need of guidance and comprehensive education. Such a political community is automatically void of any democratic or self-managing principles.

participatory institution. However, the psychiatric (and political) repression implemented in this peculiar prison is far from straightforward: as Ilić maintains in his conversation with a sceptical colleague, even though this is an institution for compulsory treatment, '[the patients] have to get re-acquainted with freedom' and be given an opportunity to choose freely to exercise their newly acquired self-discipline. In fact, Ilić's experimental ('special') treatment largely consists of his Hudolinian belief in the patients' involvement in the therapeutic process. Yet, such participation is obviously choreographed rather than spontaneous, and occurs under restrictive circumstances, ruled by both physical and psychological restraints and retributions. Moreover, Ilić seems only to be interested in the appearance of freedom—his patients are free to choose as long as they make the right—Ilić's—choice. This coercive participation then forms the backbone of the 'special treatment'—Ilić's is fundamentally a project of re-education, of permanently altering his patients' personalities, and this process of creating 'new men and women' mirrors the broader socialist mission of psychological restructuring.

Hudolin was, unsurprisingly, rather ambivalent when it came to the issue of mandatory treatment of alcoholics and their inclusion in the clubs. On the one hand, he emphasised that clubs were 'conceived as a "grouping of friends", who suffered from the same affliction and who develop a new kind of interactions and relationships… as well as deep human understanding, friendship and love'. Seemingly, no force or coercion should have been applied to motivate patients or former alcoholics to join such communities; as Hudolin himself opined, 'alcoholics experienced enough attacks and coercion from a variety of quarters on a daily basis; the club should do the exact opposite, i.e. accept the alcoholic when everyone else rejected him [sic]'. He also referred to the clubs as examples of 'autopsychotherapy'.[29] On the other hand, Hudolin's explicit rejection of coercion was belied by his ambiguous statement that all alcoholics needed a lot of persuasion and motivation to commit fully to their treatment and recovery—and that, 'if alcoholics could be easily convinced to start therapy, clubs would not be necessary at all'.[30] In fact, according to his own admission, most alcoholics joined as a result of some

[29] Hudolin et al., 'Uloga klubova lijecenih alkoholicara', *Radovi Institute za proucavanje i suzbijanje alkoholizma*, Zagreb, 1967, 70.

[30] Hudolin, *Klubovi lijecenih alkoholicara*, 81–84.

form of direct or indirect pressure—because they were required to do so by their families or employers in order to avoid divorce/family disintegration/dismissal, or because they were mandated to do so by a state institution such as the court or the police. In that sense, most members of Hudolin's clubs at least started their treatment and attendance as a result of some sort of coercion.

Paskaljević's film was then not too far off the mark, given that all Ilić's patients were undergoing mandatory rather than voluntary treatment. Hudolin justified this by insisting on the clubs' supportive and beneficial role in spite of the forced nature of many patients' referrals—when a patient is 'under duress' to start therapy and in a difficult situation, 'this is when an alcoholic needs the club the most', probably because, as we noted before, Hudolin (and Ilić) believed that therapeutic communities could ultimately benefit patients and protect their best interests even if they were implemented and run against patients' wishes.[31] Hudolin thus claimed that, even though genuinely voluntary self-referrals were so rare, the clubs were hardly coercive or repressive in themselves, as they were not in any way influenced by the attending alcoholics' families, workplaces or state institutions, and would never intimidate, force or blackmail their members in order to achieve any therapeutic goals. At the same time, however, in his description of a disruptive club member, Hudolin clearly indicated that psychiatric institutions should rely on the police if necessary, and that such an utilisation of a repressive state institution had beneficial therapeutic effects on the patient himself.

In addition to involving patients in the therapeutic process as equals, Hudolin's programme aimed to ensure that recovered alcoholics played a crucial role in educating the broader public about the mechanisms and dangers of their former illness—a lofty aim which inspires all of Ilić's endeavours in the film, and which ultimately leads to his project's catastrophic failure. Justifying the final phase of the treatment, in which the patients are taken to a brewery to perform an educational play based on their personal experiences, Ilić argues that this is the most important therapeutic moment in their recovery. 'The patients need to feel that they are socially useful, and not rejected', he continues, emphasising the broader social role for treated alcoholics. In his final statement in this conversation, Ilic could have quoted directly from one of Hudolin's articles: '[once

[31] Ibid.

released from the clinic] they will have a positive effect on their environment. Nobody can speak with greater authority about the harmfulness of alcohol than they can'.[32] This is why Ilić makes his patients the most important actors in the educational play about alcoholism.

In Kovačević's play, which, unlike the film, focuses entirely on Ilić's and his patients' performance for a local audience, the foyer of the theatre hosting the performance sports the alcoholics' artistic works—their photographs and sculptures. This artistic approach was regularly applied by Hudolin himself, whose clinic even published an LP record with 'eight songs describing the greatest moments from the lives of alcoholics in musical composition and interpretation by alcoholics'. However, the fallacy of such patient participation and involvement is exposed in the film, when one of the alcoholics screams 'But I don't want to be cured!' in the middle of the brewery performance.

As we discussed before, Paskaljević's character combines this insistence on the patients' free creative expression with a rigid obsession with self-discipline and will. Early on, as this group discusses possible origins of their illness with Ilić, one of them defines alcoholics as 'people without will and power to resist alcohol'. Ilić offers a mantra to his confused disciples, which proves to constitute the foundation of his therapeutic creed—that 'strong will is the backbone of human character', while in his value system self-discipline remains the most important psychological and ethical trait.[33] This, too, was an important concept in Yugoslav alcohology: Djukanović confirmed that 'insufficient will was precisely a fundamental constitutive element of the illness of alcoholism', and that any successful therapeutic process needed to nurture the strength of patients' will by encouraging their 'psychosocial maturation'. According to Djukanović, alcoholics shared such feeble-willed psychological character with other psychiatric patients, and the first step in their recovery had to focus on eliminating this weakness.[34] Arguably, this was the core

[32] Hudolin et al., 'Uloga klubova lijecenih alkoholicara', 56–70.

[33] Ilic's insistence on will-power and self-control, as well as his increasingly theatrical and brutal exhibition of his own authoritarianism—combined with his obsession with Wagner's music—evoke images of fascistic dictatorships and the Nitzschean figure of *uebermensch*. In this sense, Paskaljević's critique of Yugoslav socialism goes a step further, and seems to draw a parallel between fascism and communism as different yet ultimately comparable forms of totalitarian government.

[34] Djukanović, *Alkoholizam I porodica*, 125–126.

of Ilić's therapeutic efforts as well. This is why Paskaljević's psychiatrist is primarily concerned with re-defining the concept of freedom in line with his belief in the central role of self-control in psychological recovery: in his lecture to a less than captive audience at the brewery, he explains that a man can only be free if he 'succeeds in fully controlling himself, his thoughts, wishes and feelings'. Freedom is not doing whatever we want or going wherever we wish, warns Ilić, who also, paradoxically, believes that people can be free even in prisons if they can restrain and subjugate their desires, personalities and wishes in order to achieve the rational goals they set for themselves. Ilić introduces his 'actors' to the audience as people who recovered and 'became free again' (presumably through his extremely restrictive therapeutic methods)—while at that very moment they look extraordinarily downbeat, hopeless and subservient, an image very few would associate with freedom and independence.

It is very important that Ilić sees himself as a liberator of his patients, as someone who produces free personalities while at the same time viewing discipline and repression as vital values in his endeavour. The core—and tragic—flaw of Ilić's approach to human psychology turns out to be his belief that freedom can be achieved through authoritarianism and (political and psychological) subjugation of pleasures, desires and wishes. Ilić's concept of freedom is thus founded on complex mechanisms of repression, in a similar way in which the leadership of the Yugoslav self-managing socialist society attempted to convince the population that human emancipation was indeed possible in a dictatorship—a topic which inspired a number of other artistic explorations of the relationship between politics and psychiatry in Yugoslavia. In that sense, Paskaljević's film uses psychiatry and alcohology to explore the mechanisms and failings of Tito's benign totalitarianism, while the entire Yugoslav communist society is imagined as a psychiatric community subjected to experimental forced healing. Ilić's project is one of healing people despite their wishes, leading them out of their 'unconsciousness' by repressive and authoritarian methods, forcing them into compliant behaviour, and—very importantly—into supervising one another.

This rich film offers another important insight into the relationship between (Communist) politics and psychotherapeutic techniques. The 'play' prepared by Ilic's therapeutic community—the main reason for their visit to the brewery—is conceived as an experimental psychodrama, consisting of the patients' personal stories reconstructed and performed by themselves. These performances serve as an educational tool (and a warning tale) for the audience, but also as the final test for the former alcoholics, in which they ought to prove that their personal narratives and memories are brought in line with Ilić's interpretations and expectations. The play eventually gets derailed, and the one personal narrative we get to hear is that of Jelena, the only serious, unmocked character in the film. As Jelena retells the most difficult moments of her life, when she contemplated and then attempted suicide, a brutal story of marital abuse, violence and humiliation unfolds. The audience witnesses Jelena's unspeakable pain over the loss of her children, who were taken away from her due to her alcoholism and now lived with her abusive former husband. Jelena breaks down in tears towards the end of her performance, and another patient, clearly breaching Ilić's instructions, approaches her and implores her to stop. Ilić lectures to his patients that, through performing their own lives in front of an audience, they would 'liberate themselves from fear'; however, during Jelena's monologue, it becomes clear that the psychodrama requires her to unravel completely, and to fully dissolve and humiliate herself in order to be able to re-join the society of 'sane' and free citizens.

Jelena's disturbing performance of the most traumatic moments in her life is reminiscent of the infamous self-criticism sessions, practised regularly at Communist party meetings in the USSR and subsequently throughout Eastern Europe (including Yugoslavia). Jelena is clearly required to practise self-criticism: despite a lifetime of enduring unspeakable brutality and injustice, she is expected to take personal responsibility for her 'failure of will' to resist the temptations of alcoholism and addiction. Just like innumerable Communist party members and nominees did in their own self-criticism sessions, Jelena and Ilić's other alcoholic patients were forced to retell their personal stories and painful memories constantly. This served the purpose of dissolving any boundaries between personal and public lives and achieving complete transparency before the authorities. In the process, the patients were compelled to renounce their own independence of mind, desires and personal motivations in favour of full conformity with approved and publicly acceptable narratives and interpretations.

In Communist party self-criticism sessions, personal lives were subjected to harsh scrutiny, and censure was invited from the audience. Such meetings functioned through fostering an unspecified feeling of guilt among participants and remained an important tool for cultivating uncritical conformity. In his work on the narrative structures of Soviet-era autobiographies and confessions, Igal Halfin compares these autobiographical tellings and texts with religious conversion narratives. Halfin argues that achieving the absolute self-transparency of the Party membership and the population at large was the ultimate goal of the Bolshevik leaders. In order to fulfil this aim, the Soviet authorities demanded of their subjects to engage in constant, relentless life-writing and soul-searching—potential Party members as well as those arrested on suspicion of political treason were expected to always write and re-write their own stories of conversion to Bolshevism and of past sins and betrayals, and these had a very similar overarching structure.[35] They closely resembled, Halfin believes, classical religious texts and eschatology, and all relied on narrating the moral destruction of the pre-Bolshevik or sinful personality of the writer, glorifying his or her ethical and political growth following the ideological awakening of the consciousness. These autobiographies in fact turned into stories of self-discovery.

Such practices undoubtedly invoked the religious imagery of confession, redemption and salvation. However, they could also be read as politicised therapeutic situations and highly scripted instances of self-analysis, aimed at exploring various layers of the participants' psyche and their different sets of motivations. In that sense, Paskaljević engaged with one of the most psychiatrically informed forms of Communist self-fashioning, casting a proper psychiatrist in the role of the Communist Party itself, and charging him with the task of crafting official narratives of his patients' lives and imposing them on his therapeutic community. However, Jelena's confessional performance fails to develop into a story of self-discovery—she never manages to share with the audience her own moment of conversion, nor any experience of personal, moral and psychological growth in the course of her therapy with Ilić. It is only her suffering, humiliation and psychological destruction that comes to the fore in her narrative; Ilić's 'revolutionary' methods manifestly stop short of facilitating Jelena's psychological 'rebirth' and salvation, and only bring about deep confusion and, ultimately, mental breakdown.

Even before the release of Paskaljević's film, Yugoslav cinema had already taken up the theme of the contradiction between political authoritarianism and the democratic promise of workers' self-management very avidly. Some of its best films, especially from the so-called Black Wave in

[35] Igal Halfin, *Terror in My Soul: Communist Autobiographies on Trial*, Cambridge: Harvard University Press, 2003.

the 1960s and 1970s, dealt with various failures of the socialist utopia to bring about the emancipation and full self-realisation of all citizens, and constantly addressed this unbridgeable gap between state regimentation and personal happiness. Paskaljević thus contributed to a long cinematic tradition of exploring the psychology of and avenues for individual liberation, creativity and freedom of choice in the context of Marxist dictatorship.

Yugoslavia's legendary film director and the Black wave's most prominent auteur Dušan Makavejev focused in his films on precisely such clashes between individual liberties and repressive modes of behaviour promoted by the state/society. Makavejev's core concern was with the erosion of creativity but also of moral integrity and social values which might result from these repressive conflicts and contradictions. As Herbert Eagle argued, these films 'probe the principal dichotomy between liberated individual consciousness and various forms of alienation and repression (ideological dogmatism, determinism, institutionalised rigidity and elitism), thus reflecting very accurately the major concerns of the Yugoslav Marxist humanist thinkers, who have declared themselves against all forms of authoritarianism and domination and have criticized those institutions of power, authority and socialization that are by their very nature alienating'.[36] It should be added here that many of these concerns of the Yugoslav humanist thinkers and philosophers were shared by the psychiatric and psychoanalytic professions (as we saw in Chapter 3): in that sense, Makavejev's films tackle some of the core questions regarding the relationship between psychiatry/psychoanalysis, authenticity and liberation, which exercised the country's 'psy' practitioners and clinicians throughout the socialist period. Moreover, Makavejev's films often refer, directly or indirectly, to psychiatric debates, concepts and personalities, emphasising thereby the tight link between his political project and the 'psy' disciplines. In fact, psychoanalytic and psychotherapeutic approaches are often invoked in Makavejev's films to point towards alternative political futures and models of psychiatric/political citizenship.

[36] Herbert Eagle, 'Yugoslav Marxist Humanism and the Films of Dušan Makavejev', in David W. Paul, ed., *Politics, Art and the Commitment in the East European Cinema*, New York: St. Martin's Press, 1983, 132.

Makavejev's critically acclaimed films such as *Man is not a bird* (1965)[37] and *Love affair, or the case of the missing switchboard operator* (1967)[38] explore dysfunctional love stories in which one (usually male) partner's attempts at psychological re-education of and domination over the other prevent the main characters from achieving personal liberation, emancipation and authenticity. In both of these films, the narrative structure is strikingly similar: a passionate love affair develops between a free-spirited woman and an honest yet dangerously rigid man. This setting allows a much broader conflict to play out through the increasingly desperate actions of the characters: one between repressive models of thought and behaviour, and free individual praxis. It is the former that always prevails because it is wholeheartedly supported—and rewarded—by the (Yugoslav) state.

Man is not a bird brings together Jan Rudinski, a Stakhanovite worker—an engineer who behaves like a true relic of Stalinist labour, obsessing about efficiency and commitment, and nurturing Stalinist ideas about uniformity and duty to the state ('your seriousness will be the death of you', his colleague admonishes him)—and a joyful, free-spirited and sexually liberated young woman, local hairdresser Rajka, whose affections turn out difficult to be constrained by Jan's expectations and inflexibility. Torn by uncertainty and jealousy, he demonstrates aggressive, rigid and controlling tendencies, and, despite being extremely decent and personable, acts as a force of repression towards both his colleagues and his romantic partner. Moreover, through his personal and professional relationships, he represents an outmoded model of political citizenship. In a particularly important conversation with an overly gregarious fellow worker, Rudinski declares gravely that 'man is not a bird'—a sentence which serves as the title of the film precisely because Makavejev regularly uses 'flight' as a metaphor for human aspiration to unfettered freedom and spontaneity. As the film unfolds, the sentence is sadly proven to be true in Rudinski's case—he remains unable to overcome the constraints of his own repressive psychological structures, and to take a 'flight'. In the final scene, having attacked and scared Rajka off, he leaves the town,

[37] *Covek nije tica*, 1965, dir. Dušan Makavejev.

[38] *Ljubavni slucaj ili tragedija sluzbenice PTT-a*, 1967, dir. Dušan Makavejev.

and the camera's long shot portrays him as dwarfed, defeated and overwhelmed: as Goulding notes, 'he has been rewarded for his work but has lost an opportunity to open his life to spontaneity, tenderness, and joy'.[39]

The film contains a very important—and entertaining—segment on hypnosis, which runs throughout the narrative and connects different aspects of the story and different characters; this segment also reinforces the link between sciences of the mind and political control (and liberation). The small industrial town in which the love affair unfolds also hosts Roko, introduced as the youngest hypnotist in Yugoslavia. Roko takes part in a local entertainment fair, and organises well attended and obviously fascinating sessions, in the course of which he demonstrates the power of his ability to control and re-direct other people's minds by hypnotising groups of volunteers and inciting them to feelings and actions which have no grounding in the real world. As he instructs during the experiment, while in a 'deep hypnotic sleep, you will follow all my orders'. Moreover, '...under hypnosis, [man] can carry out the most complex commands, including murder'. It is, therefore, this authoritarian model of citizenship that hypnosis represents and is ideally suited to support. This is in fact the final sentence in the film—Roko literally has the final word—and it is followed by a distant shot of Jan Rudinski, a product of precisely such authoritarian thinking, walking away from the town, and from his former lover, across a bleak landscape of the factory's expansive yard. In addition, hypnosis produces citizens who can be perfect informers and who would be unable to hide anything from the state's aspiring totalitarian eye: 'a person under hypnosis tells all and keeps no secrets'.

One of the supporting female characters in the film explicitly compares hypnosis with the oppression and manipulation which she experiences in her abusive patriarchal marriage. In fact, speaking with one of her girlfriends, she declares her decision to leave her husband by saying, 'No more hypnosis'. In her own moment of recognition and personal liberation, she sees herself in those people at the fair who volunteered to be hypnotised, and draws a not so subtle parallel between mind manipulation and patriarchal/repressive politics: 'you shut up and do everything he [the husband] tells you – that's hypnosis. You look, but you've got no eyes. You go where his thoughts order you'. Importantly, she also

[39] Daniel Goulding, 'Makavejev', in Goulding, ed., *Five Filmmakers*, Bloomington: Indiana University Press, 1994, 215–218.

observes that not only her husband but 'all officials' in their bleak industrial town are comparable to the hypnotist. As Goulding rightly notes, it is particularly striking that she, the most oppressed character in the film, is also seemingly the only one who sees through hypnosis and calls out its political meanings and consequences.

At the very beginning of the film, Roko offers a long speech denouncing the social evils of popular 'delusions' and superstition, convincing his audience that 'magic is absolute nonsense, you must fight it'. He effectively juxtaposes superstition with modernity and scientific progress, and situates himself (and the discipline of hypnosis) as a representative of precisely such progress and modernity, and an opponent of backwardness. The Yugoslav socialist psychiatric profession fought a protracted and bitter battle against superstition and popular beliefs in black magic as part of the state's commitment to modernisation—just like it aggressively fought the evils of alcoholism. Very tellingly, Makavejev lets hypnosis—with all its implications of manipulative control and its aim to paralyse its 'patients' active consciousness—stand in the stead of psychiatry. While the film puts it forward as an unlikely symbol of socialist modernity and scientific progress, hypnosis remains an insidious political technique which prevents the development of liberated, authentic and fully engaged citizens. It is only if citizens can see through its harmful goals that they can grow out of the repressive institutions and undermine the power of the establishment. In that sense, hypnosis is constructed here as an ethically and politically ambivalent representative of modernity—as well as of the state, which opposed religious beliefs and superstition among the population while using its powers of psychological manipulation for ultimately repressive political ends, inducing fear and undermining individual liberties (and love relationships).

A very similar story plays out for the unlikely couple in *Love affair*: while Isabella, a young working Hungarian woman from Belgrade, evokes a sense of anarchic, complete freedom and practises sensual liberation, she is held back by Ahmed, a character strikingly similar to Jan Rudinski, whose rigid and inflexible model of behaviour ultimately leads to the extinguishing of Isabella's entire existence. Like Rudinski, Ahmed is a highly regarded professional—sanitary inspector—with an essential role in the modernisation of the Yugoslav socialist state: rat extermination. Even though he is a caring and committed partner, Ahmed the rat exterminator appears to completely misunderstand Isabella's autonomy and unencumbered approach to life. In the film, Isabella's cheerful and unconventional demeanour is juxtaposed with Ahmed's increasingly rigid and close-minded psychology. Ultimately, in this love relationship, utopian hopes of personal happiness and fulfilment face a repressive model of behaviour and an inability to overcome personal psychological inhibitions.

It is in Ahmed's professional identity—as an expert in rat extermination—that some of Makavejev's most important political criticisms are reflected. The film's segment on rat extermination consists of a 'mockumentary', which aims to delineate the civilisational and political significance of this endeavour, and its enormous role in making Yugoslavia's socialist future possible. The mockumentary's language on rats and the state's actions against them is overwhelmingly militaristic, and consequently absurd, in its tone: rats are referred to as 'huge armies' who 'conquered' large sections of Eurasia; the public is criticised for not properly appreciating 'the threat posed to mankind by rats' and 'it is still unclear who will rule the Earth in a hundred years: people or rats', while the rat extermination department is described as 'the advance guard of the human race' waging a 'fierce battle'. The anti-rat disinfection campaign—presented as the centrepiece of socialist modernisation—is regimented, aggressive and staged to the point of ridiculousness, while the voice-over recalls a struggle against fascist hordes. But the 'repression' and violence of the state's project is thrown in stark relief when images of dead rats are immediately followed by a silent projection of a Yugoslav children's poem, which tells a story of a poisoned rat from a strikingly different perspective, and, using comical children's language, elicits deep concern and sympathy for the rat's pain and suffering.[40]

The political aspect of Makavejev's take on rat extermination comes through most strongly a few scenes later, when Ahmed brings home a music record gifted to him by his colleagues from the GDR. When he plays the song on his new gramophone, its grandiose and triumphalist tones, as well as belligerent lyrics, clash with Isabella's simple and honest joyfulness: this clash is further emphasised as the camera follows her movements around the garden while the song is playing in the background. The song which so impresses Ahmed and bemuses Isabella ('what's that, for God's sake?', she exclaims) is 'The march of time', an East German political hymn composed by Hanns Eisler, the author of

[40] Dusan Radovic, 'Pesma o parcovu'.

the GDR's national anthem, in 1957 to Vladimir Mayakovski's lyrics.[41] The song in itself encapsulates the fundamental contradiction which Makavejev notes at the heart of the Yugoslav socialist experiment: the conflict between humanist Marxism and genuine democracy of workers' self-management on the one side, and repressive, regimented state institutions (or projects) on the other. The song refers to a possible future of freedom and contentment in a benign, life-asserting verse—'You promise, oh country, a future of joy, since the commune is at the door'—but quickly follows this with aggressive motives and messages, such as the invocation 'country of countries, make an assault, crush to death the rotten vermin', indicating that the utopian future of happiness and personal freedom is, ironically, only to be achieved through destruction and eradication. Importantly, this reference to enemies as vermin almost duplicates the language used in the mockumentary to describe Ahmed's rat extermination projects. In that way, Makavejev draws a parallel between Stalinist expressions of political enmity and repression, and Ahmed's professional identity: the state project of rat extermination is thus likened to an authoritarian, rigid and rather soulless political outlook, indicating that the Yugoslav state, ideology and institutions reward and sustain repressive models of behaviour but fail to encourage free individual praxis despite the official rhetoric of self-management. While both the song and Yugoslav state projects celebrate progress and an unprecedented 'march of times' in Eastern Europe, they sacrifice freedom and individual autonomy in the process.

Immediately after the scene in which Ahmed plays his record, Isabella offers her own music of choice—she sings for him a lively but gentle and sentimental traditional Hungarian song, an expression of her own authentic interests and tastes rather than a choice conditioned by political expectations and pressures. In contradistinction to Eisler's composition, Isabella's folk song warns against rigidity and thirst for punishment or revenge—'A man is not made out of wood, sometimes he can stray'—and focuses on free sexual love, which embarrasses then irritates Ahmed. It is perhaps not by accident that folk songs serve as symbols of freedom and joy in both Makavejev's and Paskaljević's films: in both, folk music is an authentic popular choice, the type of music truly felt and enjoyed by

[41] Goulding, 'Makavejev', 223.

the 'people', which is then stifled and replaced by foreign (interestingly, in both cases German) artistic creations.

Moreover, there is a further connection between the two films: Paskaljević and Makavejev ridicule the Yugoslav state's flagship modernisation projects—the 'fierce struggles' against alcoholism and against rats. In that way, psychiatric patients diagnosed with alcoholism and rats both emerge as core targets of socialist modernisation and civilising campaigns, which were meant to advance and benefit societies, and yet became objects of the critical directors' ridicule and harsh critique precisely for their self-righteousness and repressiveness. In that context, rats and alcoholics both seemed to function almost as counter-points to political authoritarianism, and the two films worked to elicit sympathy towards these unlikely symbols of resistance and liberated thinking.

Just like *Man is not a bird* refers directly to the sciences of the mind through its recurring fragments on hypnosis and psychological manipulation, *Love affair* engages with Professor Aleksandar Kostić, an elderly and good-humoured Belgrade sexologist, who talks directly to the camera about his work in several segments interspersed throughout the film. In fact, Kostić's monologue about the importance of acknowledging our interest in sex opens the film and introduces early on one of Makavejev's central themes—the relationship between sexual repression and political authoritarianism, and the importance of sexual liberation for achieving personal freedom and happiness in socialism. In his opening statement, Kostić diagnoses the Yugoslav society as a sexually repressed one: 'Sex is more whispered about than spoken openly', and proceeds to discuss sexual awareness and human sexuality as essential aspects of everyday life and as vital to a variety of social activities.

While Kostić was not a Freudo-Marxist—Makavejev's later films would become closely allied with that philosophical-political strand—his scholarly work focused on promoting a much more liberal and normalising approach to (heteronormative) sexuality, and he argued against genitocentric understandings of sex and sexual identity: for Kostić, sexuality was not confined to genital organs, but pervaded 'all of man's organism, and all his bodily and spiritual values and manifestations'.[42] In line with Freudo-Marxism, moreover, he viewed modern Western societies as much more sexually repressive than earlier civilisations. Importantly for

[42] Aleksandar Kostić, *Seksualno u nasoj narodnoj poeziji*, Belgrade and Zagreb: Medicinska naucna knjiga, 1978, vi.

this discussion, Kostić's research emphasised a fundamental distinction between oral folk poetry and 'high culture' in terms of sexual liberation, arguing that the former had a healthier, much less conservative and more affirmative attitude towards describing and integrating sexual activities. In his book titled 'The sexual in our oral poetry', Kostić noted that, through this form of art, 'our people expressed all the force and fundamental nature of their instinctual life'.[43] Therefore, like in the case of folk songs versus more 'civilised' or politically appropriate types of music, open expressions of sexuality are here linked to political independence, personal freedom and autonomy, and to authentic folk traditions. Even though some film critics see the segment on Kostić as primarily ironic or even mocking, it is important to keep in mind the provenance of his lifelong research, which addressed some of the core themes in Makavejev's filmography, and at least partly explained Kostić's prominent participation in *Love Affair*, even though the esteemed professor was by no means a Marxist or even particularly progressive in his views on family structures and gender roles.[44]

Makavejev's films were national and international critical successes, widely celebrated as some of the most important art house films in Europe's twentieth century. Their intellectual core consisted of a particularly innovative and complex political criticism—according to Eagle, Makavejev's films gave an artistic expression to Yugoslavia's Marxist humanist thought and its perceptive critique of the many ways in which the country's experiment with revolutionary practices of workers' self-management did not live up to its lofty promises. Moreover, both of the above-described films explored the most pressing political dilemmas of 1960s and 1970s Eastern Europe by focusing on the complexities of the human psyche, and '[related] individual psychological factors to social and political behaviour'.[45] What makes these films particularly important for understanding the broader significance of 'psy' concepts and disciplines in Yugoslavia is their exploration of psychological roots of political problems and aberrations, and their search for psychological/psychoanalytic

[43] Ibid., v–viii.

[44] See, for instance, Kostić, *Higijena braka*, Belgrade: Naucna knjiga, 1955.

[45] Herbert Eagle, 'Yugoslav Marxist Humanism and the Films of Dušan Makavejev', 131–148.

interpretive frameworks for revolution and liberation. Makavejev's political criticism of the Yugoslav system comes from a firmly Marxist position, and both *Man is not a bird* and *Love Affair* emphasise the inability of the Yugoslav state and social institutions to foster and reward individual psychological development and emancipation. Moreover, just like the new generation of Yugoslav psychotherapists and psychoanalysts in the 1960s and 1970s, Makavejev aimed to demonstrate that a true political revolution could not proceed without a revolutionary change in human consciousness and psychology. In that sense, his films were intellectually very close both to the core values in the socialist tradition of psychoanalysis and psychotherapy in Yugoslavia, and to the work of humanist Marxist philosophers and social scientists gathered around Yugoslavia's dissident Praxis group.

The film which articulated the director's belief in the close relationship between politics and psychotherapy most forcefully was also his most well-known, and the last one he was allowed to make in socialist Yugoslavia—*WR: Mysteries of the Organism*.[46] In it, the leading personalities of the psychoanalytic movement, Sigmund Freud and Wilhelm Reich (the *WR* from the film's title), are explicitly linked to the Yugoslav revolutionary project (as well as other Communist experiments around the world), while psychiatric and psychotherapeutic practices and theories become symbols for both political authoritarianism/totalitarianism and emancipatory revolutionary politics. *WR* offered the sharpest and most articulate critique of ossified bureaucratism, dogmatism and Communist cults of personality, but also made dangerous and provocative connections not only between Yugoslav and Soviet versions of socialism, but also between different forms of political authoritarianism in Communism, fascism and US militarism.[47]

Unsurprisingly, the film initiated a heated and polarised political discussion in Yugoslavia as soon as it was released. Even though it premiered at the Cannes Festival to great international acclaim and some positive domestic reviews, and subsequently went on to receive several major international awards, its Yugoslav license to be screened in cinemas was quickly revoked, amid increasingly loud complaints that the film offended both

[46] *WR: Misterije organizma*, 1971, dir. Dušan Makavejev.

[47] See Lorraine Mortimer, *Terror and Joy: The Films of Dušan Makavejev*, Minneapolis: University of Minnesota Press, 2009.

the Communist revolution in Yugoslavia and the image of the Soviet Union. As a result of the sustained pressure from the Association of the veterans of the Second World War (SUBNOR), which declared *WR* a veritable 'political diversion', the film received an administrative ban two months after its release. In the next sixteen years, the film was not available to Yugoslav audiences—for instance, it was not included in the programme of the 1971 Pula Film Festival—but its themes, artistic strategies and political messages were still widely debated in the press and in many grassroots political organisations, so that its ban paradoxically reinforced its public presence and visibility. In many ways, the film marked a significant change in the cultural politics of the Communist Party of Yugoslavia, as its ban announced a symbolic victory of a much more rigid and restrictive approach to the Black Wave cinema.[48]

This incredibly complex film consists of several wildly different yet related thematic strands, which Makavejev combined in a provocative montage in order to create a 'network of cross-references, associations, and above all contradictions'. As both Pavle Levi and James Roy MacBean have noted, Makavejev's use of montage as a technique primarily aimed to destabilise and call into question what might have appeared as established truths, and to offer an array of alternative directions and interpretations for his films' core themes, ideas and affects.[49]

The film is a homage of sorts to Wilhelm Reich, one of Freud's erstwhile collaborators and an exceptionally controversial Marxist psychoanalytic thinker, whose refusal to conform fully to the precepts of any of the broader ideological or disciplinary movements he belonged to—such as the psychoanalytic profession or the Communist Party—made him particularly appealing as a symbol of ideological freedom and independence. For Wilhelm Reich, the issue of suppression of individual sexuality held foremost political significance, as an ideological and sociological tool for protecting the interest and dominance of the ruling class. It followed from this, then, that an open and unmitigated expression of mature sexuality was the only strategy for undoing both individual and societal authoritarian and class structures, and for achieving personal (political) liberation. Makavejev broadly subscribed to Reich's theories

48 Radina Vucetic, *Monopol na istinu: Partija, kultura i cenzura u Srbiji sezdesetih i sedamdesetih godina XX veka*, Belgrade: Clio, 2016, 292–299.

49 James Roy MacBean, 'Sex and Politics: Wilchelm Reich, World Revolution, and Makavejev's WR', *Film Quarterly*, 1972, 25:3, 2–13; Levi, *Disintegration in Frames.*

of sexual repression and illiberalism as the core causes of political deviation and authoritarianism, and used Reichian language to explore the issue of personal freedom, happiness and fulfilment in revolutionary societies.[50] While Reich arguably had few open followers among Yugoslav psychotherapists, the Yugoslav psychiatric and psychoanalytic profession as a whole shared a lot with the radical psychotherapy movement (as discussed in Chapter 3), whose core principles were inspired by Reich and other Freudo-Marxist thinkers. Moreover, *WR* featured Freud himself quite prominently and explored the overall importance of psychoanalysis for Communist revolutions and their promise of individual happiness and emancipation. In other words, this film outlines most explicitly the close relationship between the 'psy' disciplines and political praxis (and ideology) and argues for the importance of psychotherapeutic and psychoanalytic principles for understanding humans as fundamentally political beings.

In a very important strand of his montage, Makavejev uses a 1946 Soviet film *The Pledge*, which depicts Stalin in a triumphalist and monumental style, and subversively intercuts Stalin's fictional monologues about the success of the Bolshevik revolution with different kinds of footage, most notably with highly distressing scenes from a Nazi documentary about psychiatric hospital patients. As Stalin lectures about the USSR's inauguration of the bright new socialist order, we see a nurse tube-feeding an unconscious (most probably medicated) psychiatric patient; Stalin eventually returns on the screen continuing with his pledge to follow the ideological legacies of Lenin, but this is followed by an even more gruesome scene of a helpless restrained psychiatric patient experiencing what was evidently an extremely painful and distressing application of ECT. In this montage, Stalin appears as the symbol of Soviet political authoritarianism and of the quashed revolutionary promises, but these associations are depicted through references to psychiatric abuse and violence. For Makavejev, oppressive psychiatric systems of practice and theory—in which patients are stripped of rights and input, and cannot participate in their own recovery as autonomous and free agents—serve as perfect metaphors for political totalitarianism as a whole.

This link between repressive psychiatric and political practices is multifaceted and could be read in an even more damning light: abusive 'psy'

[50] Mortimer, *Terror and Joy: The Films of Dušan Makavejev*, 160–161.

disciplines produce citizens accustomed to absolute obedience and incapable of attaining revolutionary consciousness. This was, as we saw in Chapter 3, one of the core concerns of Yugoslav socialist psychiatry and psychotherapy, which was founded on the idea that a successful political revolution would be fatally undermined by a counter-revolutionary, dogmatic and authoritarian psychiatric discipline. In that sense, for both Makavejev and Yugoslav psychotherapists, psychiatry had a particularly important political role to play. As in this particular montage, an illiberal psychiatry served to reinforce a repressive regime in a fundamental way and sabotaged a genuine revolution of consciousness by preventing patients from using therapy to achieve self-knowledge and personal development. Although the psychiatric documentary footage which Makavejev uses comes from a Nazi film-maker, it immediately evokes the international concerns raised at this time about the abusive potential of Soviet psychiatry and its central role in implementing punitive policies against prominent dissidents. The suggested ideological closeness between Soviet communism and fascism/Nazism (and their respective psychiatric professions) is constructed in other ways in the same montage sequence: as Stalin walks, Nazi flags unfurl under his feet, and the added soundtrack is the well-known German song *Lili Marlene*, which became very popular among Axis soldiers in the Second World War and was commonly played on the Nazi-controlled Radio Belgrade (and other Nazi propaganda radio stations).

The relationship between broader political structures, individual psychological profiles and personal fulfilment is further explored in the film's highly entertaining fictional strand, in which a young Yugoslav Reichian revolutionary attempts to develop a romantic and sexual relationship with an exemplary Soviet citizen and ice-skating champion Vladimir Illich. When we first meet Milena, she is deeply frustrated by the regressive sexual and gender politics of the Yugoslav revolutionary proletariat (and the Yugoslav state). She famously proclaims that 'the October Revolution failed when it rejected free love', and that socialism 'must not exclude sensual pleasures from its programme'. Moreover, sexual abstinence is not only unhealthy and unnatural, Milena lectures her gathered neighbours and fellow workers, it is also 'counter-revolutionary'. In her flat, which she shares with her sexually liberated friend Jagoda, photographs of Freud and Reich take up central positions, and both thinkers appear to look with pleasure and approval upon Milena's revolutionary proclamations, and some very joyful sexual activity between Jagoda and a young military man.

Milena's Reichian revolutionary beliefs come to a test when she attempts to influence Vladimir and encourage him to explore passion and sensual love. For his part, Vladimir is a fairly card-board character, mouthing Stalin's and Lenin's words and Soviet political slogans. Very early on in Milena and Vladimir's budding relationship, Jagoda asks him about Soviet views on personal happiness; as a Reichian would expect, Vladimir appears deeply confused by this notion, and finally says that 'there is no difference between personal happiness and the happiness of the entire people and the state', the Soviet Union reportedly 'abolished that difference'. The misunderstanding between the Yugoslav Reichians and the model citizen from the USSR only deepens from here on, as it becomes clear that Vladimir Illich (Lenin?) cannot conceive of a psychological or sensual existence of an individual outside the collective and its rigorous norms.

This caricature of Soviet totalitarianism serves to emphasise the Freudo-Marxist critique of state socialism in the USSR, but also to argue that the roots of this political deviation of the Bolshevik revolution are to be found in individual psyches and their stunted development. In the film's extraordinary finale, Vladimir Illich uses his ice skate to behead Milena in the course of a passionate sexual encounter, as he is unable to control this unexpected outburst of sexual energy and to prevent it from turning into lethal violence. Illich—who, in the film, mouths Lenin's own words about the dangerous effects of music, passion and emotions on the 'nerves' and political commitment of a revolutionary—cannot escape his repressive psychological framework, and his sexual rigidity and illiberalism translate into aggression, irresistible proclivity to authoritarianism in personal relationships as well as extreme political intolerance. Immediately before the beheading, as Illich completes his condemnation of music, human warmth and kindness in favour of political violence, the film cuts back to *The Pledge* and Stalin's peroration in Lenin's honour—the film thus arguably draws a sign of equality between the legacies of Lenin and Stalin, reflecting on the inability of either Leninism or Stalinism to accommodate true personal sexual liberation and related political emancipation. Importantly, the excerpt which shows Stalin celebrating Lenin is immediately followed by another distressing image of a psychiatric patient:

political authoritarianism and oppression are inextricably linked to mental illness and psychological breakdown.

Milena seems like a perfect illustration of Reich's conclusion that 'sexually awakened women, affirmed as such, would mean the complete collapse of the authoritarian ideology' because male patriarchal supremacy and enslavement of women remained the foundation of any authoritarian social and political regime.[51] In her struggle to reform the mentality of both 'backward' Yugoslav proletariat and a representative of the Soviet state socialist model, Milena embodies the idea, proposed as well by the Yugoslav psychotherapeutic community at the time, that a genuine revolution along the lines of workers' self-management is impossible without a prior revolution in people's minds, their family structures and sexuality. 'You love all of mankind', says Milena to Vladimir, 'but you are incapable of loving... one single living creature...you are as lovely as a revolution, you told me, but you couldn't endure being touched by that same "revolution"'. In the end, Makavejev concludes that the 'psy' disciplines are the most important companions of any truly humanist Marxist revolution—a conclusion he clearly shared with the Yugoslav psychotherapeutic profession and with radical psychotherapeutic communities and associations around the Western world. For Makavejev, just like for the country's mental health clinicians, any Marxist revolutionary project started with a re-definition of the notion of an ideal socialist citizen and a radical reformation of the population's authoritarian and repressive psychological structures and dispositions.

According to Pavle Levi, Makavejev's films explored the relationship between individual freedom and institutionalised/socialised forms of repression not only through their content, but also engaged with these issues in innovative ways through their very cinematic form. Makavejev's unique approach to montage—the effect of 'overlapping shapes'—introduced interpretive uncertainty and placed his viewer in the position of a free creative subject, who chose his or her ideological and intellectual alignments and autonomously produced the films' artistic and ideological 'truth' in the context of a plurality of possible meanings and story lines. As Levi remarked, Makavejev's films brought together a complex and often incoherent variety of images, soundtracks and ideas

[51] Wilhelm Reich, *The Mass Psychology of Fascism*, Farrar, Straus and Giroux, 1980, 107.

and supplied viewers with bewildering juxtapositions, emotional associations and intellectual contradictions, precisely in order to invite them to engage productively with the cinematic content based on their own beliefs, experiences and prejudices.[52] In that way, the director encouraged the 'viewer to define his or her own position vis-à-vis this ideological bundle', and conceived of the viewer 'as precisely that individual whose complete freedom he [advocated]'.[53] This constituted a true 'cinematic critique of ideology', and achieved a democratic 'destabilisation' of cinematic or ideological meanings, preventing any possibility of singular or straightforward interpretations.[54] For Levi, this approach aimed to create a completely different kind of spectator based on a new model of political citizenship, and was in line with the ideological project of Yugoslavia's most significant (and internationally renowned) political dissident group, Praxis.

The Praxis group mainly consisted of young sociologists, anthropologists and philosophers from the Universities of Belgrade and Zagreb, who engaged in political and philosophical critique of the Yugoslav socialist realities and drew inspiration from Karl Marx's early humanist writings.[55] For Praxis intellectuals, as we will see in the final section of this chapter, the core aim in reforming the deficiencies of Yugoslav socialist institutions and their dogmatism was the creation of autonomous creative individuals, who could avail themselves of unfettered freedom of activity and expression: 'freedom is possible only when man is truly the subject, the *creator*, of his own fate, and not a mere object over which power is exercised', wrote one of Praxis's leading philosophers Ljubomir Tadić. A political alternative to the government of autocratic 'reified bureaucracy' was only attainable through a 'consciousness of man's real power and ability to shape the conditions of his personal existence and the forces that threaten to engulf him'. Moreover, every individual's fulfilment and realisation of their own needs and potentials were only possible through

[52] Levi, *Disintegrating in Frames*, 29–35.

[53] Ibid., 31.

[54] Ibid., 31.

[55] Mihailo Markovic, 'Marxist Philosophy in Yugoslavia: The *Praxis* Group', in R.T. De George and J.P. Scanlan, eds, *Marxism and Religion in Eastern Europe*, Fribourg and Munich: Sovietica, 1976, vol. 36, 63–89.

such free and creative praxis, through which both the world and citizens could be transformed and revolutionised.[56]

In Levi's reading, Makavejev's montage technique requires viewers to become precisely such free creative subjects. In that way, his films became part of Praxis' humanist revolutionary project (and *praxis*), and they also served as an important thematic link between the political project of the Yugoslav socialist 'psy' sciences and the dissident group's theoretical outlook, effectively combining the two groups' preoccupations and interpretive frameworks. As we will see below, the ideological aims of Praxis intellectuals had a lot in common with the Yugoslav psychotherapeutic and psychoanalytic profession's understanding of their own tasks and societal roles. Just like Makavejev's films and Yugoslav psychoanalysts, Praxis discussions focused on the importance of revolutionising and transforming the human psyche as a fundamental step towards achieving a democratic Marxist society and fulfilling the promise of workers' self-management, and they engaged with psychoanalytic and psychotherapeutic concepts in order to formulate their critique of political authoritarianism and repressiveness.

Praxis Intellectuals and Their Critique of the Revolution

By the 1960s and 1970s, therefore, this radical discourse of freedom, creativity and individual self-realisation spread beyond the artistic circles, and came to inspire the philosophy of those dissidents and critics of Yugoslav realities who emphasised the failures and insufficiencies of reform Communism. Yugoslavia's fairly pluralistic socialist system was nevertheless vulnerable to authoritarian political turns and decisions of the Party and state elites. But this dynamic and changing society also bred new, highly politicised intellectual elites, who, encouraged by the reformist impulses of the 1960s, began to shed critical light on the actual achievements and applications of the self-managing system, and paid particular attention to the theme of individual freedoms, alienation, self-realisation and emancipation. In the summer of 1968, Yugoslavia was

[56] Ljubomir Tadić, 'Bureaucracy—Reified Organization', in Mihailo Markovic and Gajo Petrovic, eds, *Praxis: Yugoslav Essays in the Philosophy and Methodology of the Social Sciences*, Dordrecht: D. Reidel, 1979, 297.

shaken by widespread student protests, which clamoured against the 'red bourgeoisie' and the degeneration of socialist self-management.[57]

But several years before that, a number of distinguished intellectuals inspired by the 'new left', critical theory and Sartre's existentialism, formed a unique political dissident group—Praxis—which sharply criticised new forms of alienation and political hierarchies emerging in socialist and self-managing Yugoslavia.[58] Throughout the 1960s and 1970s, members of the Praxis group shook the political and social scene in Yugoslavia with their daring analyses of early Marxian writings, and their calls for the emergence and development of a fully autonomous and politically engaged public opinion in Yugoslavia. They insisted on the possibility of developing a genuinely democratised and humane Marxist community, which would extend to all its members a full opportunity for their complete realisation as human beings. Even more importantly, the core Praxis discussions focused on defining the social and political obstacles to this humanistic development, such as the authoritarianism and hierarchical nature of the overly bureaucratised Yugoslav socialist state and Communist Party.[59] The Praxis' philosophical elaborations of the conditions for the social creation of a fully emancipated Marxist citizen corresponded to an enormous extent to the project that Yugoslav psychoanalysts were setting up for themselves. These emerging critical political discourses were often stimulated by psychiatric and psychoanalytic writings on the creation of a free, liberated socialist individual. Indeed, the language of Yugoslavia's Europeanised child psychiatrists and psychoanalysts resembled the political symbolic and rhetoric of the Praxis group in particular.

The Praxis group opposed the orthodox Marxists' exclusive focus on the theories of surplus value and historical materialism, and proposed instead that the oft dismissed humanistic element was key to understanding Marx's philosophy. The Praxis project thus aimed to recuperate this humanist strand and to re-define Marxism as the 'philosophy of man,'

[57] Calic, *Geschichte Jugoslawiens im 20. Jahrhunert*, 286–292; Madigan Fichter, 'Yugoslav Protest: Student Rebellion in Belgrade, Zagreb, and Sarajevo in 1968', *Slavic Review*, 2016, 75:1, 99–121.

[58] Oskar Gruenwald, *The Yugoslav Search for Man: Marxist Humanism in Contemporary Yugoslavia*, South Hadley: Bergin and Garvey Publishers, 1983.

[59] Rudi Supek, 'Some Contradictions and Insufficiencies of Yugoslav Self-Managing Socialism', in Markovic and Petrovic, eds, *Praxis*, 249–272.

centred around the notion of praxis as a 'universal, free, creative and self-creative activity', and a sole way for humans to achieve and maximise their internal creative potential. Most importantly, Praxis intellectuals called for a persistent and permanent constructive critique of all the emerging socialist institutions in Yugoslavia, inviting citizens to reflect on 'the complex question of a suitable form of a social, economic and political system which would enable man with certain intrinsic potential to reach the highest level of self-realization'.[60] What they faced in the Yugoslav context was a rather underdeveloped agricultural society, in the midst of fast-paced industrialisation and urbanisation led by an authoritarian, top-down modernising Communist bureaucracy.

Importantly, Praxis discussions zoomed in on the failings and deficiencies of the Yugoslav self-managing system. As one of the group's most prominent members, Gajo Petrović, observed, even in those states 'where there were efforts to realize a genuinely human society, the inherited forms of inhumanity were not defeated and deformations emerged that did not exist earlier'.[61] In its internationally acclaimed journal and a series of very popular summer schools, Praxis was determined to define and analyse the social and political obstacles to this humanistic development in Yugoslavia: key among such obstacles were the authoritarianism and hierarchical nature of the overly bureaucratised Yugoslav socialist state and Communist Party. Moreover, Praxis philosophers certainly had a lot to say about the psychological underpinnings of revolutionary activity, as well as about possible counter-revolutionary affinities of an unreformed national psyche: 'The traditional collective psychological disposition to glorify, to adore, to be always ready for a new myth and a new cult of personality should be replaced by an attitude of criticism and resistance ... to any authoritarian pattern of behaviour'.[62] For Praxis intellectuals, it was precisely those conditions that the new generation of child psychoanalysts identified as supremely pathogenic in the family context which could actually cripple human beings in a political sense and arrest their development as democratic citizens. These dissident Marxists emphasised

[60] Ziga Vodovnik, 'Democracy as a Verb: New Meditations on the Yugoslav Praxis Philosophy', *Journal of Balkan and Near Eastern Studies*, 2012, 14:4, 433–452.

[61] Gajo Petrovic, 'Cemu Praxis?', *Praxis: Filozofski casopis*, September 1964, I:1, 3.

[62] Mihailo Marković, 'Human Nature and Present Day Possibilities of Social Development', in Paul Kurtz and Svetozar Stojanović (eds), Tolerance and Revolution, Belgrade: Philosophical Society of Serbia, 1970, 101.

the need to tear down the distinctions between state and civil society, and to replace the alienated conditions of bureaucratised socialism (rigid state and party structures) with self-managing institutions. In this process, the main enemy would be the mentality of obedience and absolute compliance to authorities, fostered in Yugoslavia's political culture according to Praxis, as well as in the country's overly patriarchal families according to child psychoanalysts.

One of the most important—and lasting—legacies of the Praxis project was its exceptional international intellectual network of stellar collaborators, contributors and followers. Some of Europe's most prominent left-wing and critical theory intellectuals, such as Erich Fromm, Herbert Marcuse, Gyorgy Lukacs, Jürgen Habermas, Leszek Kolakowski, became regular contributors to Praxis's philosophical journal and participated in the increasingly internationally renowned Korcula summer school (1966–1974). Herbert Marcuse and Erich Fromm in particular became frequent guests of the Praxis project, with Marcuse playing an extremely important role in the summer school's ambitious theoretical and philosophical work.[63] The intellectual profile of these reputed participants sheds some light on the role of psychoanalysis in Praxis' philosophical discussions: Marcuse's and Fromm's interest in the interrelationship between Marxism and psychoanalysis affected Praxis' own understanding of humanist Marxism to an important extent. Throughout the 1960s and 1970s, Yugoslav Praxis intellectuals debated the importance of Freud's philosophy for furthering the revolutionary project of European and Yugoslav socialism, and for Marxist liberation of the individual. In that sense, through Marcuse, Fromm and their Yugoslav followers, psychoanalysis remained one of the focal points of the new left in Yugoslavia.

While this was often a divisive point, with critical voices questioning Freud's place alongside Marx, Hegel or Nietzsche in the pantheon of great European thinkers, Praxis intellectuals remained deeply interested in the potential of psychoanalysis to contribute to the development of a vision of a 'non-repressive civilisation', and to provide both psychological and philosophical guidance on the subject of revolutionising the stifling bourgeois society and overcoming alienation.[64] In Praxis discussions, the

[63] Filip Kovacevic, 'Marcuse in Yugoslavia', *Radical Philosophy Review*, 2013, 16:1, 205–222.

[64] Danilo Pejovic, 'Filozofija i psihoanaliza (epilogue)', in Herbert Marcuse, ed., *Eros i civilizacija*, Zagreb: Naprijed, 1965, 227.

notion of the ultimate liberation of human creative potentials in a free society rid of (political and psychological) repression was tied up with psychoanalytic ruminations.[65] Consequently, there were close personal connections and overlaps between Praxis and the psychoanalytic profession—Nevenka Tadić and one of Praxis's most prominent philosophers Ljubomir Tadić were married to each other, for instance, and a number of intellectuals, such as Zagorka Pesic, Vladimir Jakovljević, Nevenka Tadić, straddled the two camps, combining psychoanalytic, anthropological and sociological insights in their research.[66]

Moreover, as Branislav Jakovljević claims in his study of the effects of the theory of self-management on cultural and artistic practices, 'part of the reason Marcuse and other reformist Marxists kept coming to Korčula was that in Yugoslavia their ideas were not confined to street protests, but had at least some chance of filtering up to the highest levels of institutional politics'.[67] Among other things, the above-described activist psychoanalysis was one such direct link between intellectual work and high politics, and, along with the theories of alienation and self-management, constituted an 'avenue of this traffic between critical theory and state politics'.[68] Socialist Yugoslavia may have been the only country in Europe (and even the world) in which the liberation politics of psychoanalysis overcame the narrow confines and limited social impact of philosophical texts, and became everyday clinical practice, supported by the state's core political principles (and funding).

Reflecting on the relationship between the political turmoil in the 1960s and psychoanalysis, Vojin Matić echoed Praxis philosophers by criticising the Yugoslav society for its reported preservation of 'niches of coercion': in their own niche (and family was certainly one of them), everyone was allowed to terrorise their subordinates and to live his or her dictatorial potentials/fantasies while the supposedly self-managing society

65 Branka Brujic, 'Moze li se Frojdovom meta-psihologijom utemeljiti povjesnu buducnost', *Nase Teme*, June 1966, 6, 1125–1137.

66 Zagorka Pesic-Golubovic, 'Vladimir Jakovljević (1925–1958)', 6–7; Pesic-Golubovic, 'Culture as a Bridge Between Utopia and Reality', in Markovic and Petrovic, eds, *Praxis*, 167–186.

67 Branislav Jakovljević, *Alienation Effects: Performance and Self-Management in Yugoslavia, 1945–1991*, Ann Arbor: University of Michigan Press, 2016, 120.

68 Ibid.

remained blind. In Matić's opinion, it was within families that violent societal structures needed to break first, in order for democratising tendencies to eliminate the psychological 'need for authority' and to enable the development of truly humanist Marxist individuals.[69] As we already saw in Chapter 2, Matić identified family as the bastion of state violence, which carried 'the greatest potential for violence', and traditionally produced conformist citizens, loyal members of the community who would never seriously challenge the authorities: 'the parent, as an elemental educator in conformism, is the person on whom the state can always rely'.[70] Drawing heavily on Marcuse's concept of 'surplus repression', Matić criticised the current state of affairs, in which 'parents start[ed] practising violence from the very birth [of the child]', and primarily relied on fear in their child-raising practices in order to 'raise the child in conformity with the demands of the authorities'.[71] Educated in such a repressive spirit, many people learnt to 'identify with the aggressor' in childhood, and were now experiencing a genuine 'fear of freedom' in the Frommian sense. 'Humanity was slowly recovering from state violence', Matić opined, as well as from 'moral masochism' and 'internal identification with the aggressor'—the core personality traits which made dictatorships and violent authoritarianisms possible, even necessary and supported by the population: 'Self-management is now starting to replace this identification with the aggressor, but many are still trying to abuse it, even unconsciously, to fulfil their lingering need for coercion'. Therefore, Matić offered self-management as a remedy of sorts for the pathologies of authoritarian personality.

Just like psychoanalysts regularly used explicitly political references and metaphors, some Praxis intellectuals adopted the language and concepts of the 'psy' disciplines to describe the goals and dangers of their vision of the path towards genuine socialism, and their arguments and concerns mirrored those of promoted by the progressive psychiatrists and psychoanalysts. University of Belgrade philosophy professor Ljubomir Tadić argued that any government's understanding of political power in exclusively Hobbesian terms constituted a veritable 'political pathology', and

[69] Matić, 'Izmene dinamike odnosa prema autoritetu i njene posledice u klinickoj psihologiji', *Psihologija*, 1977, 13:2, 9.

[70] Ibid., 9.

[71] Ibid., 8.

that this pathology was best expressed in the government's use of the concept of the 'masses', whose capacity for rational participation in public affairs was allegedly null.[72] As argued above, it was precisely this type of multifaceted and universal political participation of all citizens that Vojin Matić had in mind when he advised parents of his patients on how to raise children: as another Praxis philosopher clarified, 'a society is socialist to the extent that it opens possibilities for the free creative development of every man'.[73] Ljubomir Tadić similarly argued for a system which would advance the 'coming of age' of its citizens, and reject 'paternalistic guardianship', which had no place in a true socialist democracy.[74] Instead, Tadić claimed that any democratic Marxist society would need to respect the autonomy of the public opinion, and combine the ideals of a true community (solidarity, empathy, dignity) with unrestricted individual freedoms. This insistence on the communal ideal of the Greek polis as the right social context for developing unalienated and fully realised Marxist individuals also figured prominently in psychiatric and psychoanalytic discussions of the time.[75]

Perhaps unsurprisingly, the political turmoil around *Praxis* was reflected in psychiatric and psychotherapeutic debates. In her article on the problems of adolescence and family, Zagreb psychologist Martina Zmuc-Tomori described adolescents' roles and interventions in their families in overtly political terms, which strongly resonated with the turbulent 1960s and 1970s political developments in Yugoslavia. In fact, the adolescent was the revolutionary, someone who upset the hitherto predominant and settled value systems of the family, which Tomori argued was equivalent to a micro-society. Her article was published in 1974, when the conflict between the state and the Praxis group was coming to a head (in 1975, their journal was finally banned, while eight professors of the Belgrade University were forced to leave their positions), and in this context, the language Tomori chose to analyse the complex relationships within families was highly reminiscent of the political discussions

[72] Ljubomir Tadić, 'Moc, elite i demokratija', *Praxis*, 1970, 1:2, 71–74.

[73] Gerson Sher, *Praxis: Marxist Criticism and Dissent in Socialist Yugoslavia*, Bloomington: Indiana University Press, 1977, 129.

[74] Ljubomir Tadić, *Poredak i sloboda*, Belgrade: Kult, 1976, 76.

[75] Ibid., 286.

at hand. In the world of family psychoanalysis, it was in fact the rebellious and often repressed or harshly criticised adolescent who took up the social role played by Praxis—or by the student protesters of 1968—in the broader context. Tomori claimed that 'if we look at the family as a whole…we will understand that [the adolescent] transforms its dynamic completely. The adolescent is the carrier of new values within that whole. He persistently attempts to re-shape the existing system of power and dominance, the system which had already been balanced and confirmed in a family with pre-adolescent children'.[76] Therefore, frequent conflicts between parents and their adolescent children were not only normal, but were also fully understandable in terms of political power-sharing and negotiations. Moreover, one of the leading Slovene psychologists of the time Lev Milcinski argued that the adolescent's behaviour was bound to be much more shocking to the parents if they were 'firmly tied to the rigid patterns of the conventional society, and had already envisaged a place for their son or daughter in an institutionalised social structure'.[77] Similarly, one of the core sources of the adolescent's psychological conflicts was their disillusionment with their own parents, in whom they had once seen near gods.

In much the same way, one could add, the Praxis group expressed their own disillusionment with the formerly unassailable heroes of socialism, including Tito himself, the ultimate father figure, but also Marx and Lenin, who could now be criticised and revised in Praxis's academic meetings and writings. The peculiar language and value systems of Yugoslavia's psychoanalysis thus ultimately came to be tightly intertwined with critical discourses of humanist Marxism. As Tomori concluded, adolescents 'woke their families up from their ideological dormancy and remind them of some of their long forgotten principles'—just as Praxis and the protesting students reminded Yugoslavia's official Communist ideologues of some clearly forgotten principles of early Marxist humanism and ideals of individual emancipation. Finally, 'the adolescent could take a lot away from the family, but could give a lot to it as well', a warning, perhaps, to

[76] Matina Zmuc-Tomori, 'Problemi adolescencije i porodica', *Anali Zavoda za mentalno zdravlje*, 1974, 1, 171–177.

[77] Lev Milcinski, 'Psihiatricni pogledi na narkomanije', *Revija za kriminalistiko i kriminalogijo*, 1972, 3, 151–157.

the overly bureaucratised Yugoslav authorities to heed the voice of the rebels.[78]

* * *

'Psy' disciplines played an exceptionally important role in socialist Yugoslavia's non-medical discourses. Psychoanalytic, psychiatric and psychotherapeutic ideas spread beyond hospitals and consulting rooms, and informed a variety of social, cultural, artistic and political conversations in socialist Yugoslavia. In certain ways, this was not significantly different from how the theme of psychiatry, psychiatric care and psychiatric professions was depicted in mainly dissident literary and artistic production in the rest of the socialist bloc—the discipline and its institutions served to represent political oppression and authoritarianism, while the trope of psychiatric patients as the only free, creative and ethical persons, confined in a repressive and corrupt hospital, was regularly employed. In Yugoslavia as well, the theme of psychiatry and abusive psychiatrists was utilised to critique the corrupt (and dysfunctional) system of 'benign authoritarianism' and to question the sincerity of the state's promises of genuine workers' self-management and direct democracy. The theme of alcoholism and the psychiatric moral panic around it proved particularly conducive for such cinematographic and literary interpretations and processing. But the interrelationship between 'psy' disciplines and the broader socio-cultural sphere in Yugoslavia went beyond these references to psychiatry as a microcosm of political oppression, and psychoanalytic and psychotherapeutic concepts, techniques and paradigms also fundamentally informed a radical Marxist critique of the failures and shortcomings of the Yugoslav version of self-managing socialism. This happened in both artistic and political fields, as 'psy' disciplines provided the language as well as the overall interpretive conceptual framework to formulate an effective political and cultural criticism from the left of Yugoslavia's complex, overly 'bureaucratised' and authoritarian regime. Moreover, the section on Praxis also demonstrated that this relationship between 'psy' disciplines and the non-medical sphere was not unidirectional—it was not that psychoanalytic and psychotherapeutic concepts were merely used and re-contextualised by critical artists, film-makers or philosophers. Quite to the contrary, and as we already

[78] Tomori, 'Problemi adolescencije i porodica', 177.

saw in Chapter 3, 'psy' professional were also deeply engaged with some of the core political and ideological concerns inherent in a revolutionary Marxist society, and the most significant debates of critical Marxist sociology and political philosophy came to inform the psychoanalytic and psychotherapauetic language, theory and clinical practice. In that sense, Yugoslavia's 'psy' disciplines were far from apolitical—they developed into a dynamic and autonomous intellectual and professional field not because they managed to distance themselves from political influences but precisely because they viewed themselves as closely allied with the revolutionary and emancipatory political project. This reminds us that there were many ways in which mental health sciences could be 'politicised' in socialism, and a profound political influence of Marxism did not always mean political subjugation and manipulation.

CHAPTER 7

Epilogue: War Trauma and the Breakup of Yugoslavia

Yugoslavia's socialist psychiatry was indeed a rich and complex field; one which combined a large variety of theoretical approaches, engaged in brave forms of clinical experimentation and maintained a complicated and exciting network of international collaboration. However, the socialist period was marked by an important psychiatric absence—of any substantial discussions about 'war trauma' and psychological effects of the Second World War on Yugoslav soldiers and the civilian population. This was surprising for many reasons, not least because the Yugoslav population was exposed to extreme violence during the war, experiencing one of the most brutal occupation regimes in Nazi-controlled Europe and a bloody civil war. Moreover, the narrative of the Yugoslav people's immense suffering and courageous and ultimately victorious Communist-led resistance became the most important founding block of the socialist country's political identity, and the postwar regime's core legitimising strategy. Still, it transpired that a long and in-depth engagement with psychological consequences of such suffering did not necessarily boost the national narrative, which ultimately focused on triumph, perseverance and courage rather than distress and mental breakdown.

In 1971, Slovene psychiatrist Janko Kostnapfel spoke about the tasks and achievements of war psychiatry in peacetime and wartime at the Third Congress of Yugoslav medical doctors. In his introduction, he made a

A. Antić, *Non-Aligned Psychiatry in the Cold War*, Mental Health in Historical Perspective, https://doi.org/10.1007/978-3-030-89449-8_7

passing reference to the lingering psychological effects of the Second World War among his patients: 'Memories of the horrors of the last war are still very fresh. From our patients of younger and middle generations we often hear horrible stories about the war every day'. Kostnapfel concluded that this was not at all surprising, given that Yugoslavia lost about 10% of its prewar population, or about 1.7 million people: 'just that number tells us about the emotional difficulties of their surviving family members'.[1] What was surprising, however, was that Kostnapfel's reference was one of the very few mentions of any war-related emotional distress of the Yugoslav population among socialist psychiatrists. But even this extremely rare allusion to the problem was rather brief: Kostnapfel quickly moved on to discuss war psychiatry in more general terms, noting that the 'negative social consequences' of the war appeared to be much worse in the rest of the world. Despite this scarcity of information, Kostnapfel's presentation offered an important (and unprecedented) insight into the workings of Yugoslavia's postwar psychiatric clinics: they were reportedly inundated by traumatic narratives of the Second World War and by patients who were still experiencing severe war-related psychological distress.

But if that was the case, why wasn't there any public discussion of this pervasive issue? Why did Yugoslav psychiatrists not publish more on their research into the psychological consequences of the war and their approaches to therapy and healing? While these questions remain difficult to answer, it did appear that the socialist narrative of glorious war victory and subsequent revolutionary transformation did not easily incorporate individual and collective accounts of loss, suffering and psychological distress. Even though Yugoslavia's 'psy' professions were so systematically involved in transnational expert networks throughout the Cold War, the country played virtually no role in the international discussions on violence and traumatisation from the 1960s on, and in that respect, it was no different from the rest of the socialist bloc.

In the aftermath of WWII, Yugoslavia was a ravaged country: its human and material losses at the end of the war were higher than in any of the warring countries except for Poland and the USSR. Years of brutal occupation and an even more brutal civil war, fought on ethnic and ideological grounds, left the economy in ruins, so that the immediate

[1] Janko Kostnapfel, 'Rat i mir sa stanovista psihijatrije', *Zbornik III lekara Jugoslavije*, Ljubljana, 1971, 281–282.

postwar period was marred by the scarcity of basic foods, materials and housing options. Even more devastating than material destruction was the tremendous psychological impact of the war: there was hardly a family untouched by the mass murder and incarceration of civilians, and, well into the postwar, many were still waiting for information on their loved ones. Tens of thousands witnessed unprecedented crimes and cruelty.[2]

And yet, the country's flourishing psychiatric—and psychoanalytic—profession had little to say about possible long-term psychological effects of such extreme violence, personal loss and dislocation. At the first postwar Yugoslav neuropsychiatric congress in 1946, leading Croatian psychiatrist Bosko Niketić briefly acknowledged the immense psychological suffering ('much sadness, worry, uncertainty and fear') to which the country's population had been exposed, and enumerated the unspeakable atrocities many had witnessed—'mass shootings, hangings, slaughters... loss of almost all family members, and waging a resistance war in the most difficult circumstances imaginable'. Nevertheless, Niketić concluded his discussion of such harmful psychological disturbances and their possible consequences in the very next sentence, stating that, fortunately, the Yugoslav peoples had 'persevered in their struggle' despite this, and that all their mental anguish had been 'crowned'—and presumably cured—by the ultimate triumph of the anti-fascist forces.[3] Niketić and the other congress speakers then proceeded to discuss Yugoslavia's peacetime psychiatry and its future tasks.

To my knowledge, only two trauma-related issues were discussed for a brief period after the end of the war. Dr Nikola Nikolić, survivor of the infamous Ustasha concentration camp Jasenovac, published a book on the psychological and medical aspects of camp experiences based on his observations of his fellow inmates and coined the term 'horrorosis' (*hororoze*) to indicate that a completely new diagnosis was needed to describe and

[2] Jozo Tomasevich, *War and Revolution in Yugoslavia, 1941–1945: Occupation and Collaboration*, Stanford: Stanford University Press, 2001, 744. Although figures remain contested, total human losses are taken to exceed 1,5 million in the entire country (Bogoljub Kocovic, *Zrtve Drugog svetskog rata u Jugoslaviji*, London: Nase Delo, 1985, 172–180). The Yugoslav Reparations Commission estimated material losses at over 9 billion US dollars, which included over 20% of residential housing destroyed or heavily damaged, around 60% of livestock killed or plundered, and over 19 million tons of grain and other crop taken out of the country between 1941and 1945 (Tomasevich, *War and Revolution in Yugoslavia*, 715).

[3] Bosko Niketić, 'Otvaranje konferencije', *Narodno zdravlje*, 1946, 2:3, 4–5.

understand the effects of such brutal torture and incarceration.[4] Nikolić's concept of unique Yugoslav psychoses and neuroses did not catch on, and its discussion largely remained limited to his manuscript.

On the other hand, another specifically Yugoslav illness did receive more sustained public, political and psychiatric attention, because it affected the military. Towards the end of the war, the resistance army was plagued by an unnerving and mysterious phenomenon, referred to as 'partisan neurosis' or 'partisan hysteria', which required collaboration with psychiatrists and psychotherapists knowledgeable about the concept of 'war trauma'.[5] The Yugoslav form of soldiers' neurosis was soon discussed in terms of national and ideological exceptionalism: most psychiatrists and military doctors who encountered it defined it as a uniquely Yugoslav psychological disorder, fundamentally different from instances of battle exhaustion and anxiety common in the British and US armies. It was only diagnosed in Communist resistance soldiers and was indeed the opposite of battle fatigue or any kind of demoralisation: 'partisan hysteria' was not an expression of the soldiers' desire to withdraw from the frontlines (it only appeared at the very end of the war, once the most dangerous and deadliest battles had been finished), but in fact reflected the affected partisans' exceptional commitment to their war tasks, their heightened willingness to fighting. The new disorder consisted of violent and potentially harmful epileptiform seizures which simulated wartime battles and attacks. The seizures could occur at any moment and under any circumstances, usually when there was audience—in the middle of a conversation, at lectures or meetings, while driving or riding a car, in front of superiors, for example.[6] Two of Yugoslavia's leading interwar psychiatrists and psychoanalysts, Hugo Klajn and Stjepan Betlheim, were charged with running a clinic specialised for the mentally distressed partisan soldiers in the former psychiatric hospital in Kovin, in northern Serbia. This experiment ended quite quickly and unceremoniously, as Klajn and Betlheim could not handle the reportedly aggressive

[4] Nikola Nikolic, *Jasenovacki logor smrti*, Zagreb: Nakladni Zavod Hrvatske, 1948.

[5] For a more detailed analysis of partisan hysteria, see Antic, *Therapeutic Fascism*, chapter 5.

[6] Hugo Klajn, *Ratna neuroza Jugoslovena*.

and increasingly unruly behaviour of their patients, many of whom refused to obey authority or even give up their weapons and wartime mores.[7]

Given its public, performative and highly disruptive character, 'partisan hysteria' attracted a lot of attention at the end of the war, and 1945 saw a flurry of psychiatric publications on the topic, including by Klajn and Betlheim, as well as a host of military doctors and psychiatrists. But after this initial surge of psychiatric (and political) interest, the theme of 'partisan hysteria' all but disappeared from psychiatric journals and monographs. Klajn's book on the topic was shelved for ten years (considered suspicious for its 'Freudianism' but arguably also because it zoomed in on severe psychological disorders and emotional difficulties of members of the victorious and heroic resistance army), and only came out in 1955, by which time Klajn had left clinical practice.[8] In 1957, a group of Zagreb-based psychiatrists, led by Betlheim, conducted a follow-up study of wartime neurotic patients, aiming to inquire into their adaptation to civilian life in the course of ten or so years after the end of the war. The psychiatrists concluded that in the majority of cases the former partisans had suffered from 'superficial neurosis' that did not harm deeper layers of their personality, and consequently they faced no larger problems reintegrating into the postwar society.[9]

In other words, 'partisan hysteria' did not seem to have left any deeper wounds in Yugoslav society: the former neurotics apparently shed their neurotic condition fairly quickly and were able to adapt to the peacetime circumstances without major disturbances. Kostnapfel reiterated this view, dedicating three sentences to this major challenge for postwar psychiatry, and concluding that only 1% of Yugoslav soldiers had succumbed to neurosis in 1945.[10] By the end of the 1950s, 'partisan hysteria' was thus completely cured, and it was reportedly far from a widespread phenomenon to begin with. There consequently appeared no reason to think of Yugoslav partisans in terms of war trauma or psychological distress.

[7] Betlheim and Lerotic, *Stjepan Betlheim: Radovi, pisma, dokumenti*, 12.

[8] Eduard Klain, 'Uspomene Prof. Dr Huga Klajna na njegovie prve kontakte sa psihoanalizom', *Psihoterapija*, 1999, 29, 217–221.

[9] Stjepan Betlheim et al., 'Adaptacija ratnih neurotika', *VSP*, 1957, 9, 508–509.

[10] Kostnapfel, 'Rat i mir sa stanovista psihijatrije', 283–284.

In 1947, both Nikolić and Niketić recognised the need for a new social psychiatry to help Yugoslavs make sense of the extraordinary deprivations, grief and agony caused by the war. Although, as we saw, Yugoslavia did develop a formidable discipline of social psychiatry, this profession largely focused on other issues and did not fulfil the mission set out for it at this early meeting. However, Yugoslavia's postwar psychiatrists unfortunately got another opportunity to engage with the problem of war-related psychological stress in their clinical practice.

In the late 1980s, Yugoslavia went through a series of political and economic crises, as the political leaderships from its six republics attempted to agree on a plan to reform and reimagine the federation. In 1990, both Slovenia and Croatia held national referenda at which a vast majority voted in favour of independence. Bosnia's independence referendum followed in 1992 with similar results. In the spring and summer of 1991, a series of conflicts broke out between the local Slovene and Croat territorial defence and police units on one side, and the Yugoslav People's Army on the other. The Yugoslav People's Army, which intervened to prevent secession, increasingly came under the influence of the Serbian political leadership, quickly lost its multi-ethnic character and was pitted against the other republics. In Croatia and Bosnia, the local Serbian populations refused to accept the referendum results and, encouraged and supported by the Serbian leadership, staged armed rebellions.[11] On Bosnian soil, this turned into a brutal conflict, in which the Bosnian Serb army in particular targeted non-Serb civilians with some of the most gruesome forms of violence, including the first genocide on the European territory since the end of the Second World War.[12] The wars of Yugoslav secession generated hundreds of thousands of civilian refugees and displaced persons—Bosnian Muslim civilians headed to relative safety in Croatia, Croats from the Serb-dominated territories were forced to leave their homes and find alternative accommodation, while a large number of Croatian Serbs were expelled to Serbia at the end of the conflict.

Yugoslav psychiatrists on all warring sides were by no means passive observers as they witnessed the violent breakup of their country in

[11] For more information, see Baker, *The Yugoslav Wars of the 1990s*, Basingstoke: Palgrave Macmillan, 2015.

[12] Lara Nettelfield and Sarah Wagner, *Srebrenica in the Aftermath of Genocide*, Cambridge: Cambridge University Press, 2014.

1991–1995. As they worked to help restore the psychological health of thousands of civilians and combatants who had experienced (or inflicted) unspeakable horrors, they were the sole generation of European psychiatrists who engaged with the problem of 'war trauma' twice in their professional careers.

In 1993, Belgrade's flagship Institute for Mental Health marked its thirtieth anniversary under less than auspicious circumstances. On that occasion, one of its leading psychiatrists Jovan Bukelić noted that the Institute was first established with the help and support of the Yugoslav WWII veterans' associations 'in order to help soldiers from the Second World War get over their invisible but grave psychological wounds'.[13] Bukelić thus explicitly linked the Institute to the psychiatric challenges of the Second World War, and, moreover, established a direct relationship between the two conflicts fifty years apart, as he emphasised that 'history was repeating itself' and that the Institute was once again setting up centres for dealing with war-related stress and trauma all over Serbia. Importantly, the Institute's war-related origins had been rarely discussed in public throughout the socialist period, and it was not in any way obvious from its publications, research and clinical projects that its work had been focused on treating the Second World War's emotional and psychological aftermath. In the 1990s, however, Bukelić spoke about the 'holy duty' of psychiatrists to help cure the tragic effects of wars on vulnerable populations and effectively reformulated the Institute's mission in terms of its supposedly longstanding engagement with postwar trauma.[14]

In my interviews with Nevenka Tadić, Ksenija Kondic and Svetomir Bojanin in 2014, I asked each of them about their professional engagement with the concept of war traumatisation at the beginning of their careers in the 1950s and 1960s.[15] They all responded that this was not something that preoccupied them at the time, other than indirectly through their work with orphans homed in state institutions. But whenever I raised the issue of possible psychological effects of the Second World War on their patients, these experienced psychiatrists brought our conversations to the 1990s wars instead: it was then rather than in the

[13] Jovan Bukelic, 'Institut za mentalno zdravlje, 1963–1993', in Predrag Kaličanin et al., eds, *Stresovi Rata*, Belgrade: Institute za mentalno zdravlje, 1994, 13–20.

[14] Ibid., 19.

[15] Interviews with Nevenka Tadić, Svetomir Bojanin, Dusan Popovic and Ksenija Kondic, January–February 2014, Belrade, Serbia.

aftermath of 1945 that they were called on and had an opportunity to work on war-related emotional distress and psychological trauma among refugees, children, former soldiers, survivors of torture and imprisonment. This was also when socialist psychiatrists' interest in Klajn's and others' research on partisan neurosis resurged: the 1990s saw a continuation of the discussion of Yugoslav soldiers' neurosis from the 1940s, as Klajn's and Betlheim's work was recontextualised in the brutal circumstances of the wars of Yugoslav succession.

In the early 2000s, reflecting on his experience of working with Serbian refugees from Croatia who were forcibly mobilised upon their arrival in Serbia in 1995, a young Serbian psychoanalyst and psychiatrist Vladimir Jović referred admiringly to Klajn's rather sensitive and 'complex' writings. According to Jović, Klajn's explorations provided an invaluable guiding light for interpreting war trauma of the 1990s: 'Following the end of the recent wars [in Yugoslavia], military psychiatrists could say that Klajn's understanding of war neurosis was of tremendous help'.[16] Moreover, for the first time since the late 1940s, the Yugoslav psychiatric community now started considering the contributions of other participants in the post-WWII discussion about war trauma or 'partisan hysteria'. Klajn's nuanced and understanding analysis was juxtaposed with military psychiatrist Josip Dojc's much harsher take on the affected partisans' medical and moral status. As Jović reported, Dojč conceived of the war traumatised in rather narrow terms—as either 'hereditarily burdened' neurotics or malingerers. Instead of therapy, Dojc recommended 'most energetic disciplinary and pedagogical measures'.[17] For Jović and his colleagues, Klajn's interpretation certainly appeared much more relevant, not only because of its more empathetic approach but also because it primarily relied on psychoanalytic insights to make sense of the Yugoslav soldiers' mysterious condition. It was indeed so helpful that a 1994 edited volume on war psychiatry and psychotherapy, 'Stresses of War', inspired by Serbian psychiatrists' experiences of treating traumatised soldiers and survivors of the 1990s war, reprinted the most important sections of

[16] Vladimir Jović, 'Posttraumatski poremecaj u socijalnom i politickom kontekstu devedesetih', in Zeljko Spiric, ed., *Ratna psihotrauma srpskih veterana*, Belgrade: Udruženje boraca rata Republike Srbije od 1990. godine, 2008, 381.

[17] Ibid., 384.

Klajn's discussion of WWII partisan neurosis.[18] For the authors of the volume, parallels were obvious and self-explanatory.

In Croatia, leading psychiatrist and coordinator of the national mental health section during the 1990s war Eduard Klain published his reminiscences about Hugo Klajn on the occasion of the latter's death in 1996 and re-printed an interview he had conducted with the esteemed Belgrade psychoanalyst in 1975. In his recollections, Klain insisted on drawing direct parallels between 1945, when Hugo Klajn worked with Yugoslav partisan soldiers, and 1995, when Eduard Klain handled mental health difficulties of Croatian soldiers and other war-affected sections of the population. According to Klain, even though the two of them had to deal with very different types of government, 'neither regime considered working with war-traumatised soldiers with benevolence'.[19] In the immediate aftermath of WWII, Klajn was given ample resources to develop a specialised ward for partisan 'hysterics' and encouraged to practice psychoanalysis, but his resulting monograph—still a landmark study of war trauma in Eastern Europe—was published with a staggering ten-year delay, as it was not immediately approved by the ideological commission of the Communist Party's Central Committee. Klain proposed that the problem with the monograph was only partly in its 'Freudian' approach, which was ideologically questionable in 1945. The extreme political sensitivity of psychiatric work with victorious soldiers was an equally important issue: 'both then and today it was widely considered that our warriors were heroes who could not possibly have psychological difficulties'. Apparently hinting at his own more recent problems with the Croatian authorities, Klain added that 'people who used to stand for certain ideas... tend to change completely when they come to power'.[20] It is unclear whether Klain felt politically constrained in any way in his attempts to publish on Croatian soldiers' experiences of war trauma and its medical treatment, but his belief that his and Klajn's situations were comparable was truly striking, especially given the widely divergent ideological contexts of 1945 and 1995. In any case, Croatia's leading psychoanalytic journal *Psychotherapy* followed Eduard Klain's

[18] Bukelic, 'Prof. Dr Hugo Klajn: Ratna neuroza Jugoslovena', in Kaličanin et al., *Stresovi Rata*.

[19] Eduard Klain, 'Sjecanja na Huga Klajna', *Psihoterapija*, 1999, 29, 209–215.

[20] Ibid., 213.

piece and interview with Hugo Klajn with an English-language selection of excerpts from the latter's book. This was the first time the monograph was discussed in Yugoslav psychiatric literature since 1955, and the first time it had ever been translated into English for international audiences.

There were other, more concrete continuities between the 1940s and 1990s. It was not only that psychiatrists suddenly started discussing Yugoslav theories and research on the psychological effects of the Second World War. In some cases, WWII-related distress entered psychiatric encounters and consulting rooms much more directly and literally. In 1992, Vlado Jukić and Vasko Muacević presented the case of a 64-year old patient, whom they diagnosed with PTSD in December 1991, but the diagnosis was based on the patient's participation in the Second World War (as he did not take part in any military activities in 1991). Namely, he joined the partisan resistance army in 1941 and experienced a series of highly distressing events which included imprisonment, torture and mock execution. After that, the patient suffered from a number of psychological difficulties throughout the 1950s: 'insomnia, fear, anxiety… dark, depressive thoughts, forced memories of wartime horrors', etc. The most persistent symptom was a dream, in which the patient had to relive the mock execution. However, after intense psychotherapy in Zagreb, all these emotional struggles reportedly disappeared, only to get 'reactivated' 28 years later, when the war in Croatia began in the summer of 1991.[21]

According to Jukić's and Muacević's description, the dream was the first symptom to return, accompanied by familiar feelings of hopelessness, anxiety and 'betrayal'. Importantly, the psychiatrists emphasised the political aspect of this PTSD reactivation: the patient reported that he 'felt particularly bad when he looked at the former military barracks, which he used to visit in the past', but which now became the symbol of the Serb-controlled Yugoslav People's Army and its aggression against Croatia. The patient apparently also felt the need to emphasise that his renewed psychological distress did not come out of any 'nostalgia for the past, nor fear of the new non-communist authorities [in Croatia] (he used to be a communist, and head of the WWII veterans' association…)'.[22] These final political remarks served as a conclusion of sorts, as the authors added no

[21] Vlado Jukić and Vasko Muacevic, 'Posttraumatski stresni poremecaj', in Eduard Klain, ed., *Ratna psihologija I psihijatrija*, Zagreb: Glavni Sanitetski Stozer, 1992, 33.

[22] Ibid., 33–34.

further analysis to the case presentation. But the sense of psychiatric and diagnostic continuity between the two wars was striking: this patient's condition was seen as no different from any other instances of PTSD in soldiers who took part in the 1991 war (and in fact, his case presentation was preceded by a much more 'regular' case of a young active policeman who experienced 'combat stress reaction' following a close encounter with enemy soldiers)—it was only its exceptional 'chronicity' that set it apart. But in this way, the psychiatrists constructed the patient as a loyal Croatian partisan, who, even though he used to be a Communist and member of the old Yugoslav People's Army, was indeed no different than the Croatian patriots defending their state in 1991. The diagnosis of war trauma or, more universally, PTSD thus served to reconcile two different ideological poles within the Croat nation: the patient noted in the end that he was now the head of a new veteran association which included all Croatian soldiers, both partisans and homeguards, who fought on the Axis side in WWII.

The 1990s were also the first time Yugoslav psychiatrists and psychoanalysts spoke about the issue of transgenerational trauma originating in the Second World War. In particular, several authors emphasised the likely traumatisation of some high-ranking officers of the Federal Army, who had lived through extreme psychological distress as children in war-torn Croatia or Bosnia. For instance, Eduard Klain speculated about the destructive power of such 'transgenerational memories' of extreme violence, which could now be triggered and re-activated: 'surviving members of these groups have always remembered awful scenes of separation, such as the killing of their parents in front of their eyes, or the fierce dragging away [of] a child from his mother when she was taken to a concentration camp'.[23] Once such feelings and memories were transmitted within families or wider ethnic groups, they could become dangerous fuel for inter-ethnic hostilities, and a fertile ground for violent nationalist propaganda. For people living in Yugoslavia at the time, these were only thinly veiled references to the Serbs' collective memories of the Second World War Ustasha campaign against their community in the Independent State of Croatia, seeing as the 1980s and 1990s were marked by the Serbian political leadership's and intelligentsia's mobilisation and manipulation of precisely such memories and anxieties.

[23] Eduard Klain, 'Yugoslavia as a Group', *Croatian Medical Journal*, 1992, War Supplement 1, 11.

Importantly, psychiatrists now argued that that the traumatic experiences of WWII could not be irrelevant in the context of yet another armed conflict, and expected them to haunt Yugoslavs and their families. As Miro Jakovljevic noted in 1992, '[the notion of] massacre is in the collective memory of the Serbs, and therefore they are themselves inclined to committing massacres'.[24] Serbian psychiatrists agreed that a 'reactivation' of transgenerational traumatic memories in some Yugoslav citizens of Serbian ethnicity could lead to various psychopathological reactions, including aggressive behaviour.[25] In the immediate aftermath of WWII, however, such concerns were not aired publicly, nor were they in any way figuring in psychiatric or psychoanalytic professional debates.

War and Child Psychiatrists

As we have seen in Chapter 5, while Yugoslav child psychotherapists remained an extraordinarily active, productive and innovative profession throughout the socialist period, they did not have much to say about the psychological difficulties of children survivors of the Second World War. In the 1950s and 1960s, war orphans would occasionally receive some limited clinical attention as part of broader studies on the mental health of children who lived in collective accommodation. But after John Bowlby's notable WHO- and UN-funded exploration of the circumstances of Yugoslav children and orphans, and the war's effects on their mental health, the attention of the Yugoslav psychiatric and psychotherapeutic community shifted elsewhere, to different child populations and their peacetime problems.[26] As psychiatrist Nikola Vulf noted in 1994, the first systematic investigation of this topic was only contemplated in 1981, almost forty years after the end of the war, and even this was at the initiative of an American research organisation interested in a comparative study of European child survivors. This attempt did not materialise

[24] Miro Jakovljevic, 'Psychiatric Perspectives of the War Against Croatia', *Croatian Medical Journal*, 1992, War Supplement 2, 10–17.

[25] Milanko Čabarkapa, *Psiholoski faktori stresa u borbenim aktivnostima*, PhD Dissertation, University of Belgrade, 1996, 52.

[26] John Bowlby, 'Materinska briga za dijete i duševno zdravlje: prilog Svjetske zdravstvene organizacije programu Ujedinjenih nacija za zaštitu djece bez doma', Zagreb: Zastita Zdravlja, 1953.

immediately, and it was only in 1987 that Vulf began a process of identifying and interviewing Jewish child survivors of the Second World War in Yugoslavia.[27]

His clinical explorations, interviews and analysis were completed within two years, but the study was first published in Serbo-Croatian in the early 1990s, when the country was plagued by yet another war in which children were exposed to unspeakable brutality. In fact, Vulf's article appeared in a volume titled *Stresses of War*, which primarily focused on the psychological suffering of various groups of civilian victims in the 1990s, and headed a section on 'war trauma' in Serbian children in Croatia and Bosnia. Vulf himself emphasised that his research on WWII survivors was particularly important at that moment because 'lessons of the past could contribute to a better understanding of the current and future problems of the children affected by this awful and reckless war', as well as help predict what kinds of difficulties present-day children could experience as adults as a result of their wartime experiences.[28]

Overall, Vulf's conclusions were rather optimistic—most of his interviewees seemed to have adapted reasonably well to peacetime circumstances and managed to lead outwardly successful lives. But here again, the psychological trauma of the Second World War was described as in danger of being reawakened by the outbreak of violence in the 1990s. Vulf argued that his interviewees started re-experiencing a variety of psychological and somatic symptoms—nightmares, fear and anxiety—'under pressure of the current events and the civil war in our homeland'.[29] Bukelić noted this explicitly in his introduction to Vulf's article but chose to focus on Serbian rather than Jewish victims: 'war consequences for children from the Kozara mountain [where the Axis forces killed or sent to concentration camps thousands of Serbian civilians in 1942] are still being felt, despite a long phase of ideological taming. Some fears are now being reactivated, leading to delirious horrors and nightmares'.[30] In Bukelić's reading, therefore, even though Second World War traumas were not

[27] Nikola Vulf, 'Jevrejska deca proganjana u ratu – 40 godina kasnije', in Kaličanin et al., *Stresovi Rata*, 49–59.

[28] Ibid., 49–50.

[29] Ibid., 59.

[30] Bukelic, 'Deca I stresovi rata', in Kaličanin et al., *Stresovi Rata*, 44.

properly addressed under socialism for ideological reasons, these 'psychological scars were often invisible wounds that never healed'. This then did not bode well for possible 'unpredictable long-term consequences' of the psychological stresses faced by children in the 1990s.

Even more importantly, Vulf's descriptions of WWII survivors' distressing childhood experiences, such as witnessing the death of parents or their public humiliation, separation from parents, expecting one's own death, were strikingly similar to what children had to confront in the 1990s war, and these more recent ordeals were narrated in subsequent chapters of *Stresses of War*. In that way, the editors of the volume drew a direct parallel between Jewish children's extreme suffering in WWII, and the traumatic circumstances of Serbian children in the war-affected areas in the 1990s.

In the articles that followed, some of the most distinguished Serbian child psychotherapists and psychoanalysts described their own experiences working with children refugees from Croatia and Bosnia, who escaped to Serbia in the period 1991–1995. It was primarily these children's separation from close family members that caused psychological difficulties: separation usually meant that male family members (most often fathers) remained on the frontlines and only saw their children irregularly, but many refugees experienced or directly witnessed their parents' death or wounding, and were themselves exposed to violence. In one case, a six-year-old boy lived in collective refugee accommodation in Belgrade and did not know where his parents were, while an adolescent saw his parents getting murdered, and was then separated from his brother and grandparents upon their arrival in Serbia.[31] Another fifteen-year-old was diagnosed with psychosis one day after she saw her uncle's throat cut.[32] Children often suffered multiple and repeated separations in the course of their journeys and search for safety, and psychiatrists worried that such experiences might fundamentally change those young people's behaviour and personality structures. Just like Vulf's interviewees, child refugees also frequently witnessed their own parents' or other adult role models' humiliation or fundamental ethical disorientation. In the process, many children's identification figures were irretrievably lost,

[31] Nenad Rudic et al., 'Deca I mladi u izbeglistvu I kolektivnom smestaju', in Kaličanin et al., *Stresovi Rata*, 84.

[32] Svetomir Bojanin and Veronika Ispanovic-Radojkovic, 'Adolescenti I stresovi rata', in Kaličanin et al., *Stresovi Rata*, 78.

which led to confused or perverted value systems: 'the war suddenly revealed these persons as completely different beings, unfamiliar and dangerous'.[33] Finally, 'the theme of death pervaded their reality'—the experience of being close to violent death sometimes led to most severe psychotic breakdowns in children, as death 'threatened to become their life's core preoccupation'.[34]

In these poignant accounts of children's suffering, psychiatrists regularly emphasised the psychological difficulties of those young refugees who came from ethnically mixed families. While in the past they could proudly claim Yugoslav identity or simply ignore the thorny issue of national belonging, this now became a seemingly insurmountable obstacle—psychiatrists wrote about such children's 'crisis of identity' as well as of familial loyalty. In the case of Filip, a fourteen-year-old boy with a Croatian mother and Serbian father, psychiatrists reported that the main trauma stemmed from his parents' 'nationalist-ideological conflict:' Filip recounted that the worst wartime 'event' he experienced was his parents' constant blaming of each other and each other's ethnicity for the outbreak of the war.[35] On the other hand, even these accounts of children's mental health problems were used in support of the narrative of Serbian victimhood. Although these articles rarely made any explicit political statements, in case after case a picture emerged of a multitude of reported microaggressions and humiliations experienced by the Serbian minority in Croatia. A fifteen-year-old girl from Croatia, whose one parent was Serb, told her psychiatrists that she still received offensive and threatening letters from her former friends in her hometown, and spoke about having been harassed and mocked at school before escaping to Serbia. When asked why, 'surprised that we even had to ask and assuming that this was self-understood, she said that it was due to the fact she was Serb'.[36] Another girl remembered her Croatian maternal uncle, whom she had always adored and respected but whose behaviour became increasingly erratic and hostile at the beginning of the war, as he tried to convince her mother

[33] Ibid., 79–80.

[34] Ibid., 78–79.

[35] Veronika Ispanovic-Radojkovic, Svetomir Bojanin, Nevenka Tadić, and Nenad Rudic, 'Zastita mentalnog zdravlja dece I mladih – zrtava rata u bivsoj Jugoslaviji (1991–1993)', in Kaličanin et al., *Stresovi Rata*, 63–64.

[36] Vida Rakic et al., 'Psihosocijalne reakcije I poremecaji dece I mladih u izbeglistvu', in Kaličanin et al., *Stresovi Rata*, 70.

to leave her Serb father 'and save the child'. This was the family's main motivation to leave their home and come to Serbia.[37]

PTSD and National Legitimation Strategies

The outbreak of the war in Yugoslavia appeared to have given an impetus to psychiatrists to start discussing recent developments in international classification systems in their field and to comment rather extensively on the current diagnostic standardisation trends in psychiatric epidemiology. The sudden appearance of PTSD in psychiatric and political discussions in the early 1990s prompted a large number of specialist articles explaining the historical development of the diagnosis and its criteria, and the political struggle for its inclusion in the American Psychiatric Association's DSM-III in 1980. As mentioned above, this was also the time when the concept of war trauma was elaborated in great detail, and a lot of attention was paid to different conceptualisations and clinical treatments of war-related psychological disorders throughout the twentieth century. While Yugoslav psychiatrists seemed to be superficially familiar with the description of and discussions about PTSD in the US context (as it was further developed in the revised version of DSM in 1987), their clinical practice was formally guided by an alternative diagnostic and classification system, the WHO's International Classification of Diseases (ICD), which only included PTSD as a separate nosological entity in its tenth edition in 1990.[38] For those reasons, it appeared that both the lay public and the psychiatric profession needed more expert guidance when it came to understanding and diagnosing PTSD, as well as developing appropriate therapeutic strategies.

As Vlado Jukić, one of the most prominent psychiatrists in post-socialist Croatia and long-time head of the country's main psychiatric hospital, noted in one of his articles in 1992, the meaning and relevance of PTSD were rather vague to most of the Croatian public until 1991, but he could already predict then that this would become the country's most serious psychiatric problem.[39] Other psychiatrists discussed

[37] Svetomir Bojanin et al., 'Adolescenti I stresovi rata', 80.

[38] Vladan Starcevic, 'DSM-IV: Nov product iz radionice za proizvodnju psihijatrijskih klasifikacija', *Psihijatrija Danas*, 1994, 26:2–3, 211–218.

[39] Vlado Jukić, 'Klinicka slika posttraumatskog stresnog poremecaja', *Socijalna psihijatrija*, 1992, 20, 187–197.

the DSM's and ICD's comparative strengths and weaknesses, but noted the importance and reliability of such international efforts at standardisation and universalisation, which made particular diagnoses and clinical treatments valid in different cultural contexts. At this time, it was particularly important for the Yugoslav psychiatric profession to demonstrate its (thoughtful) acceptance of and participation in these global trends by contributing to such critical professional discussions. For a group of experts used to such intense international collaboration, the imposed isolation of the war years presented an added frustration, and they invested significant efforts in maximising their international reach and maintaining their professional contacts outside of Yugoslavia.

But the intensification of their discussions of international standardisation strategies at this time also served another purpose: as we will see below, internationally recognised psychiatric entities and diagnoses validated national suffering in transnational circles and lent it scientific legitimacy. As Serbian psychiatrist Marko Munjiza argued in 1994, universal and standardised classification systems such as the ICD played a crucial role in developing a psychiatric *lingua franca*, which enabled 'different interested parties ... to understand each other, share experiences and join forces' in their efforts to improve the treatment and outcomes of mental ill health.[40] In the context of the wars of Yugoslav succession, such goals assumed even greater significance, as the Croatian and Serbian sides in particular vied for the status of the victim, and the international language of psychological trauma was used to substantiate such claims.

As anthropologist Goran Dokić demonstrated in his interviews with Croatian psychiatrists, before 1991 PTSD was considered an 'exotic disease', only encountered in textbooks and theoretical discussions. But with the start of the wars in the 1990s, both Bosnia and Croatia became prime sites for humanitarian psychiatry and international trauma advocacy and intervention programmes.[41] By 1994, there were already 185 such projects operating in the two countries, and a range of international humanitarian aid agencies tasked with the protection of refugees and civilian war victims developed and funded extensive psychological

[40] Marko Munjiza, 'Dijagnosticki kriterijumi u psihijatriji', *Psihijatrija Danas*, 1992, 24:3–4, 257–266.

[41] Goran Dokic, *Psychosocial Transition in a Postsocialist Context: PTSD in Croatian Psychiatry*, MA dissertation, University of Victoria, 2005.

counselling programmes for war-affected populations.[42] Institutions such as the European Community Task Force, the WHO, UNICEF and UNHCR emphasised the primary importance of psychosocial interventions over other forms of aid and placed PTSD and mental health of 'traumatised' populations at the centre of their own extensive activities in war-torn Yugoslavia.[43] WHO mental health consultant Soren Buus Jensen agreed with Jukić that 'post-traumatic stress is going to be the most important public health problem in the former Yugoslavia for a generation and beyond', estimating that over 700,000 people in Croatia and Bosnia were afflicted by severe traumatic experiences.[44] In framing their own psychosocial involvement in the wars of Yugoslav succession, these international actors promoted PTSD as an unproblematic, largely context-free and cross-culturally applicable medical concept.[45]

In the Croatian context, the frequency of diagnosing PTSD was directly related to the rising number of trauma-focused seminars and other educational programmes for psychiatric staff at the beginning of the war. A significant part of these educational efforts was indeed funded by the international organisations involved in trauma advocacy, but the Croatian government also invested enormous resources in training both general practitioners and mental health experts in what they referred to as the core principles of the 'war psychiatric minimum'. Throughout the war, this was a very important aspect of the work of the Croatian government's Medical Corps Headquarters' (*Glavni Stozer Saniteta*) mental health section.[46] By his own confession, by 1992 Vlado Jukić had already given more than ten seminars on PTSD to Croatian medical personnel.[47]

[42] Inger Agger, Sanja Vuk, and Jadranka Mimica, *Theory and Practice of Psychosocial Projects Under War Conditions in Bosnia-Herzegovina and Croatia*, Brussels: ECHO and the European Community Task Force, Psychosocial Unit, 1995.

[43] Paul Stubbs, 'Transforming Local and Global Discourses: Reassessing the PTSD Movement in Bosnia and Croatia', in David Ingleby, ed., *Forced Migration and Mental Health: Rethinking the Care of Refugees and Displaced Persons*, New York: Springer, 2006.

[44] Quoted in S. Kinzler, 'In Croatia, Minds Scarred by War', *New York Times*, 9 January 1995.

[45] K. Allden, T. Franciskovic, J. Lavelle, M. Mathias, K. McInnes, R.F. Mollica, and L. Moro, *Harvard Trauma Manual: Croatian Veterans Version*, Cambridge: Harvard Program in Refugee Trauma, 1998.

[46] Eduard Klain, *Kako sam prozivio domovinski rat*, Zagreb: Croatian Medical Journal, 1996.

[47] Jukić, 'Klinicka slika posttraumatskog stresnog poremecaja', 187.

But if the involved international aid organisations and programmes conceptualised their PTSD interventions as a depoliticised expert field, the development of subsequent local discourses of war trauma in both Croatia and Bosnia was deeply shaped by, and reflected, the complex politics of war memory and national legitimation.

In Croatia, the political usefulness of turning to the DSM and its relatively new take on war-related disorders became clear early on. According to Dokic's ethnographic research in Belgrade, Serbian veterans of the 1990s believed that their Croatian and Bosnian counterparts were in a much more enviable position and that their status in post-socialist Croatia resembled much more clearly that of much celebrated post-WWII Yugoslav partisan soldiers.[48] Indeed, veterans of the Homeland Defence War, as the conflict was officially termed in Croatia, received symbolic and material benefits which were unparalleled anywhere else in the post-Yugoslav context.[49]

The numbers of Croatian veterans who claimed disability pensions, in large part on the basis of the PTSD diagnosis, rose throughout the 1990s during the leadership of the nationalist wartime president Franjo Tudjman. But this trend did not change with Tudjman's departure in 2000; quite to the contrary, the first decade of the new millennium saw the most dramatic leap in approved veteran pensions.[50] In fact, in 2000 the Croatian Ministry of Defence commissioned and published a report about the incidence and most important features of PTSD among Croatian soldiers, concluding that as many as 40% of veterans could be suffering from some form of PTSD, and that the existence and availability of effective programmes of professional psychosocial support had a decisive role to play in lowering this figure.[51] Disabled Croatian veterans, moreover, have had a more inclusive benefit package than their counterparts in Germany, the UK, the US and Israel. Their pensions have remained higher than Croatian citizens' average income, and they have

[48] Goran Dokic, 'States of Victimhood and Irreparable Losses: Serbian Veterans of the Post-Yugoslav Wars', *Glasnik Etnografskog Instituta SANU*, 2017, 1, 104–105.

[49] Mladen and Vanessa Pupavac, 'Trauma Advocacy, Veteran Politics and the Croatian Therapeutic State', *Alternatives: Global, Local, Political*, 2012, 37:3, 199–213.

[50] Ibid., 201–202.

[51] Zoran Komar and Herman Vukusic, 'Post-Traumatic Stress Disorder in Croatian War Veterans; Incidence and Psychosocial Features', Zagreb: Ministry of Defence of the Republic of Croatia, 2000.

enjoyed a long list of additional privileges, such as 'health insurance rights, education allowances, priorities related to university enrolment, allocation of rooms in student halls of residence, free textbooks, priorities related to leasing commercial properties, various import duty and tax exemptions and administrative levies, and free shares in privatized companies'.[52]

Just like socialist Yugoslavia used official histories of the partisan resistance movement in the Second World War as its core strategy of political legitimation, the nationalist account of Croatia's victorious defensive war against Serbian aggression became the foundational narrative of the post-socialist Croatian state. Croatia's Homeland war veterans, therefore, assumed their natural place in the pantheon of national heroes, and were celebrated by successive political governments which sought to nurture their loyalty and support. As Vanessa and Mladen Pupavac have noted, attempts to limit resources spent on veteran pensions, or to make the process more transparent, have on the whole been unsuccessful, and remained a risky political strategy.[53] It is the status of war veterans as proclaimed founders of the newly independent Croatian state that made the concept of war trauma and the diagnosis of PTSD so prominent in Croatia's political circles. Moreover, it was this global paradigm of trauma and traumatisation that made it possible for Croatia to protect the key constituency of veterans from the internationally imposed demobilisation and cuts to the state's military budget.

In Bosnia, which was affected by the war even more tragically and ended it as a highly dysfunctional divided state, local veterans' situation was significantly more ambiguous and precarious—despite what Serbians soldiers might have believed. Bosnian veterans could claim and receive material and symbolic recognition in different entities according to their own ethnicity: Bosniac and Bosnian Croatian fighters in the Federation of Bosnia-Herzegovina, and Bosnian Serb soldiers in the Republic of Srpska. But the Bosnian state narrative of the war was similarly divided and internally contradictory, which meant that the political and social status of those who fought in the war could not be straightforward, nor could their contributions be commemorated, celebrated or rewarded in an unproblematic way. Moreover, the postwar Bosnian state experienced

[52] Goran Dokic, 'States of Victimhood and Irreparable Losses', 97–110; Pupavac and Pupavac, 'Trauma Advocacy, Veteran Politics and the Croatian Therapeutic State', 202.

[53] Pupavac and Pupavac, 'Trauma Advocacy, Veteran Politics and the Croatian Therapeutic State', 207–208.

unprecedentedly severe financial pressures, which further complicated veterans' ability to claim rewards for their military efforts or compensation for their disability. Very importantly, because of the local legislation, the diagnosis of PTSD was rather difficult to use as grounds for veterans' disability.

During the war and in its immediate aftermath, Bosnian politicians spoke of the state's duty to honour those who fought for its independence by providing a range of benefits for disabled and unemployed veterans, and for families of fallen soldiers. This was not significantly different from the Croatian case, at least in the Federation entity: certain influential political forces in Bosnia sought to secure and nurture veterans' political and electoral support in exchange for economic benefits, and, according to Jessie Hronesova, veterans used this opportunity and 'formed powerful pressure groups, drawing on extensive political and economic resources'.[54] Just like in Croatia, veterans were also to be given preferential treatment in medical, educational and employment contexts. However, in a country whose essential services and infrastructure were rapidly deteriorating, most never managed to avail themselves of such possibilities. By the end of the 1990s, these privileges had 'proved to be largely illusory', and so had the veterans' heroic status.[55]

In Bosnia, as in Croatia, the key international financial actors such as the IMF and the World Bank exerted increasing pressure on relevant state institutions to reduce public spending, and in particular focused their campaign on veterans' payments, which they portrayed as financially deleterious, socially harmful, and largely corrupt and non-transparent. For various reasons, Bosnian politicians were less successful than their Croatian counterparts in protecting veterans' associations and families from such cuts, although certain soldiers did continue to receive sizeable remunerations, which primarily depended on their political networks and connections.[56] As Jaroslav Klepal demonstrated, such a negative assessment of the broader societal effects of veterans' pensions and disability

[54] Jessie Hronesova, 'Might Makes Right: War-Related Payments in Bosnia and Herzegovina', *Journal of Intervention and Statebuilding*, 2016, 10:3, 339.

[55] Xavier Bougarel, 'The Shadow of Heroes: Former Combatants in Post-War Bosnia-Herzegovina', *International Social Science Journal*, 2006, 58:189, 479–490.

[56] Jaroslav Klepal, 'The Only Thing I "Earned" in the Damned War Was PTSD'. Reconsidering Veteran Sociality and Politics in Bosnia and Herzegovina', *Southeast European and Black Sea Studies*, 2018, 18:4, 489–507.

payments was not exclusive to the neoliberal international organisations, but they were nevertheless exceptionally influential in shaping the relevant discourses in Bosnia, not least because the Bosnian state was in an extremely difficult financial situation, and its officials apparently saw no alternative but to agree to the mandated reductions in welfare spending in order to secure essential loans and arrangements. The narrative of veterans' benefits as harmful to Bosnia's economic and political recovery undermined the symbolic status of veterans as national heroes and was experienced by their families as deeply humiliating. Following the WB and IMF campaign, even the federal authorities and media began focusing on the reportedly high incidence of illegally awarded veteran disability pensions—in fact, a typical veteran was portrayed as having malingered or misreported his injuries in order to draw permanently on the state's depleted welfare resources.[57]

The public spending and military pension reforms introduced by the Bosnian state further limited veterans' access to benefits and reduced the amount of disability payments. Moreover, it was only the veterans' bill of 2004 that listed PTSD as grounds for disability, and only if it was officially diagnosed before 1997 (this was then opposed—without success—by both veterans' associations and a number of Bosnian psychiatrists, who rightly argued that, by definition, symptoms of PTSD could emerge years, even decades, after one's exposure to traumatic events).[58] In a country in which the WHO deemed in 1996 that more than a third of the entire population suffered from 'post-trauma stress disorders', most veterans with war-related psychological difficulties were excluded from the benefit system. Those who did secure access to disability payments generally received meagre and constantly dwindling sums.

In the meantime, Bosnian psychiatrists estimated that, in the early 2000s, over 50% of the Sarajevo population still suffered from some form of PTSD: almost eight years after the war, the prevalence remained high, while the 'disorder became chronic and more severe'.[59] Moreover, Bosnian mental health researchers warned of the high incidence among

[57] Ibid., 495–496.

[58] Ibid., 500–501.

[59] Ljiljana Orus et al., 'Posttraumatic Stress Disorder Among Women After the War in Sarajevo: A Rationale for Genetic Study', *Bosnian Journal of Basic Medical Sciences*, 2004, 4:1, 50.

the country's ex-combatant population of particularly complex post-traumatic psychological disorders, in which patients with PTSD developed a range of other mental illnesses such as depression, alcohol and drug abuse, as well as different kinds of personality disorders conditioned by extreme traumatic events.[60] Finally, veterans suffering from such complex forms of PTSD were reportedly much more likely to engage in delinquent and criminal behaviour, and more likely to develop debilitating physical illnesses as well.[61] According to an internal survey by one veterans' association in Tuzla in 2006, no members managed to obtain disabled veteran status based on a PTSD diagnosis although over 60% had symptoms during and after the war. Moreover, over a half lived below the poverty line, and over one-third were still unemployed more than ten years after the war.[62]

Therefore, while the military achievements of Bosnian veterans were regularly honoured in certain nationalist political circles, their public status as well as material and social circumstances remained precarious. As the financial reforms demonstrated, they were far from 'untouchable'. Overall, in the context of a deeply divided society suffering from mass unemployment and severely limited public resources, large sections of the public could perceive veterans as a reactionary, violent, corrupt social group made up of extreme nationalists.[63]

However, even in Croatia, where the dominant narrative of veterans' glorification and heroism was much more powerful, the explicit politicisation of PTSD, multiple contradictions within the national narrative about traumatised soldiers, and mounting concerns about corruption and abuses in the veterans' pension system complicated this discourse. Mental health professionals were still markedly uneasy about the obvious and increasing entanglements between the medical diagnosis and political rhetoric, and observed how the medicalisation of veterans' social and

[60] Ifeta Licanin and Amir Redzic, 'PTSD and Comorbidity', *Bosnian Journal of Basic Medical Sciences*, 2002, 2:1–2, 57–61.

[61] Milan Stojakovic, 'Forenzicko-psihijatrijska vjestacenja posttraumatskog stresnog poremecaja', *Psymedica*, 2011, 2:1–2, 10–19.

[62] Quoted in Klepal, 499–500.

[63] Hronesova, 'Might Makes Right', 350; Larisa Kurtovic, '"Who Sows Hunger, Reaps Rage": On Protest, Indignation and Redistributive Justice in Post-Dayton Bosnia-Herzegovina', *Southeast European and Black Sea Studies*, 2015, 15:4, 639–59.

economic problems could easily lead to re-traumatisation.[64] Even those psychiatrists close to the government could express ambivalent attitudes towards soldiers diagnosed with war-related psychological problems.

The earlier disagreement between Hugo Klajn and Josip Dojc was replayed albeit in more moderate terms. On the one hand, in the Croatian public discourse, the diagnosis of PTSD (and other war-related injuries) was treated with significant respect.[65] The foundational narrative of the newly independent post-socialist Croatian state, after all, rested on the military commitment and achievements of these men, as well as on the wartime suffering of Croatian civilians. On the other hand, there were very influential voices in Croatian psychiatry who reminded the public that 'premorbid personality' was an extremely important factor in the emergence and persistence of pathological reactions to stress. Vlado Jukić concluded in 1993 that 'according to multiple indicators, a great majority of the psychotraumatised in this war would not develop PTSD, despite having experienced traumas which went beyond "common human experience"', while those who did develop PTSD symptoms would be able to overcome them within six months. According to Jukić, the main contributing factor to this rather positive outcome was deemed to be a healthy premorbid personality, i.e. no prior personal history of mental illness nor any 'constitutional predilection' for psychopathology.[66] Even though he did note that 'more grave stressors led to chronic forms of PTSD', he still argued that 'predisposition' was central to the gravity of the clinical picture of PTSD and to more serious impairments in patients' social functioning. In other words, PTSD was decidedly not a normal person's reaction to abnormal circumstances. After all, 'almost 80% of patients with PTSD fulfil the criteria for at least one or two additional psychiatric diagnoses'.[67] In that sense, for Jukić PTSD always likely signified an already psychologically impaired personality, especially if the symptoms were serious, socially disruptive and long-lasting, and marked by the patient's general maladaptation.

[64] Dokic, 'Psychosocial Transition in a Postsocialist Context', 75–80.

[65] Ljiljana Moro et al., 'Potpora radne sredine I obitelji kod posttraumatskog stresnog poreemcaja', *Socijalna psihijatrija*, 1992, 20, 233–240.

[66] Vlado Jukić, 'Posttraumatski stresni sindrom I paranoidnost', *Socijalna Psihijatrija*, 1993, 21, 52.

[67] Vlado Jukić, 'Klinicka slika posttraumatskog stresnog poremecaja', 195–196.

Moreover, like Dojc, early in the war Jukić was also concerned about the supposedly highly harmful phenomenon of 'rent neurosis' among Croatian soldiers and cautioned his colleagues about those 'veterans' who might claim to suffer consequences of wartime suffering without ever having taken part in the war (he referred to this as the Munchausen syndrome).[68] In this reading, even if soldiers with PTSD were not deemed constitutionally 'burdened', their clinical diagnosis could still betray deeper issues with their personality and ethical value system. At the beginning of the war, Jukić and psychoanalyst Eduard Klain warned that PTSD would likely be the most common disorder among those soldiers who, at least subconsciously, experienced ambivalence regarding their participation in the war. Writing about soldiers with physical wounds and their psychological attitudes to their impaired condition, they identified one type of reaction, which was reportedly extremely rare—'feelings of relief and exceptional satisfaction ... for not having to return to the frontlines'. It was from the ranks of such soldiers—who looked forward to escaping fighting and possible death without being deserters or malingerers—that 'war neurotics were most commonly recruited'.[69] Therefore, suffering from PTSD and 'war neurosis' could indicate a soldier's lack of commitment—a conclusion decidedly not in line with the international (particularly US) diagnostic tendencies and interpretations. On the other hand, Jukić continued in the tradition of a significant group of Yugoslav military psychiatrists—at the end of the Second World War, Dojc mockingly referred to partisan neurosis as *Auslands-mania*, because those soldiers diagnosed with war neurosis were initially evacuated to the liberated territory in Italy, behind the partisan frontline. For Dojc, there was little more to the concept of war neurosis than these pusillanimous soldiers' desire to remove themselves from difficult battles.[70]

In a similar vein, other psychiatrists wrote of Croatian veterans' resistance to treatment and healing, and identified their 'need for compensation' as an important obstacle to therapy. Such a need was reportedly generated by 'narcissistic regressive' personality changes in some veterans, who demanded 'admiration and all their requests to be fulfilled'. While

[68] Ibid., 195.

[69] Vlado Jukić and Eduard Klain, 'Psihicke poteskoce ranjenika I zrtava rata, sa posebnim osvrtom na PTSP', *Klinicka medicina*, 1992, 1:1, 79–86.

[70] Josip Dojč, 'Inozemstvo-Mania, nova zarazna bolest!', Arhiv Sanitetske sluzbe Ministarstva odbrane, R-202.

this reading certainly did not dismiss veterans' psychological disorders as malingering, it partly relied on Dojc's and Jukić's interpretations, and the authors warned that veterans' narcissistic expectations could affect therapists as well as the broader society and governmental institutions, and lead to veterans' continued dependence on others (as was arguably already happening in postwar Croatia).[71]

This complex and ambivalent discourse about Croatian soldiers' PTSD revealed a major tension in Croatian psychiatric discussions about the psychological consequences of the war. On the one hand, there was a strong politically motivated tendency (and pressure) to view soldiers who fought in the 1990s war as heroes of almost superhuman courage and commitment (as Jukić testified, wounded soldiers most often burnt with desire to go back to fighting).[72] On the other, PTSD was an extremely useful and internationally recognised concept to document the enormous suffering inflicted on the Croatian society by the aggressors. Perhaps better than any other individual debate, clinical and political discussions around PTSD demonstrated a fundamental contradiction at the heart of Croatia's official war narrative: a clash between its self-perceptions as a victim and as a glorious victor. As James Gow and other researchers have noted, Croatia sought to gain international legitimacy, sympathy and support by presenting its state institutions and population as victims of the 'barbaric' Serbian aggression.[73] In that sense, the globally accepted framework of trauma and PTSD was perfectly appropriate to validate such claims of national victimhood and (well documented) suffering, and it consequently permanently reshaped Croatian psychiatry. However, domestically, the Croatian wartime and postwar government tended to eschew victimhood narratives, and instead justified its own claim to power by fostering national pride in Croatia's political and military triumph in the war.

Veterans embodied this irresolvable contradiction: their status as invincible national heroes was often undermined by their position as medical (even worse—psychiatric!) patients. Jukić's writings in particular seemed to demonstrate these unspoken contradictory assumptions very well. At

[71] Vlasta Stalekar and Leonida Akrap, 'Otpori proradi ratne trauma I gubitaka', *Socijalna psihijatrija*, 2000, 28, 113–116.

[72] Jukić and Klain, 'Psihicke poteskoce ranjenika I zrtava rata', 81.

[73] James Gow, *The Serbian Project and Its Adversaries: A Strategy of War Crimes*, London: Hurst, 2003, 236–240.

the same time, veterans' privilege and social benefits could only be preserved if they agreed to the patient role within the framework of psychological trauma. Moreover, given that PTSD was defined and developed in the context of the US military defeat in Vietnam, and was primarily used to describe and diagnose American soldiers who were perceived to have fought an unjust and unethical war, it was in an important sense entirely inappropriate for the postwar Croatian context. Croatia's veterans with PTSD were celebrated as heroes with unblemished records who won an honourable defensive war, and this further complicated both political and psychiatric narratives of trauma and veterans' benefits.

Despite their extremely privileged social position, therefore (or precisely because of it), Croatian veterans hardly evoked exclusively positive reactions, and critical discourses could take different forms. It seemed that, just like in 1945, the psychiatric encounter with war-traumatised soldiers from the 1990s wars could be exceptionally explosive and volatile. Hugo Klajn and Stjepan Betlheim raised grave concerns about their own and their patients' safety at the Military-hygienic centre in Kovin in 1945 because some 'partisan hysterics' refused to disarm and also reportedly stole and hid knives from the hospital kitchen to assault the psychiatrists.[74] In 1990s Croatia, psychiatrists soon started writing about the increased potential of soldiers with PTSD to cause disruption and physical violence, and exacerbate general social relations. Such concerns over the aggressiveness and volatility of traumatised soldiers replicated the post-WWII anxieties over the unstable figure of a neurotic hero.

As many psychiatrists testified, wartime Croatian hospitals were indeed potentially dangerous places, not because they could have been attacked by the enemy forces but because of some of the ill soldiers' reactions. At the beginning of the war, many soldiers reportedly feared that they would not be physically safe in hospitals, and refused to give up their weapons while receiving treatment. This resulted in explosive situations, in which anxious soldiers kept their guns in hospital rooms, and 'there was great resistance' to the order that arms could not be brought into medical institutions.[75] Moreover, 'the wounded insisted that only "reliable and tried"

[74] Klajn, *Ratna neuroza Jugoslovena*, 78–82.

[75] Aleksandar Maletic, 'Psihoterapija psihickih ratnih traumi', *Socijalna psihijatrija*, 1992, 20, 213–214.

colleagues – volunteers and professional soldiers of the Croatian Army – should guard them'.[76] This was reportedly a drawn-out and intense conflict, certainly reminiscent of the post-WWII situations in Yugoslav hospitals, where psychiatrists such as Nadezda Jevtić, at Belgrade's 'Laza Lazarević', blamed partisans for wreaking havoc on the hospital order and putting everyone's lives in danger.[77]

As psychoanalyst Muradif Kulenović noted in 1996, 'the socially most intrusive patients are those with war-related wounds... the most challenging and difficult problem remains the case of active war participants diagnosed with PTSD, who, due to the nature of their illness, most often cause grave misunderstandings, uncontrolled aggressive incidents, and at times physical assaults on medical staff'. Kulenović recounted a colleague's experience with such a soldier in a small-town hospital. The soldier, who was permanently physically injured in the war, returned home and received adequate material help as well as medical care, but refused to be seen by any medical doctors, and never came to the hospital himself. Instead, he demanded that a variety of analgesic (pain-relieving) medications be prescribed and delivered to him without any medical examinations or reviews. When a new doctor arrived, she initially refused to keep up this regime and asked to see the patient first. After that, the patient visited her once in the hospital and threatened to kill her with his rifle 'from his room, which was right across from her consulting room'.[78]

It is striking that Kulenović's language when referring to this soldier was also, perhaps unintentionally, mirroring the post-WWII discourses about partisan hysterics. Namely, Yugoslav psychiatrists of the 1940s increasingly concluded that 'partisan neurosis' was almost exclusively diagnosed in very young, uneducated and immature ('primitive') soldiers, who used it to express their frustration with peacetime requirements and limitations. While Kulenović's reading was less ideologically complex, he did emphasise the 'backward nature' of the patient's home region, which was then reflected in his attitudes and educational levels: 'the patient came from the interior of Croatia, which is less economically developed and

[76] Jukić and Klain, 'Psihicke poteskoce ranjenika I zrtava rata', 81–82.

[77] Archive of Serbia, G-222, F-120, files 20888, 20890.

[78] Muradif Kulenović, 'Balintove grupe u poslijeratnom razdoblju Hrvatske', *Psihoterapija*, 1998, 28:1–2, 77.

backward in a social and cultural sense'.[79] Moreover, the patient was indeed very young, only in his twenties well after the end of the war, so he was in many ways reminiscent of the figure of the partisan hysteric from fifty years ago.

This inability of many veterans to control their aggressive impulses and establish a productive therapeutic relationship with their psychiatrists was emphasised time and again in postwar Croatia. Veterans with diagnosed PTSD increasingly became a highly problematic and disruptive presence both in a variety of social contexts and in therapeutic settings. Vedran Bilic wrote of a patient who 'hated his wife so much that he constantly plotted her murder' but refused to get treatment for this destructive relationship. Another veteran nearly strangled his wife after an argument—he reportedly described in some detail how her face 'had gone blue'—the woman was only saved after their daughter interfered, while others declared seemingly proudly in group therapy that their wives and other family members were afraid of them and did not dare criticise them in any way.[80] Three Zagreb-based psychotherapists noted the difficulty of integrating veterans in wider groups of patients for the purposes of art therapy: 'those groups which contained more than four PTSD participants suffered from a disruption of the entire group dynamic' due to the 'rigidity of their symptoms, long exposure to traumatic experiences, failure of therapy, rent neurosis motives'.[81]

Importantly, as we will see below, the corresponding literature on PTSD among Serbian veterans rarely discussed former soldiers in similar terms, as potentially aggressive and disruptive patients and citizens, and only addressed this issue in general terms. Serbian psychiatrists and a number of politically progressive NGOs in fact wrote about Serbian soldiers as victims of the state's neglect, and any tendencies to aggressive or disruptive behaviour were coached in terms of victimhood, lack of systemic support and the consequent inability of veterans to re-adapt to peacetime circumstances.

[79] Ibid., 76–77.

[80] Vedran Bilic, 'Oboljeli ucesnik rata u obitelji', *Psihoterapija*, 1998, 28:1–2, 23–31.

[81] Davor Rak et al., 'Grupni crtez kao jedan od parametara (dijagnostickih I terapijskih) kod pacijenata sa PTSP', *Psihoterapija*, 1999, 29:1–2, 127–128.

'Trauma' and Erased Memories of the War in Serbia

According to Zeljko Spiric, psychiatrist based at the chief Belgrade military hospital and editor of a rather extraordinary collection of psychiatric essays on Serbian veterans' war trauma of the 1990s, this 2008 volume was the first Serbian publication to explore specifically psychological disorders of Serbian soldiers who took part in the wars of the Yugoslav Spirić. While there were other monographs and articles which addressed the concept of PTSD in general terms, or the psychological difficulties of children, refugees or torture victims, they generally strove to maintain the focus on civilians' wartime suffering—perhaps because this topic was significantly less controversial and more likely to elicit universal agreement and sympathy. Military veterans and direct participants in the wars in Slovenia, Croatia, Bosnia and Kosovo, on the other hand, assumed a much more complex and awkward position in the Serbian society and public discourse. Their own status, social support and material benefits they were likely to draw from their years of military service were directly related to the Serbian society's collective memory of the wars and the political leadership's preferred memory narratives. But since the 1990s Serbian government officials as well as leaders of the right-wing nationalist opposition maintained that the country never took part in the war, the position of veterans who needed mental healthcare became increasingly complicated. Moreover, the outcome of the wars—negative from the official Serbian point of view—made their situation even more difficult. As Spiric noted in his analysis, 'in a majority of (victorious) states, veterans enjoyed public support and sympathy, served as an important source of national pride, and were glorified'. In Serbia, however, veterans from the 1990s became an unwelcome reminder of the national defeat (which was never officially proclaimed as such), and an 'obstacle in the process of forced repression of the [collective] memory of war losses'.[82]

Spiric described Serbia's official disregard of its war veterans as akin to the behaviour of defeated states throughout the twentieth century, and this was one of the rare moments when Serbia's participation in the war was referred to as an outright defeat. As Spiric and his fellow contributors suggested, postwar Serbia was a troubled society which never declared

[82] Zeljko Spiric, 'Foreword', in Zeljko Spiric, ed., *Ratna psihotrauma srpskih veterana*, 12–15.

either victory or defeat, never even recognised its own participation in the military activities on the neighbouring states' territories, and, even more importantly, never articulated its political (and ethical) attitude towards its soldiers' wartime behaviour. This final concern was perhaps the most important: Serbian veterans were also perpetrators of some of the gravest war crimes (including genocide) on the European soil after the Second World War, and a more involved political and psychiatric debate on the psychological consequences of the war would need to at least in part reflect on this highly uncomfortable fact. As Serbian journalist Ljiljana Mitrinović argued, 'it has not yet been said [in Serbia] whether this war, to whose victims we are supposed to build a monument, was a war of aggression or a defensive war; who the heroes and criminals were; whether it has been worth it.... We live in a country in which we are increasingly forced to listen to the truth from others because we don't want to speak about it ourselves'.[83] Quite shockingly, it was only in 2007 that the Serbian Ministry for work and social politics approved the first research project aimed at evaluating systematically the mental health status and needs of the war veterans from the 1990s, in order to (finally) design a long-term healthcare plan for this population.

In fact, the exact number of war veterans has not yet been ascertained in Serbia—researchers who engaged with this problem have estimated that there could be anywhere between 400,000 and 800,000 former soldiers.[84] The state's marked disinterest in counting and recording the names of all participants in the wars of Yugoslav succession was further reflected in most veterans' inability to claim social security support and any material benefits except in a small number of cases when long-term medical disability was medically proven. Moreover, for many disillusioned veterans, the glaring absence of symbolic acknowledgement was even more harmful, as the entire political leadership which entangled the country in a series of wars now renounced their responsibility for both the wars and those who fought in them: 'contrary to the general opinion how veterans were only interested in material rewards, most of the soldiers' narratives revolved around the loss of dignity and the lack of

[83] Ljiljana Mitrinovic, NIN, 16 January 2003 (2716).

[84] Vladan Beara, Predrag Miljanovic, and Boris Popov, 'Zasto uopste pomagati ratnim veteranima', *Temida: Casopis o viktimizaciji, ljudskim pravima I rodu*, 2004, 7:4, 47–49.

any symbolic recognition'.[85] According to Dokić, who conducted interviews with members of a veterans' association in Belgrade, one of his interviewees admitted that he felt ashamed of his veteran status, and felt very clearly that 'everybody despises us'.[86] As Belgrade psychoanalyst Branimir Stojanović noted, 'Veteran is another name for absolute exclusions and invisibility… as long as veterans' status remains unrecognised, the state will be able to pretend there were no wars'. For that reason, Dokić was also able to conclude that, 'when compared to Croatia, PTSD was practically non-existent' in Serbia's official political discourse.[87] Veterans' claims remained on the political margins, and in this sense, the Serbian experience of the 1990s was markedly different from the state policies and attitudes towards partisan veterans in the 1940s, who became celebrated as heroes and founders of the new socialist state.

But whether they were heroes, war criminals or awkward reminders of Serbia's traumatic and unsavoury recent past, Serbian veterans were a sizeable group whose needs and health difficulties were virtually invisible to the rest of the society for the most part of the postwar decade. This did not mean that such needs and difficulties did not exist: in fact, it appeared that the very experience of invisibility confounded veterans' attempts at recovery and reintegration. As several psychiatrists and psychologists testified from their own clinical experience, the extreme political and military events of the 1990s left an indelible mark on various sections of the Serbian population, and soldiers and veterans were among the worst affected in terms of psychological health. At Belgrade's Institute of Mental Health, psychologist Vladimir Jović and his colleagues were, by the mid-1990s, seeing dozens of traumatised veterans every week (and that excluded any active military officers, who reported to a separate military hospital).[88] According to Spiric, even though the intensity of relevant 'war stressors' diminished radically in the years after 1995 (or 1999), 'the number of patients treated for PTSD did not decrease significantly'.[89]

[85] Vladimir Jović, 'Posttraumatski poremecaj u socijalnom i politickom kontekstu devedesetih', 369–386.

[86] Goran Dokic, 'States of Victimhood and Irreparable Losses', 97–110.

[87] Ibid., 105–106.

[88] Vladimir Jović, 'Posttraumatski poremecaj u socijalnom I politickom kontekstu devedesetih', 384.

[89] Spiric, 'Foreword', 13.

Moreover, PTSD often went hand in hand with additional chronic and debilitating psychiatric and somatic disorders. As we will see below, Spiric's narrative thus painted a grim picture of mass suffering endured by neglected and marginalised veterans, whose symbolic and material status in the Serbian society was simply too politically difficult to resolve.

Milanko Čabarkapa, a Serbian military psychologist who dedicated his career to researching Serbian soldiers' PTSD, wrote about the psychological and social dangers of untreated and unacknowledged war trauma in war participants: in addition to significant impairments of individual emotional, professional and familial functioning, long-term effects of unprocessed and neglected PTSD included a 'diminished capacity for democratic orientation and democratic dialogue', i.e. an erosion of those social and individual capabilities which 'enabled people to enter into associations and create their own better future'.[90] In other words, the widespread experience of PTSD in veterans was more than a clinical problem, and it seriously compromised the Serbian society's ability to move forward. In a similar vein, Spiric warned about the broader societal 'dangers stemming from the [psychological] consequences of the war' suffered by Serbian veterans, who, ten years after the end of their military engagement, experienced severe difficulties in their social adaptation (their inability to maintain family and personal relations and to take part in normal economic and professional activities did not bode well for the development of the Serbian society in general).[91]

However, while Carbarkapa's own clinical research went a long way towards shedding light on the nature of psychological difficulties of Serbian veterans, it never seriously delved into the complex ethical aspects of Serbian soldiers' war conduct and possible psychological consequences suffered by perpetrators of extreme violence against civilians. Čabarkapa interviewed hundreds of Serbian soldiers—members of the Yugoslav People's Army—who took part in the wars in Slovenia and Croatia in 1991, and aimed to determine which circumstances, events and experiences had the highest potential to cause traumatic reactions. In his 1996 doctoral dissertation and his subsequent publications, Čabarkapa focused on the difficult and extraordinary circumstances in which Yugoslavia's

[90] Milanko Čabarkapa, 'Psiholoske I socijalne posledice neizlecene ratne traume', in Spiric, *Ratna psihotrauma srpskih veterana*, Belgrade, 308.

[91] Spiric, 'Posleratna adaptacija ratnih vojnih veterana', in Spiric, *Ratna psihotrauma srpskih veterana*, 323–363.

regular army found itself at the beginning of the war, when it faced open hostility from the local population in both Slovenia and Croatia, and went through a torturous process of dissolution along ethnic lines in the midst of an escalating armed conflict.[92] In his analysis, Čabarkapa thus zoomed in on negative psychological effects of such overall political and military conditions, describing in detail the disorientation of Serbian recruits who had to witness 'mass desertion of both regular soldiers and commanders', as well as what Čabarkapa referred to as a 'betrayal by the military command and the political leadership of the country' as the army was ordered to withdraw from Slovenia.[93]

However, in his discussion of soldiers' responses in Croatia, Čabarkapa noted that the second most traumatic experience was 'seeing massacred human corpses', while one of the most significant 'events' described by his interviewees was the 'destruction of all moral values and loss of respect for personhood and the value of human life'.[94] These statements were vague enough and could be read in a variety of different ways, i.e. they did not necessarily mean that the interviewed soldiers spoke of their own army's and comrades' responsibility for the massacres and unethical behaviour. Nevertheless, Čabarkapa never clarified their implications, and they remained the sole somewhat ambiguous references which did not construct Serbian soldiers and recruits explicitly as victims of their circumstances. In his own research conducted in 2005, Spiric listed 'death of a large number of civilians' among the most intense stressful events in the war as reported by his Serbian interviewees: the characteristically ambiguous formulation (which civilians, and how were they killed?) was not elaborated any further.

In the rest of his research and analysis, Čabarkapa focused on a variety of factors which in no way touched on the issue of Serbian responsibility for war crimes and crimes against humanity: the death and wounding of other soldiers; sudden, unexpected and stealthy attacks from the enemy side (fellow Yugoslavs until recently); lack of military and fighting experience; unclear war aims and contradictory information regarding

[92] Čabarkapa, *Psiholoski faktori stresa u borbenim aktivnostima*.

[93] Milanko Čabarkapa, 'Psiholoske i socijalne posledice neizlecene ratne traume', in Spiric, ed., *Ratna psihotrauma srpskih veterana*, 30.

[94] Ibid., 32–33.

commands and course of action, etc.[95] In fact, Čabarkapa reported that most of his interviewees did not feel hostility towards the 'enemy side', defined as Slovene and Croat territorial defence organisations, local police units and the civilian population who opposed the Yugoslav People's Army in 1991. To the contrary, almost 60% of the soldiers in Čabarkapa's sample testified that they had not seen these organisations as 'enemies' at the beginning of the conflict, and that, moreover, they had at times had very good relations with their representatives and the local population. In the author's reading, the absence of any hostile emotions paradoxically led to further psychological difficulties as Serbian soldiers experienced deep confusion and ambivalence, and were, moreover, poorly motivated to fight.[96] On the other hand, their relatively positive disposition towards the enemies, claimed Čabarkapa, made it unlikely that they would struggle with aggressive impulses or feelings of hatred, or behave destructively during the conflict. In a similar vein, another group of mental health clinicinas concluded that their research subjects—a group of Serbian POWs who had been tortured in Croatian camps and prisons—still expressed an exceptionally 'mature' form of patriotism 'without hatred or any revanchist feelings towards the nation from which their torturers hailed'.[97] Not even such profoundly traumatising experiences and unspeakablly cruel treatment at the hands of their enemies could, thus, provoke hatred and aggression in Serbian soldiers.

Other psychiatrists largely joined the denialist trend: Spiric noted in passing that war veterans in Serbia experienced 'satanization', 'stigmatization' and 'disrespect' for their service coming from certain unnamed media outlets and organisations.[98] These reportedly drew on unsupported conclusions about the entire veteran population on the basis of some 'incident situations (violence, crimes, murders, suicides) in which individual soldiers took part', and because of the ongoing war crimes trials of 'individual veterans'.[99] In that sense, the belated discussion about Serbian

[95] Čabarkapa, 'Psiholoski faktori stresa u ratu na prostorima bivse Jugoslavije', in Spiric, ed., *Ratna psihotrauma srpskih veterana*.

[96] Ibid., 47–48.

[97] Branislav Petrovic et al., 'Zlostavljanje uhapsenih I zarobljenih lica', in Kaličanin et al., *Stresovi Rata*, 158.

[98] Spiric, 'Posleratna adaptacija ratnih vojnih veterana', 326–237.

[99] Ibid., 327.

soldiers' PTSD almost completely eschewed the issue of the psychological and moral status of perpetrators and failed to explore the psychological and moral burdens of a society which needed to reintegrate such perpetrators. This is not particularly surprising in the broader political and social context of contemporary Serbia, although the concept of PTSD was particularly well suited to discussing diagnosed patients in terms other than victimhood.

Moreover, even though Serbian psychiatrists such as Spiric and Čabarkapa generally presented their own profession as a victim of the broader social and political circumstances, which made it impossible for mental health scientists to plan and conduct systematic research into Serbian soldiers' PTSD, the situation was indeed much more complex than that. In the midst of extreme social divisions and political crises in 1990s Serbia, those psychiatrists who worked with war stresses played an active role in shaping the dominant political narrative. Discussions about PTSD and 'reactive psychological disorders' were omnipresent in psychiatric and medical journals throughout the war, and also dominated post-1995 psychiatric discourses. As mentioned before, the focus was on civilian victims of the wars—children, survivors of torture and prison camps, civilian refugees—and such partial psychiatric analyses relied on the perceived universal scientific value and appeal of international diagnostic categories (such as PTSD) in order to reinforce the narrative of (Serbian) innocence, victimhood and even generosity (Serbs did not hate the nation from which their torturers hailed, their patriotism was devoid of such destructive feelings). In his analysis of the applicability of ICD-X to the Yugoslav context, Kaličanin noted that 'the real circumstances in which we live in themselves constitute a stressor to which our entire nation is exposed'.[100] In that sense, such international classifications validated the suffering of the Serbian people as a whole, serving as the ultimate proof of its unjust victimisation.

Still, Čabarkapa's, Spiric's and others' work on the diagnosis of PTSD served as a powerful and uncomfortable testimony to the sheer magnitude of Serbia's and Serbian citizens' involvement in the wars in Slovenia, Croatia and Kosovo, and a reminder of the heavy psychological burden that such participation imposed on the Serbian society. Again, psychiatric debates became an unexpected forum for discussing highly controversial

[100] Predrag Kaličanin and Irida Petkovic, 'Reaktivni psihicki poremecaji prema ICD-X klasifikaciji', *Psihijatrija Danas*, 1992, 24:3–4, 285–290.

political issues and concerns which could not be addressed elsewhere. According to Spiric's analysis of over 200 questionnaires filled in by war veterans in Serbia, the military conflicts in former Yugoslavia cast a long and troubling shadow, and dramatically shaped the lives of its participants. For instance, Spric assessed that over 40% of the veterans 'probably' suffered from undiagnosed PTSD, which limited their postwar adaptation and severely impaired their efforts to rebuild their own social networks. Importantly, on average, nearly 60% of the interviewed veterans still thought about the war frequently (a decade after its end), and that number rose significantly, to 70%, for the subgroup with PTSD symptoms (who were experiencing intrusive memories and flashbacks). Moreover, nearly 30% of PTSD veterans now regretted their participation in the war, and a significant number developed a fairly negative assessment of their war activities.[101] Finally, the veterans' overall physical health, the quality of their social and family relations, as well as their ability to provide for themselves and their families deteriorated dramatically, while systematic state policies to address these problems were sorely lacking. Nearly 30% of the veterans described their own physical health as bad, while a shocking 78% believed that their material situation was bad or exceptionally bad. They were also much more likely to underperform at work, to get fined or fired, and were promoted much more rarely than before the war. In fact, unable to find solid ground in a society undergoing major structural transformations after the change of political regime in 2000, they often labelled themselves 'losers of the transition'.[102]

Vladimir Jović was one of the very few mental health clinicians in Serbia who raised the issue of collective memory of and ethical responsibility for war crimes and human rights abuses when addressing his own experiences with treating PTSD.[103] He, furthermore, noted the similarity between the situation of Serbian soldiers and that of Vietnam veterans in the US, especially with regard to the Serbian leadership's 'confusion about the wars' political aims' and the Serbian society's negative attitudes towards war participants. Through this comparison, Jović introduced the issue of war crimes and veterans as perpetrators, whose psychological

[101] Spiric, 'Posleratna adaptacija ratnih vojnih veterana', 349–453.

[102] Ibid., 354–360.

[103] Vladimir Jović, 'Posttraumatski poremecaj u socijalnom I politickom kontekstu devedesetih', 369–386.

problems were in large part caused by their own violent or destructive acts. This concern with responsibility for war crimes was likely a result of the main focus of Jović's article: the suffering of Serb refugees from Croatia and Bosnia, who were recruited against their will immediately upon their arrival to Serbia and sent back to the frontlines, usually after having been exposed to torture and harassment at one of the semi-legal 'military training camps' in the country.[104]

While, according to Jović and most of his colleagues, all Serbian veterans found themselves in difficult and unfair circumstances after the end of the war, this was obviously a particularly badly affected subgroup of soldiers, whose grievances, memories and psychological difficulties were extremely difficult to overcome. By zooming in on these refugees-turned-soldiers, Jović's research raised the issue of the Serbian state's complicity in civilian suffering almost naturally: there was no way of eschewing a discussion of the Serbian military (and paramilitary) formations' crimes against civilians and international humanitarian laws. Moreover, he explicitly referred to the Serbian military groups' most heinous crimes outside of Serbia, on the territories of Bosnia and Croatia, such as the shelling and destruction of the Croatian town of Vukovar and executions of its civilian population, the shelling of the historic city of Dubrovnik and the mass murder of civilians in the Eastern Bosnian town of Srebrenica. In his analysis, Jović critiqued the absence of any 'societal self-reflection on a national level' in Serbia, any reassessment of Serbia's status following a series of mass crimes, military defeats and humiliations, or 'any steps whatsoever towards reconciliation with the other nations against which we waged wars'.[105] Instead of taking a hard look at itself, the Serbian society continued to deny its own role in any of the post-Yugoslav carnage by ignoring the needs and the very existence of its veterans. Jović even compared the Serbian public to bystanders in the Holocaust, who knew about but remained indifferent to the fate of concentration camp inmates, even though they themselves did not commit any crimes.

In that sense, Jović's article was about the PTSD diagnosis of the entire society—those citizens who identified with the Serbian 'national interests' and criminal leadership still inhabited a grey zone and remained

104 Ibid., 384.

105 Ibid., 376–377.

dependent on a political ideology which would enable them to 'distance themselves from any considerations of war crimes' and their own moral responsibility for them. For such people, the chances of psychological recovery were rather low in Jović's diagnosis. But the problem was even larger than this group of people, and here Jović continued the practice of relying on psychoanalytic interpretive frameworks to explain the war's political effects. A majority of Serbian citizens, whether or not they supported Milosevic's belligerent regime, found it impossible to integrate the destructive experiences of the wartime (poverty, extreme fear and helplessness, humiliation) into their memory and meaningful sense of self, so they utilised the strategy of 'externalisation', 'denial' and 'projection'. In other words, a strong delineating line needed to be maintained between those who participated in the war formally, and those who did not: 'the group which contained any references to the war had to be held at a long enough psychological distance' so that any negative war-related memories or feelings could be symbolically 'deposited' in such figures and expunged from the national space. Veterans, as 'contaminated' by the war, were either expelled from the public discourse or vilified. It was very difficult for psychiatrists like Jović to help overcome such efforts at externalising the veterans' experiences, precisely because this strategy hid the most difficult truth—in a society of morally complicit bystanders, everyone was traumatised.[106]

On the other hand, there was a group of psychiatrists and psychotherapists in Serbia, largely working with children, who regularly presented themselves as neutral and even-handed observers of the war. In their research, which primarily focused on the status of mental health in Serbian refugees from Croatia and Bosnia, they regularly referred to the wars of Yugoslav succession as a civil war between three equally brutal sides, emphasising that in this conflict 'nobody was innocent but children'. All three warring parties were said to be characterised by 'religious exclusivism, which [led] us into an anachronistic medieval situation of ruthless religious wars'.[107] In one article, Yugoslav writer Ivo Andrić was evoked and quoted in the middle of a clinical analysis of child refugees and

[106] Ibid., 377–378.

[107] Vida Rakic et al., 'Psihosocijalne reakcije I poremecaji dece I mladih u izbeglistvu', 70–71.

their psychological disorders in order to make sense of the current political developments and the violent dissolution of the country. In these citations, the psychiatrists used pronouncements of a variety of Andric's literary characters to argue that the 'spirit of the Balkan man' was hopelessly and permanently tied to inflicting and suffering violence, and that the 'four faiths' coexisting in the region had since time immemorial thrived on the feelings of hatred and intolerance towards one another.[108]

In this reading, the 1990s war and its consequences, even though they were referred to as 'man-made' or 'man-intentioned', were in fact constructed as akin to natural disasters, caused by timeless and inexplicable forces of destruction. This also by necessity meant that there was no individual responsibility to speak of and very little individual agency, especially since everybody involved was reportedly equally morally bankrupt. The practical political implications of this line of thinking were obvious almost immediately: describing the case of a girl refugee, who spent some time in besieged Sarajevo before making it to Belgrade with her family, the psychiatrists noted that her boyfriend was killed by a sniper in one of the 'street fights' in the Bosnian capital.[109] In that way, the responsibility for this murder was removed from the Bosnian Serb army, which kept the city a hostage and killed and wounded over 16,000 civilians. Instead, the reference to street fights once again implied that the burden of guilt is completely diffused, and shared among all participants.

Beyond attempts at diagnosing war participants and interpreting the origins of the war in psychoanalytic terms, therefore, psychiatrists used their clinical materials and experiences to make direct political pronouncements about what was going on in the war-affected areas of the former country. In Serbian psychiatry in particular, the idea of establishing equal responsibility of all three ethnic 'sides' was very common, most likely because it undermined the narrative focused on Serbian aggression and the growing international condemnation of the Serb armies' and paramilitaries' crimes against civilians. In their 1994 paper about raped women in Bosnia, Serbian psychiatrists Slobodan Jakulic and Miomir Krstic presented the cases of ten Serb women from Bosnia, most of them raped by soldiers of the Bosnian Army, who got pregnant following the rapes

[108] Ibid., 72.

[109] Veronika Ispanovic-Radojkovic, Svetomir Bojanin, Nevenka Tadić, and Nenad Rudic, 'Zastita mentalnog zdravlja dece I mladih', 62–63.

and were subsequently referred for psychiatric examination and treatment. The article purports to explore the psychological effects of rape, but only dedicates slightly over one page to such an analysis, concluding that all patients suffered from acute reactive disorders and were likely to develop chronic PTSD because 'rape represented one of the gravest forms of psycho-physical trauma'.[110] However, most of the article was not based on this clinical material—instead, the authors used their work with raped women as an opportunity to respond to the allegations that the Serb army was engaging in a systematic rape campaign of Muslim and Croatian women. By 1994, such claims gained important international traction, and, even more significantly, they were supported by a mounting body of evidence and witness testimonies.[111]

The authors still rejected any such notions that the Serb military command ordered mass rapes and used them as a military-political strategy. Even though the Bosnian side claimed that approximately 50,000 Muslim women had been raped by that point, the Serbian psychiatrists countered this with less than convincing evidence: that the number of 50,000 was simply impossible to arrive at because 'in our culture, women won't talk of rape' unless they found themselves in extraordinary circumstances. Instead, the authors argued in line with the wartime president of the Republic of Srpska Biljana Plavsić (hardly a neutral source), that 'rapes happened on all three sides of the war, that they were sporadic' and that 'the number of rapes was approximately equal on all three sides'.[112] Of course, no clinical or statistic data were offered to support such statements, and Plavsić's pronouncements remained the only proof. The authors, furthermore, complained about the European Parliament's resolution condemning the rape of Bosnian women, as well as its public debate on this issue (in February 1993), from which Serb experts were reportedly excluded.[113]

[110] Slobodan Jakulic and Miomir Krstic, 'Silovanje kao psihotrauma u ratnim uslovima', in Kaličanin et al., *Stresovi Rata*, 161–168.

[111] See Alexandra Stiglmayer, *Mass Rape: The War Against Women in Bosnia-Herzegovina*, University of Nebraska Press, 1994.

[112] Jakulic, Krstic, 'Silovanje kao psihotrauma', 164.

[113] They might have been referring to the UNHCR resolution 'Rape and Abuse of Women in the Territory of the Former Yugoslavia', 23 February 1993, available at https://www.refworld.org/docid/3b00f03a34.html.

In other words, most of this article focused on the international debate about the emerging evidence of the Serb military officers' and soldiers' reprehensible behaviour towards Bosnian Muslim women. The authors did present their own clinical cases, but those cases, tragic and extremely upsetting as they were, formed a highly inadequate evidentiary basis for the article's core political arguments and conclusions, and in that sense, the article was deeply manipulative. It soon became clear that the psychological wellbeing and distress of the ten women were of secondary relevance, and were only addressed as a prelude to a more general defence and normalisation of the Serbian army's behaviour in the war ('every population contains approximately 5% of psychopathic personalities who are capable of committing crimes against others, and even enjoying in them'). When these women were quoted, their statements were mined for incriminating information about the enemy army: for instance, to find evidence to indicate the 'Muslim leadership's tendency to make it possible for psychopaths to rape as much as possible', or that the Bosnian army might have had a systematic plan to impregnate as many Serb women as they could.[114]

Psychoanalysis as a Tool in Political Warfare

In 1993, Serbia's leading psychiatrist and a prominent participant in debates about war trauma among the Serbian population Predrag Kaličanin gave a speech to his colleagues at the Institute of Mental Health, in which he protested the economic sanctions and political isolation imposed upon Serbia by the UN (because of the Serbian leadership's direct participation in the wars in Bosnia and Croatia). Interestingly, Kaličanin framed the sanctions as a foremost psychiatric problem, as they reportedly led to a 'grave impairment of the health of all citizens of this country', and to 'tragic mass consequences..., which inflicted enormous suffering on the already ill, and resulted in further illnesses and deaths of the innocent'. Moreover, Kaličanin used this opportunity to appeal to the international community to prevent the 'satanisation of the Serbian nation' in medical and psychiatric journals in particular.[115] Kaličanin had in mind a specific expert publication based in Croatia—the new *Croatian*

[114] Jakulic and Krstic, 'Silovanje kao psihotrauma', 163–164.

[115] Predrag Kaličanin, 'Nasilje nad zdravljem', in Kaličanin et al., *Stresovi Rata*, 5–12.

Medical Journal, whose first issue came out very soon after the start of the hostilities, in 1992, and which was only published in English, presumably primarily intended for international audiences. In its first year, particularly in its two 'war supplements' from 1992, the journal ran several articles by distinguished Croatian (and former Yugoslav) psychiatrists and psychotherapists, who used a variety of psychoanalytic concepts to understand the origins of the war, violence and aggression on the Yugoslav soil. Kaličanin objected vehemently to such interpretations, and their reliance on psychodynamic theories to demonstrate that, in Kaličanin's words, 'the Serbs were a criminal and genocidal people with cannibalistic impulses'.[116]

The Croatian Medical Journal caused a major international stir with its early psychiatric publications, although it never published anything similar to Kaličanin's above-mentioned quote. On the other hand, a group of psychiatrists and psychoanalysts, caught up in the horrific realities of war and aggression on the Croatian territory, did utilise a host of psychoanalytic principles and theoretical frameworks in rather dubious ways to diagnose sources of that aggression and pathologise the collective psyche of the Serbian people. This first came to the attention of their Serbian colleagues in 1992, when they contacted the journal's international advisory board and other international medical organisations to complain about the 'unscientific derivation of generalizations based on psychoanalysis', and 'the disqualification of entire nations…through psychiatric or rather psychoanalytic diagnoses'.[117] In the Serbian-language version of the letter, they criticised the 'reductionism and superficiality' of such psychoanalytic interpretations, and warned that 'psychoanalysis developed from studying individuals, so that its application for the purposes of understanding [collective] cultural phenomena could never be scientifically rigorous'.[118] The *Croatian Medical Journal* reluctantly published the Serbian psychiatrists and medical doctors' letter of complaint—apparently at the insistence of some of its own advisory board members—but

[116] Ibid.

[117] Marko Marusic, 'The Belgrade Letter', *Croatian Medical Journal*, 1992, 33:2–3.

[118] Predrag Kaličanin, Josif Vesel, and Dusica Lecic-Tosevski, 'Zloupotreba medicine I psihijatrije u satanizaciji srpskog naroda', in Kaličanin et al., *Stresovi Rata*, 219.

the editor apologised to the journal's readership for 'burdening' them with such an inappropriate and, he implied, inaccurate text.[119]

The peculiar case of the *Croatian Medical Journal*, and the bitter political conflict fought on its pages, signalled a tragic breakup of what used to be a formidable and internationally renowned psychiatric and psychotherapeutic profession. But it was striking and very surprising that, as these former friends and colleagues were busy realigning their medical and political loyalties with the perceived interests of their respective ethnic communities, they decided to conduct their political discussion in almost exclusively psychoanalytic terms. In the 1990s, by which time psychoanalysis had in other parts of the world largely been banished from medical practice to literature and history departments, the fractured Yugoslav psychiatric community still held on to it as the core interpretive framework to make sense of the extreme violence plaguing their former country.

'We may state freely that war is often started by sick political minds that have created a sick collective political consciousness and culture', wrote Zagreb-based psychiatrist Miro Jakovljevic in his article about 'psychiatric perspectives on the war against Croatia'.[120] This tendency to view the political conflict in 1990s Yugoslavia as an issue of collective psychiatric pathology set the tone for the two war supplements of the *Croatian Medical Journal*. According to Vladimir Gruden, from the Zagreb University's Department of Psychological Medicine, the sources of the war were in the Serb nation's 'enormous aggressive energy', and their predominant 'regressive psychic tendencies', understood in the Freudian sense as '[closeness] to [one's] own uncontrolled impulses' and 'diminished capacity for sublimation'. Gruden and most other contributors to the war supplement referred to Serbian folklore, national mythology, political choices as well as everyday life and customs in order to substantiate their diagnoses: 'In Serbs, regressive tendencies can be recognized in their inclination toward oral and other bodily pleasures... Their business partners are frequently surprised by this regressiveness when attempting to establish usual business communication with them'. On the other

[119] Marusic, 'The Belgrade Letter'.

[120] Miro Jakovljevic, 'Psychiatric Perspectives of the War Against Croatia', *Croatian Medical Journal*, 1992, War Supplement 2, 10–17.

hand, Croatians—as representatives of the superior Western civilisation—were characterised by an excellent ability to sublimate, and this provoked the Serbs' hatred, envy and guilt. Moreover, the Serb nation was diagnosed with a collective 'paranoid condition' and described as being 'at the level of schizoparanoid position in the development of personality' as a result of such a deeply embedded regressive orientation.[121] In this interpretation, the Serbs' disintegrated self was then projected onto the Croats, which could explain the Serbs' violent and destructive impulses towards Croatian territories and citizens. Eduard Klain argued in a similar vein that, in relation to the Croats, the 'Serbs often [had] the complex of inferiority, because they [were] aware of their lower level of civilization and culture'.[122] All these psychoanalytic theories and concepts were thus mobilised to demonstrate the Serbian nation's supposedly deeply ingrained propensity to violence, destruction and irrationality.

But the Croats (and other Yugoslav peoples) got their occasional collective diagnoses as well on the pages of the *Croatian Medical Journal*, although these diagnoses were generally framed in more positive or neutral terms. Unlike Gruden, Klain noted regressive psychological tendencies in the Croatian nation, too, but argued that they did not encourage violent or aggressive forms of behaviour because they were 'closer to the depressive position'. For that reason, Croats were psychologically inclined to feelings of guilt and religious feelings rather than to destructive reactions and 'paranoid projections'.[123] In Jakovljević's reading, Croats developed narcissistic psychological mechanisms in the aftermath of the first free elections in 1991, in which a non-communist political option won. But this narcissistic tendency did not indicate anything particularly damning about the fundamental characteristics of the Croatian collective—it led to 'benevolence and naivety' as the Croats strongly identified with 'the great democracies of the world' and underestimated the dangerous 'barbarism and primitiveness' of their Serbian enemies.[124]

[121] Vladimir Gruden, 'Psychologic Sources of the Serbian Aggression Against Croats', *Croatian Medical Journal*, 1992, War Supplement 2, 6–9.

[122] Eduard Klain, 'Yugoslavia as a Group', *Croatian Medical Journal*, 1992, War Supplement 1, 3–13.

[123] Ibid., 5.

[124] Jakovljević, 'Psychiatric Perspectives', 14–15.

In these discussions about the psychological roots of the Yugoslav wars, psychiatrists utilised yet again their discipline's evolutionary narrative of primitivism, 'barbaric' societies and modernisation. As this book has argued, the psychiatric profession in Yugoslavia framed their own tasks and broader societal mission in terms of a 'civilising mission' from the very beginning. Throughout the twentieth century, they aimed to take active part in discussions about the Yugoslav society's cultural, political and social modernisation, emphasising their own expertise in the mechanisms of human psyche and behaviour, and promoting their own role in modernising the population's 'mind'. In different historical and political contexts, the meaning and specific aims of such a psychiatric civilising mission could change quite radically, but this narrative of the profession as the prime national moderniser remained a constant. It is hardly surprising, then, that it got its final twist in the psychiatric-political discussions of the 1990s. In the *Croatian Medical Journal's* war supplements in particular, the civilising mission of psychoanalysis was explored to its fullest (and most problematic) potential.

While Gruden certainly had very few affirmative things to say about the collective Serbian psyche, in the spirit of self-criticism he did note that Croats did share a part of the blame for the way in which the Yugoslav conflict evolved over the preceding months. Relying on developmental psychology and psychoanalysis, he established that the Serbs, as a regressive collective actor—comparable to a child—could not help themselves without the guidance of 'persons or a group who had achieved a certain degree of sublimation', and who was on a higher level of civilisational development. It was up to the Croats to perform this corrective function and aid their Serbian neighbours (as well as Croatia's Serbian citizens), who were 'incapable of achieving maturity' and needed to be led out of their infantile phase into collective adulthood. Unfortunately, wrote Gruden, instead of taking this educational and civilisational process seriously, and acting with 'strictness and resoluteness' towards the Serbian child-nation, the Croats 'respected their regressive demands' in both Yugoslav states.[125] Gruden also faulted Serbian political leaders, many of whom were psychiatrists and were aware of their nation's need for maturation, but still failed to act in a responsible manner.[126]

[125] Gruden, 'Psychologic Sources of the Serbian Aggression Against Croats', 9.

[126] It is important to note here that Croatian psychiatrists and psychoanalysts were by no means alone in engaging in such acts of collective diagnosing and pathologisation.

This psychoanalytic rhetoric was clearly inspired by evolutionary colonial tropes. As we discussed in Chapter 5, Yugoslav socialist psychiatry and psychoanalysis made a significant contribution to global transcultural psychiatry. In his meticulous investigations, Vladimir Jakovljević, for instance, challenged some of the most important assumptions of Western colonial (and early post-colonial) psychiatry, and complicated West European psychiatrists' interpretations of the African (or 'primitive') psyche. Perhaps unsurprisingly, such nuanced approaches were substituted in the 1990s with a much cruder framework, within which practitioners did not reflect on the problematic nature and colonial origins of many psychiatric and psychoanalytic concepts used. As we saw above, in these early Croatian debates the 'Serbs' assumed the position of 'primitive' non-European societies, and constant reminders that Croats belonged to the Western civilisation further reinforced this argument. Moreover, the terms primitivism and barbarism were used and applied to the Serbian nation uncritically, without any indications of the significant colonial historical baggage which such concepts carried within and outside the psychiatric profession.

For instance, Klain insisted that the Serbian war against Croatia demonstrated 'destructive aggression of the archaic type, found in primitive people' such as African tribes and that the Serbs' 'behavioural patterns [corresponded] to the most aggressive fantasies of a child in a schizoparanoid position'.[127] In his analysis of the 'sociobiological' underpinnings of Serbian behaviour in the war, Croatian psychologist Árpad Barath described the Serb military actions as belonging to the 'category of aggressive and predatory behaviour of decorticated animals', primarily because it was marked by hatred and 'rage', which was 'more easily elicited with decorticated than with normal animals'. And while the Croatian people were characterised by reason, civilisation and notions of personal responsibility, the cruelty and barbarism of Serbian soldiers could

We have already seen that Serbian psychiatrists such as Jović could rely on psychoanalytic frameworks to analyse wartime and postwar group dynamics in the Serbian society, but there were other examples much more akin to the *Croatian Medical Journal*. In 1996, for instance, Milanko Čabarkapa diagnosed Croats with a 'complex of historical inferiority and running away from their south Slavic origins', Serbs with a complex of 'unrequited love and narcissism', while other, smaller Yugoslav nations were deemed to be suffering from a complex of 'unclear identity' which led to secessionism (Čabarkapa, *Psiholoski faktori stresa u borbenim aktivnostima*, 54).

[127] Klain, 'Yugoslavia as a Group', 12.

only be understood in the context of 'crowding', i.e. a collective, undifferentiated mindset in which nobody bore any individual responsibility and 'bestial' and violent collective actions were possible.[128]

* * *

In the 1990s, the Yugoslav psychiatric profession faced unprecedented challenges, which both undermined its revolutionary socialist legacy and temporarily boosted its local political significance. As the country saw extreme violence unfolding on much of its territory, the notion of war-related psychological trauma rapidly rose to significance in both political and psychiatric contexts, and the diagnosis of PTSD became the primary framework through which to discuss the memory of the war and its broader social consequences. In that sense, psychiatry was again at the very centre of some of the most sensitive political debates, and fractured psychiatric narratives closely reflected a range of social, political and cultural tensions, anxieties and controversies. Very importantly, Yugoslav socialist psychiatrists were probably the only group of postwar European psychiatrists who had a dubious privilege of dealing with war-related psychological stresses twice in their career. As we saw in this chapter, the silence that quickly settled around discussions of war trauma in aftermath of the Second World War was finally broken in the early 1990s, when psychiatrists in different parts of war-torn Yugoslavia began reflecting on the psychological consequences of the extreme violence and dislocation of the 1940s, and considered at some length the Yugoslav population's experiences from nearly fifty years ago. Some of the most important publications from the immediate post-WWII era were revisited in the 1990s, partly as an attempt to find professional precedents and guidance for dealing with large numbers of soldiers and civilians who lived through extreme experiences, and partly to draw (politically expedient) parallels between the 1940s and 1990s.

And while psychiatrists' work on trauma and PTSD strangely re-energised the mental health professions and brought attention to their political significance in the newly formed, ethnically delineated post-Yugoslav states, the breakup of the socialist country had a devastating

[128] Arpad Barath, 'Towards Understanding the War in Croatia During 1990–1991: Sociopsychologic Perspectives', *Croatian Medical Journal*, 1992, War Supplement 2, 18–25.

effect on the overall status of this group of experts. Yugoslav socialist psychiatry was a formidable, rich and highly innovative clinical and research field. As we saw earlier in this book, the profession and its practitioners were renowned in the European and global contexts, and they developed diverse and extensive networks of international contacts, which crossed the conventional Cold War political boundaries and enabled dynamic, experimental and in many ways revolutionary developments. With the outbreak of the war, psychiatrists almost everywhere in former Yugoslavia experienced a long period of professional isolation from their international networks, as well as of extreme uncertainty and economic deterioration. Whether it was due to international political sanctions (Serbia), violent disruptions and military activities (Bosnia and Croatia), or depleted material resources and devastated infrastructure, Yugoslav psychiatrists found themselves cut off from what they considered their natural professional environment, and struggled to make their voices heard beyond the borders of their new countries. Unable to travel and to access international psychiatric literature, they looked for other ways: several psychiatric journals in Serbia and Croatia decided in the early 1990s to publish all of their proceedings in English in an attempt to make their research more accessible to international audiences, and they strove to include foreign colleagues in their editorial boards. In some ways, they did succeed, and this was also the time when some international mental health practitioners grew increasingly interested in Yugoslavia, and internationally funded trauma advocacy programmes offered local clinicians some limited opportunities for transnational collaboration and international exposure. But overall, this was but a shadow of their erstwhile achievements, reputation and influence.

Even more importantly, what they wrote in their new English-language journals was not as innovative and internationally relevant. In many ways, psychiatric discussions of PTSD reinforced dominant nationalist political narratives and justifications, reflected collective ethical blind spots of their respective national groups, and often served to substantiate political constructions of national victimhood. Once members of a revolutionary, progressive and emancipatory profession, Yugoslav psychiatrists now used openly colonial and orientalist frameworks to write about each other's ethnicities, and engaged in dubious efforts to pathologise entire national collectives and deny 'their own' groups' responsibility for violence, aggression and war crimes.

However, one important legacy of the socialist period remained: even throughout the 1990s, psychoanalysis remained an exceptionally important analytical framework for analysing the origins of violence and ethnic hostilities, and for exploring the mechanisms of broader group dynamics and interactions in Yugoslavia. In one of the most memorable examples of this tendency, Eduard Klain explained the rise of anti-Communism after Tito's death as the 'devouring during the totemic meal of the father who left them without offering them some fixation or referential point of support'.[129] Serbian psychiatrist Radomir Samardzić ended his article on PTSD in Serbian prisoners of war and victims of torture with an extended discussion of Freud's and Einstein's well-known exchange on the origins of human propensity for aggression,[130] while a 1993 issue of the Croatian journal *Psihoterapija* opened with Freud's response to Einstein.[131] Even if their methods and some of their conclusions were questionable, this was a remarkable development, and perhaps the only original contribution of post-Yugoslav psychiatry. After the end of the war, psychoanalytic paradigms remained influential, and post-Yugoslav clinicians relied on them to discuss the lingering psychological consequences of the war (particularly notable in this context was the prominent Balint group gathered around Zagreb's Muradif Kulenović), or to make sense of the inability of post-Yugoslav societies to acknowledge their own moral responsibility for violence and crimes committed in the war.

[129] Eduard Klain, 'Yugoslavia as a Group', 13.

[130] Radomir Samardzic, 'Ratno zarobljenistvo I tortura', in Spiric, ed., *Ratna psihotrauma srpskih veterana*.

[131] Sigmund Freud, 'Zasto rat?', *Psihoterapija*, 1993, 23:1–2.

CHAPTER 8

Conclusion

As this book has demonstrated, a study of socialist psychiatry can offer unique and very important insights into the social, cultural and political history of Yugoslavia and its multiple Cold War engagements and internationalisations. This profession's increasingly dynamic involvement with the revolutionary ideas of personal emancipation and radical democracy in the context of socialism and workers' self-management made Yugoslav psychiatry into an explicitly political site, where ideological discussions were often indistinguishable from therapeutic or medical interventions. Moreover, such close engagements with Marxism and political ideology did not necessarily mean that Yugoslav psychiatrists became subordinated to the state's authoritarian government and executioners of its demands for political compliance—quite to the contrary, the profession's most prominent theoretical and clinical work aimed to challenge the concept of unquestionable authority in both family and society, and to encourage self-expression and active disobedience for the purposes of dismantling existing hierarchies and patriarchal institutions.

In that sense, Yugoslav psychotherapy and psychoanalysis from the 1950s tended to style themselves as handmaidens of revolution and progressive politics rather than of political repression. However, the Yugoslav socialist psychiatric practice also encapsulated one of the core contradictions of that society: despite the unprecedented social, cultural

A. Antić, *Non-Aligned Psychiatry in the Cold War*, Mental Health in Historical Perspective,
https://doi.org/10.1007/978-3-030-89449-8_8

and even political liberalisation following 1948, the regime continued with a variety of authoritarian practices and violent repression of political dissidents. Within psychiatry, such tendencies manifested themselves in an exceptionally clear manner. As we have seen earlier in the book, Yugoslav psychiatric institutions could be involved in both progressive, anti-hierarchical emancipatory praxis and repressive authoritarian activities, and the profession itself was marked by this surprising coexistence of such contradictory engagements. Moreover, this demonstrated how some of the most significant emancipatory concepts and frameworks in both socialism and psychotherapy could be implemented and used for repressive purposes. A comparative analysis of Yugoslav psychiatry's emancipatory and authoritarian activities thus offers an insight into one of the most fraught aspects of the Yugoslav socialist state and society.

Finally, while Yugoslavia was certainly not the only socialist state that took part in technical assistance and knowledge exchange missions with the global South, but it was the only one to send psychiatric experts to the decolonising world. They, as this book has also shown, worked to develop a specifically Marxist and socialist approach to transcultural psychiatric research and demonstrated how important and innovative East European contributions to the decolonisation debate could be. Even more importantly, their involvement in global transcultural psychiatry indicated that socialist psychiatry's project of personal emancipation and reinforcement of 'revolutionary personalities' was truly cross-cultural—the psychiatric efforts to revolutionise the 'backward' and traditional Yugoslav population were directly linked to the transcultural psychiatric project of transforming and revolutionising the decolonising world. Just like psychiatry has provided an exceptionally fitting lens to explore the contradictory coexistence of emancipatory and repressive impulses in the Yugoslav society, it also demonstrates the fraught nature of Yugoslavia's anti-colonial stance: while transcultural psychiatrists such as Jakovljević did offer an important critique of the lingering colonial frameworks in postwar global psychiatry, his embrace of some of the same problematic colonial models and concepts exposed the limits of Yugoslavia's non-aligned and anti-imperial exceptionalism. This book has, therefore, demonstrated how the politics and ideology of non-alignment bred contradictions, challenges and tensions in broader cultural and social spheres beyond foreign policy, and how such contradictions were addressed and attempted to be resolved in the psychiatric and political spheres.

Yugoslav 'psy' sciences experienced multiple internationalisations and globalisations in the post-WWII period. These transnational connections—with West, East and South—remained at the centre of this book. They determined Yugoslavia's political and psychiatric profile and shed new light on the international history of Cold War Europe. The 'psy' disciplines were among the most thoroughly and consistently internationalised (and Westernised) professions in Cold War Yugoslavia and Eastern Europe. Because of this, they provide a window onto the complications of Cold War internationalism, offering an opportunity to rethink postwar Europe's internal dynamics. This book has told an alternative, pan-European narrative of the post-1945 period, demonstrating that, in the Cold War, there existed sites of collaboration and vigorous exchange between the two ideologically opposed camps, and places like Yugoslavia provided a meeting point, where ideas, frameworks and professional and cultural networks from both sides of the Iron Curtain could overlap and transform each other. These exchanges were relevant beyond the psychiatric profession: they concerned strategies for ideological and political 're-education', construction of the 'new socialist person', and the mental health of children and youth, who were seen as the future of nations East, West and South. The histories of Yugoslav and West European 'psy' sciences were deeply entangled during the Cold War, and ideas about the human mind and pathology, as well as professional experiences and practices, were regularly exchanged across the Iron Curtain. Yugoslav psychiatrists engaged with Western schools of psychotherapy and psychoanalysis with a view to reforming what they perceived as backward and authoritarian Balkan societies, families and individuals, and creating new social relationships more conducive to a genuinely democratic Marxist society.

Psychiatry and Revolution

Both domestically and in the international context of non-alignment, the concept of revolution was central to the development and self-perception of the Yugoslav 'psy' sciences. One of the most important changes to come out of the Second World War and the socialist revolution of 1945 was the profession's move away from the reductive organicism of traditional psychiatry, and their increasing inclination to consider the role of sociological, cultural and political factors in patients' personal histories. For Marxist practitioners, this was of the utmost ideological and clinical importance: a psychiatric framework that reduced psychological conflicts to biological, chemical or neurological explanations removed any potential for social critique or engagement, and undermined Marxist psychiatrists' ability to relate their work to broader socio-political trends and objectives.[1] But in the immediate aftermath of the war, psychiatrists' relationship to the multiple disruptions caused by the revolution was ambivalent. In 1944 and 1945, a rapidly growing number of 'war neurotics' among the victorious partisan resisters caused major concern for both the Communist political leadership and the psychiatric profession. Mental health professionals linked the outbreak of war hysteria to the disruptive potential of the revolution itself, and clearly harboured doubts about the positive outcome of the reform and radical social change they were experiencing.

Following this turbulent period in which revolutionary changes were often seen to lead to volatile and dangerous situations, however, a new generation of psychiatrists started conceptualising 'revolution' in more positive ways, and even embraced it as one of their profession's most important goals. By the 1960s, psychiatrists and psychotherapists actively sought a major role for themselves in the realisation of the revolution on individual, family and societal planes. This was a profession many of whose members were increasingly committed to a radical social/political agenda, and whose most prominent representatives aimed explicitly to reconcile revolutionary Marxist worldview with psychotherapeutic and psychiatric practices. Many used overtly political language to frame their professional aims and experiences and turned their consulting rooms into revolutionary sites.

This was highly unusual: nowhere else in socialist Eastern Europe was psychoanalysis practised so openly and awarded such a prominent clinical and intellectual position.[2] In recent years, many scholars have challenged the proposition that East European psychiatry was fully subservient to the Soviet diktat, and developed within the rigid constraints of the materialist-organic and neurological Pavlovian framework.[3] Because of a unique

[1] Stjepan Betlheim, 'Kakav je stav lekara prema psihoanalizi', *Nas Vesnik*, 1956, 3, 204.

[2] Savelli, 'The Peculiar Prosperity of Psychoanalysis in Socialist Yugoslavia', 262–288.

[3] Christine Leuenberger, 'Socialist Psychotherapy and Its Dissidents', 261–273; B. Buda, 'Psychotherapy in Hungary During the Socialist Era and the Socialist Dictatorship', *European Journal of Mental Health*, 2009, 4:1, 67–99; Savelli, '"Peace and Happiness Await

constellation of political events, this transformation was particularly effective in Yugoslavia, where social psychiatry and psychoanalytic approaches thrived to an unprecedented extent when compared to other socialist societies.[4]

The Yugoslav political and intellectual elites promoted the concept of humanist, democratic Marxism in contradistinction to the authoritarian Stalinist model, and it required a new type of socialist citizen—one characterised by independence of mind, autonomy and self-initiative instead of blind political obedience. Such a dramatic ideological change opened up new possibilities for the psychiatric profession. A new generation of socialist psychiatrists stopped worrying about the revolution's disruptive potential, and became the most ardent promoters of radical political change and reform, increasingly preoccupied with notions of individual emancipation. Heavily influenced by the Frankfurt school, and by psychoanalytic thinkers such as Erich Fromm, Igor Caruso and Karen Horney, they developed original ideas about revolutionary psychiatry and psychoanalysis, which primarily aimed to undermine lingering authoritarian structures in social institutions (including the family), and to aid patients on their road to personal liberation and emancipated authentic existence as democratic Marxist citizens.

Historians of mental health sciences have already demonstrated that the Cold War did not prevent socialist psychiatrists' involvement in transnational collaboration with Western colleagues. Such historical analyses argue that East European psychiatry was perhaps 'socialist by default'—i.e. shaped by necessity by the socialist context—but not deeply grounded in socialist ideology and therefore not fundamentally different from its West European or North American counterparts.[5] However, as the Yugoslav case demonstrates, East European 'psy' disciplines could become radically reformed as a result of their interpenetration with Marxist intellectual frameworks, and informed by broader socialist or revolutionary principles. As Greg Eghigian argued in relation to psychiatry in the German Democratic Republic, Yugoslav psychiatrists imagined the socialist subject as a psychiatric and psychotherapeutic project—and this

Us:" Psychotherapy in Yugoslavia, 1945–1985', *History of the Human Sciences*, 2018, 31:4, 38–57.

[4] Savelli, 'The Peculiar Prosperity of Psychoanalysis in Socialist Yugoslavia', 262–288.

[5] Matthew Savelli, 'Beyond Ideological Platitudes'.

meant that the profession as a whole came to participate wholeheartedly in the development of this new type of personality.[6] This was not necessarily a sign of political authoritarianism and professional subordination: Marxist psychiatry in its Yugoslav version developed original emancipatory approaches, even on the global level, and engaged in innovative and experimental projects. This was then a specifically socialist psychiatry, although it was not necessarily abused by the Communist Party: rather, it was meant to participate in the broader political project precisely by raising a new generation of *non-conformist* citizens.

Socialist psychiatry and psychoanalysis in Yugoslavia played an exceptionally important political role and contributed to some of the core discussions of democratic socialism, workers' self-management and Marxism. In addition to participating in political repression and manipulation, socialist psychiatry also became a site for autonomous and often critical or subversive discussions about the meaning—and failures—of reform communism. Because of the country's search for an alternative Marxist system, the Yugoslav brand of East–West psychoanalysis and psychotherapy bred a truly unique intellectual framework, which borrowed from a variety of psychoanalytic and political schools of thought in order to think through a set of political and ideological dilemmas regarding the relationship between individuals and social structures. Psychoanalysis and other 'psy' disciplines played a major role in fashioning and re-thinking one of the most important socialist experiments—Yugoslavia's system of workers' self-management—in post-1945 Europe.

In socialist Yugoslavia, therefore, 'psy' disciplines became instrumental in shaping and reshaping minds and experimenting with new political ideas. Psychoanalytic and psychotherapeutic theories became increasingly important for understanding and developing the notions of socialist revolution, individual enlightenment and self-management that underpinned reform Communism. These disciplines informed not only political debates but also broader cultural, artistic and social spheres, and have remained central to understanding the history of a wide range of different phenomena in socialist Yugoslavia, such as, for instance, the country's most famous dissident group of philosophers and anthropologists, Praxis;

[6] Greg Eghigian, 'The Psychologization of the Socialist Self: East German Forensic Psychology and Its Deviants, 1945–1975', *German History*, 2004, 22:2.

broader social conceptualisations of children and childhood; or the new 'black wave' cinema of the 1960s and 1970s.

The history of Yugoslav psychiatry's complex and dynamic globalisations challenges the existing historiographical narratives of East–West exchanges which assume a largely unidirectional travel of ideas from the 'modern' West to the 'backward' or underdeveloped East. In fact, Yugoslavia was both a contested site of international collaboration and a laboratory in which some of the most progressive and experimental forms of psychotherapy were first tested and developed. In that sense, the field of Yugoslav psychiatry and psychotherapy was hardly lagging behind; to the contrary, it offered unique and innovative combinations of socialism and 'psy' approaches and often served as a model on a European or even global scale. Because of its specific political and ideological position, Yugoslav offered a unique opportunity to develop a new brand of activist, revolutionary psychoanalysis, whose goals and agendas could be supported by the (socialist) state. In the second half of the twentieth century, many activists and commentators in the West grew concerned about possible negative consequences of combining psychotherapy with radical politics, worrying that such an alliance might re-frame political oppression as an individual (and apolitical) psychological problem, which might undermine collective political action. But Yugoslav socialist psychoanalysts and psychotherapists demonstrated in an exemplary manner that the dividing line between therapy and political revolution was porous and increasingly irrelevant, and used explicitly political language to talk about individual mental health. Yugoslavia's 'psy' professionals also saw direct links between family and political structures, turning the very therapeutic encounter into a vehicle of revolutionary politics.

In Yugoslavia, the legacy of these extraordinary developments remains mixed. Following the breakdown of socialism, the psychoanalytic profession became both freer—it did not have to field occasional ideological attacks and prove the compatibility between Freud and Marxism—and more restricted in its reach—state funding decreased dramatically, and the era of free psychoanalysis came to an end. The state's political interest in psychoanalytic projects disappeared completely, together with any investment in the theory and practice of workers' self-management. The marginalisation of psychoanalysis on a global scale played an important role in these post-socialist developments. At the same time, however, the strong networks and theoretical advances achieved under socialism enabled post-socialist psychoanalysts from the Yugoslav territories to regain access to the international circles after an initial period of isolation: both the Croatian and Serbian psychoanalytic societies gained official membership of the International Psychoanalytic Association after 1991, and became among the most active and influential participants from Eastern Europe. Talented practitioners such as Tamara Popovic-Stajner, Aleksandar Vuco, Eduard Klain quickly rose to prominence in the international psychoanalytic institutions, and worked effectively on strengthening their respective national associations, and on promoting psychoanalysis in Eastern Europe.[7] Their critique of traditional and authoritarian families, and of the pernicious effects of patriarchal relations on children's and women's mental health remained current and germane to the former socialist societies in transition, especially as those societies renounced some of the most progressive social and cultural policies of the previous era and opted for social conservatism, extreme nationalism and political authoritarianism in order to build ethnically clean nation-states. As one author termed it, post-Yugoslav psychoanalysis became a 'resistance movement'—a marginal and often subversive discipline, critiquing a number of prominent social and political trends.[8]

On the other hand, as we saw in the epilogue, psychoanalysts did not always oppose or resist the politics of nationalist warmongering in the course of the wars of the Yugoslav succession, and psychoanalytic concepts were often used to inform some rather problematic political interpretations of the breakup of Yugoslavia and the extreme violence that followed. In that sense, with the death of Yugoslav socialism, post-Yugoslav psychoanalysis lost its unique link to a broader political project, but it still remained an important professional and theoretical presence, as well as a surprisingly influential political interpretive framework. Psychoanalytic professionals played a vital role in treating survivors of the 1990s wars and engaged with the dire psychological consequences of the violent breakup of the country and its painful transition to neoliberal economy.[9]

[7] Boris Kordic, 'Istorija psihoanalize u Srbiji u XX veku', *Engrami*, 2001, 33:1.

[8] Branimir Stojanovic, 'Psihoanaliza kao pokret otpora', *Danas*, 16 October 2012.

[9] Ksenija Kondić, *Kako sačuvati mentalno zdravlje porodice u izbeglištvu*, Belgrade, 2000; Tamara Stajner-Popovic, 'Childhood in a Time Tunnel', in Judit Szekacs-Weisz and Ivan Ward, eds, *Lost Childhood and the Language of Exile*, London: The Freud Museum, 2004; Ksenija Kondic, *Priručnik za primenu intervjua s decom lišenom roditeljske pratnje*, Belgrade: Cigoja, 1996; Vojislav Ćurčić and Vesna Brzev-Ćurčić, *Kako sačuvati mentalno zdravlje mladih u izbeglištvu*, Belgrade, 2000.

Moreover, it is possible, as some authors have recently argued, that the legacy of workers' self-management affected to some degree the radical political movements and grassroots initiatives in the 1990s and 2000s. Since 1991, the former Yugoslav territories saw a number of anti-regime and anti-war protests, student movements, workers' demonstrations and other experiments in direct democracy, which invited citizens to radically rethink their relationship to the post-socialist political authorities. In that sense, even though the post-Yugoslav political and economic elites quite universally dismissed the project of self-management, its principles, promoted in no small part by the psychoanalytic community, possibly continued to shape some important left-wing groups' and citizens' political experiences, and to influence the face of the new left in the Balkans.[10]

Eastern Europe and Global Psychiatry

It is, moreover, important to reconsider the role of Eastern Europe in the global history of 'psy' disciplines. If we look more closely at the Yugoslav case, it becomes clear that socialist psychiatry was neither a helpless political handmaiden nor a mere imitation of Western psychiatric techniques. It was only in Eastern Europe that a truly radical and revolutionary psychiatry received full state support instead of existing on the social and political margins, and it was practised in a range of mainstream state-funded clinical establishments. In that sense, this East European socialist experiment, in which a new activist psychotherapy became the norm, remains central to understanding the 'psy' disciplines as a tool for socio-political critique and activism in the second half of the twentieth century. In the postwar world, psychotherapy and psychoanalysis became important sites for discussing left-wing politics, political ideology and revolutionary change, and these professions' concepts and practices came to inform radical political movements, theories and actions. It is important to remember that socialist Eastern Europe was not cut off from these developments, nor irrelevant in the broader history of psychoanalytically informed political critique and experimentation. Quote to the contrary, it was probably at the centre of these processes: the sustained state investment in such a revolutionary brand of psychotherapy produced

[10] Srecko Horvat and Igor Stiks, eds, *Welcome to the Desert of Post-socialism: Radical Politics After Yugoslavia*, London and New York: Verso, 2015.

an exceptional situation in which radical political agenda dominated the entire discipline of psychoanalysis and psychiatry in a socialist country.

East European psychiatrists remained important in the global context in yet another respect—as active and original contributors to the emergence and development of postwar transcultural psychiatry and its institutions. Even though it has so far been completely written out from the global history of transcultural psychiatry and its decolonisation, East European socialist psychiatry contributed important and innovative insights to this global field of knowledge production and intervened in some of its core debates.[11] The historiography of twentieth-century global psychiatry has largely been focused on Western Europe and the broader Western world, as well as its relationship to the (former) colonial territories and their psychiatric expertise.[12] Indeed, the history of transcultural psychiatry has remained tightly intertwined with and shaped by the processes of decolonisation and the attendant major global transformations.[13]

While a lot has already been done to decentre this narrative and give voice to actors—experts, patients, family members, policymakers—from outside the Western centres of knowledge production, historians have rarely considered the East European region (and the socialist world in general) to be a significant part of this broader history, perhaps because Eastern Europe did not directly participate in colonialism and decolonisation.[14] However, as we have seen in Chapter 5, East Europeans had a lot to say about colonial oppression and were deeply interested in co-defining the major tasks of decolonisation, and Yugoslav psychiatrists

[11] Marks and Saveli, 'Communist Europe and Transnational Psychiatry'; Waltraud Ernst and Thomas Mueller, eds, *Transnational Psychiatries: social and Cultural Histories of Psychiatry in Comparative Perspective c. 1800–2000*, Newcastle upon Tyne: Cambridge Scholars, 2010.

[12] Volker Roelcke, Paul Weindling, and Louise Westwood, eds, *International Relations in Psychiatry: Britain, Germany and the United States to World War II*, University of Rochester Press, 2010; Warwick Anderson et al., eds, *Unconscious Dominions.*

[13] Waltraud Ernst, *Colonialism and Transnational Psychiatry: The Development of an Indian Mental Hospital in British India, c. 1925–1940*, London: Anthem Press, 2013; Hans Pols, *Nurturing Indonesia: Medicine and Decolonisation in the Dutch East Indies*, Cambridge: Cambridge University Press, 2018.

[14] See Pringle, *Psychiatry and Decolonisation in Uganda*; Katie Kilroy-Marac, *An Impossible Inheritance: Postcolonial Psychiatry and the Work of Memory in a West African Clinic*, University of California Press, 2019; Heaton, *Black Skin, White Coats.*

joined this conversation with particular eagerness. Precisely because they were increasingly integrated in West European networks of psychiatric knowledge exchange, Yugoslav psychiatrists quickly came into contact with the growing field of transcultural psychiatry, and were exposed to some of its most intense debates, such as controversies around the incomplete decolonisation of psychiatric theory and practice, and the establishment of global psychiatric institutions. Coming from a Marxist background, they also indirectly participated in the socialist bloc's broader scheme of technical and educational exchange with the global South, and offering a socialist alternative to the failed Western colonial project.

Through their engagement with the decolonising, non-European world, psychiatrists such as Jakovljević pioneered a transnational approach based on the idea of socialist solidarity between Eastern Europe and the decolonising world.[15] This idea of solidarity was, of course, unique to socialist psychiatrists, and it was particularly notable because it produced an alternative form of non-Western psychiatric universalism, which worked to undermine some aspects of the lingering colonial frameworks, and hierarchical and evolutionary thinking in Western transcultural psychiatry. In that sense, socialist psychiatrists' contributions significantly reshaped the landscape of postwar global psychiatry—their interpretations of the non-European 'psyche' were fundamentally shaped by their own society's geopolitical marginality, and their concerns about Yugoslavia's own progress and modernisation produced a much more optimistic understanding of the developmental potentials and modernising capabilities of the decolonising global South. Moreover, they used their global engagements to explore revolutionary societies in different parts of the world and to produce an innovative cross-cultural model of 'revolutionary personality', based on a new interpretation of the relationship between socio-cultural environment and mental illness.

Finally, socialist psychiatrists were perhaps the only group in postwar global psychiatry who viewed cross-cultural encounters as productive and non-pathological, offering an alternative reading of one of the most important and taxing phenomena in the second half of the twentieth century. In the later decades of the Cold War, it was not by accident that another Yugoslav psychiatrist, Hadzi Nikolic, became one of the most radical voices from the 'new transcultural psychiatry' field, which further

[15] Vucetic and Betts, eds, *Tito in Africa: Picturing Solidarity.*

challenged West European 'psy' practitioners' unreconstructed Eurocentric tendencies.[16] East European transcultural psychiatry can thus open up an unexpected and unique window into the socialist world's involvement with the global South and contributions to the global debates about decolonisation, modernisation and development.

Importantly, the experiences in the South decisively shaped the development of internal Yugoslav psychiatric debates, and the 'psy' profession established direct links between Yugoslavia's experiences of socialist revolution and the decolonising world's path to post-colonial modernity. They drew direct and indirect parallels between the Balkan and African populations, their cultural orientation and 'primitivism' and placed these two different but comparable peripheral regions in the same political (and psychiatric) context, drawing on their Yugoslav research to shed light on Global South concerns and vice versa. In that sense, Yugoslavia's activist revolutionary brand of psychoanalysis was a unique result of a truly global dynamic, in which psychiatrists and psychotherapists aimed to draw broader, global conclusions about the human psyche and psychological effects and aspects of revolutionary change, political emancipation, violence and modernity. This sheds crucial light on socialist conceptualisations of the human mind, and on the process of revolutionising a society through constructing a new socialist person.

Tracing the Yugoslavs' imaginations of and involvement with Africa as well as with the Western world, the book has zoomed in on possible parallels between postcoloniality and the Balkans' own global structural position, asking whether post-colonial theory can help us understand the history of the Balkans and the motivations of Balkan historical actors.[17] By looking at how Yugoslav socialist 'psy' professionals reframed the relationship between individual psyche, society, race and culture, the book has shed light on these actors' self-perceptions in a European and global context. In terms of their perceptions of their own political and cultural identity, Eastern Europe and Yugoslavia remained centrally attached to Europe and often implicated in orientalising, racist, Eurocentric and essentially colonial discourses of the white West.[18] However, this was

[16] Littlewood, 'From Categories to Context'.

[17] See Baker, *Race and the Yugoslav Region*.

[18] Diana Mishkova, 'Symbolic Geographies and Visions of Identity: A Balkan Perspective', *European Journal of Social Theory*, 2008, 11:2.

qualified by the experience and ideology of socialism, as well as, in the Yugoslav case, by the practices and discourses of non-alignment, which at times appeared to take Yugoslavia outside of Europe altogether. Moreover, even though the Balkan region might have seen itself as politically, geographically and civilisationally European (even under socialism), its historical legacy was one of imperial subjects rather than imperial rulers, and the attachment to a 'European identity' was accompanied by narratives of cultural inferiority and experiences of rejection by Europe. In that sense, non-aligned Yugoslavia's geopolitical and civilisational status was permanently unstable, and a close analysis of psychiatric discourses of socialist, Western and African psyche has demonstrated how this instability shaped the medical, cultural and political history of the region.

Despite socialist 'psy' disciplines' significant efforts to undermine colonial discourses in global transcultural psychiatric networks, 'primitivism' remained an important concept in both socialist and Western psychiatry, and it fundamentally informed Yugoslav psychiatrists' involvement in the postwar global networks of knowledge production and expertise. As mentioned above, this sheds light on some rather glaring contradictions in Yugoslavia's politics and rhetoric of anti-colonialism and solidarity with the global South. No less than their Western colleagues, Jakovljević and his socialist contemporaries still divided the world into 'civilised' and 'primitive' parts, and adopted a linear model of historical development, and of social, cultural and political progress. The socialist psychiatric profession's obsession with 'primitive' patients at home extended to its global engagements, and this struggle against social and cultural 'backwardness' became one of its most important theoretical, political and clinical tasks.

As we saw in this book, this anxiety over 'primitivism' and primitive patients marked the entire twentieth-century history of Yugoslav psychiatry and spanned the watershed year of 1945. While the socialist revolution radically transformed the Yugoslav (and East European) 'psy' professions, it did not seem to affect this particular concern in any significant respect. By foregrounding their concern with eliminating backwardness in their patients, the Yugoslav 'psy' disciplines placed themselves at the centre of a series of different political projects of modernisation. Both before and after 1945, thus, psychiatrists sought to construct their expertise in the mechanisms of the human mind, and their clinical practice as fundamental to the success of the 'civilising process'. The nature and final goals of these efforts at 'civilising' Yugoslavia's largely agricultural and socially traditional population changed rather dramatically over the course of the twentieth century—while the interwar governments (and psychiatrists) aimed to 'catch up' with Western Europe, the socialist period was focused on facilitating revolutionary leaps and radical emancipation—but the psychiatric profession's concern with primitivism, backwardness and the psychological repercussions of rapid modernisation remained an important continuity. In that sense, Yugoslav 'psy' disciplines shared some important characteristics and conceptual frameworks with Western colonial psychiatry, even when they only dealt with domestic populations, who were often viewed as culturally and socially quite distant from psychiatric practitioners. For those reasons, socialist psychiatrists' approach to the global South was perhaps predetermined by their tendency to reinforce Western colonial civilisational scales in both domestic and global contexts.

Perhaps unsurprisingly, the final unsavoury twist to this narrative of psychiatrists as civilisers came in the midst of the 1990s wars of Yugoslav succession, when post-Yugoslav psychiatric discourses resorted to much cruder notions of barbarism and primitivism in order to apportion blame for the country's demise, extreme violence and war crimes. While socialist psychiatrists attempted to reconsider and critique colonial frameworks, post-Yugoslav psychiatric practitioners of the 1990s often regurgitated some of the least nuanced colonial conceptualisations of 'primitive minds' when talking about their erstwhile compatriots and current war enemies.[19]

In conclusion, Communist psychiatry in Yugoslavia was a dynamic, complex and often autonomous field: an active participant in global discussions on post-colonial transcultural psychiatry, a regular partner to West European and American psychoanalytic schools of thought, as well as a collaborator in Soviet and other East European psychiatric projects. Moreover, while political ideology played an important part in the intellectual development of the Yugoslav 'psy' sciences, the relationship between communism/socialism and psychiatry should not be caricaturised. On the one hand, some Yugoslav psychiatrists and psychiatric institutions were instrumental to implementing the government's

[19] On psychoanalysis in the Balkans in the 1990s, and its attendant discourses of self-orientalization, see also Dusan Bjelic, *Normalizing the Balkans: Geopolitics of Psychoanalysis and Psychiatry*, Routledge, 2016.

policies of repression, discreditation and silencing of political dissidents and critics. On the other hand, the 'psy' disciplines in Yugoslavia provided a site for a genuine and critical engagement with the possibilities and limitations of Yugoslavia's brand of socialism and workers' self-management. In many ways, the political interpretations and implications of psychiatric discussions in the 1950s and 1960s matched the critical discourses of prominent dissident Marxist philosophers and scholars such as the Praxis group. The ideology of Marxism decisively shaped the Yugoslav psychiatric and psychoanalytic profession, but this did not lead exclusively to political abuse and manipulation. The originality and innovativeness of the profession in Yugoslavia precisely stemmed from its willingness to address seriously in its clinical work some of the core ideological postulates of Marxism, and explore them in ways which did not always depict the Yugoslav state in particularly positive terms. At the same time, concepts and discourses taken from socialist psychiatry and psychoanalysis informed broader social and cultural fields in Yugoslavia, so that the 'psy' disciplines, far from old-fashioned and static coercive sciences, became involved in a dynamic conversation with a variety of actors and spheres of life.

Archives and Libraries

Archive of Yugoslavia, Belgrade.

State Archive of Serbia, Belgrade.

Archive of the Neuro-Psychiatric Hospital 'Laza Lazarevic', Belgrade.

Archive of the Movement for the Protection of Human Rights, Belgrade.

National Library of Serbia, Belgrade.

University Library 'Svetozar Markovic, Belgrade.

State Archive of Croatia, Zagreb.

National and University Library, Zagreb.

State Archive of Bosnia-Herzegovina, Sarajevo.

British Library, London.

Bodleian Library, University of Oxford.

A. Antić, *Non-Aligned Psychiatry in the Cold War*,
Mental Health in Historical Perspective,
https://doi.org/10.1007/978-3-030-89449-8

Bibliography

Adler, Nanci, et al., 'Psychiatry Under Tyranny: A Report on the Political Abuse of Romanian Psychiatry During the Ceausescu Years', *Current Psychology: A Journal for Diverse Perspectives on Diverse Psychological Issues*, 1993, 12:1, 3–17.

Agger, Inger, Sanja Vuk, and Jadranka Mimica, *Theory and Practice of Psychosocial Projects Under War Conditions in Bosnia-Herzegovina and Croatia*, Brussels: ECHO and the European Community Task Force, Psychosocial Unit, 1995.

Allden, K., T. Franciskovic, J. Lavelle, M. Mathias, K. McInnes, R.F. Mollica, and L. Moro, *Harvard Trauma Manual: Croatian Veterans Version*, Cambridge: Harvard Program in Refugee Trauma, 1998.

Amnesty International, *Yugoslavia: Prisoners of Conscience*, London, 1985.

Angelini, Alberto, 'History of the Unconscious in Soviet Russia: From Its Origins to the Fall of the Soviet Union', *International Journal of Psychoanalysis*, 2008, 89:2, 369–388.

Antic, Ana, 'The Pedagogy of Workers' Self-Management: Terror, Therapy and Reform Communism in Yugoslavia After the Tito-Stalin Split', *Journal of Social History*, 2016, 50:1, 179–203.

———, *Therapeutic Fascism: Experiencing the Violence of the Nazi New Order*, Oxford: Oxford University Press, 2017.

———, 'Heroes and Hysterics: "Partisan Hysteria" and Communist State-Building in Yugoslavia After 1945', *Social History of Medicine*, 2014, 27:2, 349–371.

A. Antić, *Non-Aligned Psychiatry in the Cold War*,
Mental Health in Historical Perspective,
https://doi.org/10.1007/978-3-030-89449-8

Applebaum, Anne, *Gulag: A History of the Soviet Camps*, New York: Doubleday, 2003.

Avramović, Mihailo, *Nase seljacko gazdinstvo*, Belgrade: Stampa Sveti Sava, 1928.

Bacic, Franjo and Nikola Srzentic, *Komentar krivicnog zakona*, Belgrade: Savremena administracija, 1978.

Bacu, D., *The Anti-Humans: Student Re-education in Romanian Prisons*. Englewood, CO: Soldiers of the Cross, 1971.

Bains, Jatinder, 'Race, Culture and Psychiatry: A History of Transcultural Psychiatry', *Transcultural Psychiatry*, 2005, 16:2, 139–154.

Baker, Catherine, *Race and the Yugoslav Region: Post-Socialist, Post-Conflict, Postcolonial?*, Manchester: Manchester University Press, 2018.

———, *The Yugoslav Wars of the 1990s*, Basingstoke: Palgrave Macmillan, 2015.

Bakovic, Teodor, 'Psiholoski aspekti golootocke torture i sadistickog mucenja', in *Goli Otok (1949–1956): Radovi sa okruglog stola, Podgorica 27. juna 1995*, Podgorica: CANU, 1998.

Banac, Ivo, *With Stalin against Tito: Cominformist Splits in Yugoslav Communism*, Ithaca, NY: Cornell University Press, 1988.

Barnes, Steven, *Death and Redemption: The Gulag and the Shaping of Soviet Society*, Princeton: Princeton University Press, 2011.

Bechmann Pedersen, Sune and Christian Noack, eds, *Tourism and Travel During the Cold War: Negotiating Tourist Experiences Across the Iron Curtain*, London and New York: Routledge, 2020.

Beller, M, and J. Leerssen, eds, *Imagology: The Cultural Production and Literary Representation of National Characters*, Amsterdam: Rodopi, 2007.

Betlheim, Ruth and Gordana Lerotic, *Stjepan Betlhaim: Radovi, pisma, dokumenti, 1898–1970*, Zagreb: Antibarbarus, 2006.

Bidermann, A., *March to Calumny: The Story of American POWs in the Korean War*, New York: Macmillan, 1963.

Birn, Anne-Emanuelle and Raul Necochea Lopez, eds, *Peripheral Nerve: Health and Medicine in Cold War Latin America*, Duke University Press, 2020.

Bjelic, Dusan, *Normalizing the Balkans: Geopolitics of Psychoanalysis and Psychiatry*, Routledge, 2016.

Bloch, S. and P. Reddaway, *Russia's Politica Hospitals: The Abuse of Psychiatry in the Soviet Union*, London: Gollancz, 1977.

Bojanin, Svetomir, *Škola kao bolest*, Belgrade: Plato, 1990.

Bougarel, Xavier, 'The Shadow of Heroes: Former Combatants in Post-War Bosnia-Herzegovina', *International Social Science Journal*, 2006, 58:189, 479–490.

Brickman, Celia, *Aboriginal Populations in the Mind: Race and Primitivity in Psychoanalysis*, New York: Columbia University Press, 2003.

Brintlinger, Angela, 'The Hero in the Madhouse: The Post-Soviet Novel Confronts the Soviet Past', *Slavic Review*, 2004, 63:1, 43–65.

British Medical Association, *Medicine Betrayed: The Participation of Doctors in Human Rights Abuses*, London, 1992, 64–82.

Brown, Julie V., 'Heroes and Non-heroes: Recurring Themes in the Historiography of Russian-Soviet Psychiatry,' in Mark S. Micale and Roy Porter, eds, *Discovering the History of Psychiatry*, Oxford: Oxford University Press, 1994, 297–310.

Buda, B., 'Psychotherapy in Hungary During the Socialist Era and the Socialist Dictatorship', *European Journal of Mental Health*, 2009, 4:1, 67–99.

Buda, B., T. Tomcsanyi, J. Harmatta, R. Csaky-Pallavicini and G. Paneth, 'Psychotherapy in Hungary During the Socialist Era and the Socialist Dictatorship', *European Journal of Mental Health*, 2009, 4:1, 67–99.

Bulatovic, Marko, 'Struggling with Yugoslavism: Dilemmas of Interwar Serb Political Thought,' in John Lampe and Mark Mazower, eds, *Ideologies and National Identities: The Case of Twentieth-Century Southeastern Europe*, Budapest: CEU Press, 2004, 254–276.

Bullard, Alice, 'Imperial Networks and Postcolonial Independence: The Transition from Colonial to Transcultural Psychiatry', in Malone and Vaughan, *Psychiatry and Empire*, Basingstoke: Palgrave Macmillan, 2007.

Cabarkapa, Milanko, *Psiholoski faktori stresa u borbenim aktivnostima*, PhD dissertation, University of Belgrade, 1996.

Calic, 2010. Calic, Marie-Janine, *Geschichte Jugoslawiens im 20. Jahrhunert*, Munich: C.H. Beck Verlag, 2010.

———, *Sozialgeschichte Serbiens 1815–1941: Der Aufhaltsame Fortschritt wahrend der Industrialisierung*, Munich: R. Oldenbourg Verlag, 1994.

Carothers, John Collin, 'A Study of Mental Derangement in Africans, and an Attempt to Explain Its Peculiarities, More Especially in Relation to the African Attitude to Life', *East African Medical Journal*, 1948, 25:4, 142–166.

Chabal, Patrick and Jean-Pascal Daloz, *Africa Works: Disorder as Political Instrument*, Oxford and Bloomington: James Currey and Indiana University Press, 1999.

Chafer, Tony, *The End of Empire in French West Africa: France's Successful Decolonization?* London: Bloomsbury, 2002.

Chisholm, Brock, 'The Psychiatry of Enduring Peace and Social Progress (The William Alanson White Memorial Lecture)', *Psychiatry*, 1946, 9, 3–20.

Ćurčić, Vojislav and Vesna Brzev-Ćurčić, *Kako sačuvati mentalno zdravlje mladih u izbeglištvu*, Belgrade, 2000.

Cvetkovic, Srdjan, 'Ko je ovde lud? - primeri političke (zlo)upotreba psihijatrije u SFRJ', *Istorija 20. veka*, 2013, 2, 145–163.

Davico, Oskar, *Crno na belo*, Belgrade: Prosveta, 1962, 20.

David-Fox, Michael, *Showcasing the Great Experiment: Cultural Diplomacy and Western Visitors to the Soviet Union, 1921–1941*, New York: Oxford University Press, 2012.

Decarvalho, R. J. and Ivo Cermak 'History of Humanistic Psychology in Czechoslovakia', *Journal of Humanistic Psychology*, 1997, 37:1, 110–130.

Dedijer, Vladimir, *Izgubljena bitka J. V. Staljina*. Belgrade: Prosveta, 1969.

Delille, Emmanuel, 'On the History of Cultural Psychiatry: Georges Devereux, Henri Ellenberger, and the Psychological Treatment of Native Americans in the 1950s', *Transcultural Psychiatry*, 2016, 53:3.

Diawara, Manthia, *In Search of Africa*, Cambridge: Harvard University Press, 1998.

Djokic, Dejan, *Elusive Compromise: A History of Interwar Yugoslavia*, New York: Columbia University Press, 2007.

Djukanovic, Borisslav, *Alkoholizam i porodica*, Belgrade: Privredna stampa, 1979.

Dokic, Goran, 'States of Victimhood and Irreparable Losses: Serbian Veterans of the Post-Yugoslav Wars', *Glasnik Etnografskog Instituta SANU*, 2017, 1, 97–110.

———, *Psychosocial Transition in a Postsocialist Context: PTSD in Croatian Psychiatry*, MA dissertation, University of Victoria, 2005.

Dowbiggin, Ian, *The Quest for Mental Health: A Tale of Science, Medicine, Scandal, Sorrow, and Mass Society*, Cambridge: Cambridge University Press, 2011.

Duancic, Vedran, *Geography and Nationalist Visions of Inter-War Yugoslavia*, Basingstoke: Palgrave Macmillan, 2020.

Duraković, Lada and Andrea Matošević, eds, *Socijalizam na klupi: Jugoslovensko društvo u očima nove postjugoslovenske humanistike*, Pula and Zagreb: Srednja Europa, 2013.

Eghigian, Greg, 'The Psychologization of the Socialist Self: East German Forensic Psychology and Its Deviants, 1945–1975', *German History*, 2004, 22:2.

———, 'Was There a Communist Psychiatry? Politics and East German Psychiatric Care, 1945–1989,' *Harvard Review of Psychiatry*, 2002, 10:6, 364–368.

———, 'Care and Control in a Communist State: The Place of Politics in East German Psychiatry,' in Marijke Gijswijt-Hofstra, et al., eds, *Psychiatric Cultures Compared: Psychiatry and Mental Health Care in the Twentieth Century*, Amsterdam: Amsterdam University Press, 2005, 183–199.

Erlich, Vera, *Family in Transition: A Study of 300 Yugoslav Villages*, Princeton: Princeton University Press, 1966.

Ernst, Waltraud, *Colonialism and Transnational Psychiatry: The Development of an Indian Mental Hospital in British India, c. 1925–1940*, London: Anthem Press, 2013.

Ernst, Waltraud and Thomas Mueller, eds, *Transnational Psychiatries: Social and Cultural Histories of Psychiatry in Comparative Perspective c. 1800–2000*, Newcastle upon Tyne: Cambridge Scholars, 2010.

Etkind, Alexander, *Eros of the Impossible: The History of Psychoanalysis in Russia*, Routledge, 1997.

Fassin, Didier, 'Ethnopsychiatry and the Postcolonial Encounter: A French Psychopolitics of Otherness', in Warwick Anderson, Deborah Jenson, and Richard Keller, eds, *Unconscious Dominions: Psychoanalysis, Colonial Trauma, and Global Sovereignties*, Duke University Press, 2011.

Fichter, Madigan, 'Yugoslav Protest: Student Rebellion in Belgrade, Zagreb, and Sarajevo in 1968', *Slavic Review*, 2016, 75:1, 99–121.

Frosh, Stephen, *For and Against Psychoanalysis*, Abingdon: Routledge, 2006.

Galmarini-Kabala, Maria Cristina, 'Psychiatry, Violence, and the Soviet Project of Transformation: A Micro-History of the Perm Psycho-Neurological School-Sanatorium', *Slavic Review*, 2018, 77, 307–332.

Gibianskii, Leonid, 'The Soviet-Yugoslav Split and the Cominform', in N. Naimark and L. Gibianskii, eds, *The Establishment of Communist Regimes in Eastern Europe, 1944–1949*, Boulder, CO: Westview Press, 1997.

Goulding, Daniel, ed., *Five Filmmakers*, Bloomington: Indiana University Press, 1994.

Goulding, Daniel, *Liberated Cinema: The Yugoslav Experience, 1945–1991*, Bloomington: Indiana University Press, 2002.

Gow, James, *The Serbian Project and Its Adversaries: A Strategy of War Crimes*, London: Hurst, 2003.

Grant, Bruce, 'Siberia Hot and Cold: Reconstructing the Image of Siberian Indigenous Peoples', in Galya Diment and Yuri Slezkine, eds, *Between Heaven and Hell: The Myth of Siberia in Russian Culture*, New York: St. Martin's Press, 1992.

Gruenwald, Oskar, *The Yugoslav Search for Man: Marxist Humanism in Contemporary Yugoslavia*, South Hadley: Bergin and Garvey Publishers, 1983.

Hadzi-Nikolic, Caslav, *Kad se vidi ono sto se ne vidi: Samani i halucinogeni*, Belgrade: Itaka, 2004 (reprinted).

Halfin, Igal, *Terror in My Soul: Communist Autobiographies on Trial*, Cambridge: Harvard University Press, 2003.

Harsch, Donna, *Revenge of the Domestic: Women, the Family, and Communism in the German Democratic Republic*, Princeton: Princeton University Press, 2007.

Heaton, Matthew, *Black Skin, White Coats: Nigerian Psychiatrists, Decolonization, and the Globalization of Psychiatry*, Athens: Ohio University Press, 2013.

Herman, Ellen, *The Romance of American Psychology: Political Culture in the Age of Experts*, Los Angeles: University of California Press, 1995.

Herzog, Dagmar, *Cold War Freud: Psychoanalysis in an Age of Catastrophes*, Cambridge: Cambridge University Press, 2016.

Horvat, Srecko and Igor Stiks, eds, *Welcome to the Desert of Post-Socialism: Radical Politics After Yugoslavia*, London and New York: Verso, 2015.

Hoskovcová S., J. Hoskovec, A. Plháková, M. Sebek, J. Svancara, and D. Voboril, 'Historiography of Czech Psychology', *History of Psychology*, 2010, 13:3, 309–334.

Hronesova, Jessie, 'Might Makes Right: War-Related Payments in Bosnia and Herzegovina', *Journal of Intervention and Statebuilding*, 2016, 10:3, 339.

Hudolin, Vladimir, *Klubovi lijecenih alkoholicara*, Zagreb: Jumena, 1982.

Ierunca, V., *Fenomenul Pitesti*, Bucharest: Humanitas, 1990.

Jakovina, Tvrtko, *Americki komunisticki saveznik: Hrvati, Titova Jugoslavija i SAD 1945–195*, Zagreb: Srednja Europa, 2003.

———, *Treća strana hladnog rata [The Third Side of the Cold War]*, Zagreb: Fraktura, 2011.

Jakovljevic, Branislav, *Alienation Effects: Performance and Self-Management in Yugoslavia, 1945–1991*, Ann Arbor: University of Michigan Press, 2016.

Jakovljevic, Vladimir, *Neuravnotezena porodica*, Belgrade: Centar za obavestavanje roditelja, 1961.

———, *Neuravnotezena porodica*, Belgrade: Centar za obavestavanje roditelja, 1961.

———, *Prilozi za Socijalnu Patologiju*, Belgrade: Sloboda, 1984.

Joravsky, David, *The Lysenko Affair*, Chicago and London: University of Chicago Press, 1986.

Kalicanin, Predrag, et al., eds, *Stresovi Rata*, Belgrade: Institute za mentalno zdravlje, 1994.

Karge, Heike, *Der Charme der Schizophrenie. Psychiatrie, Krieg und Gesellschaft im serbokroatischen Raum*, Berlin: De Gruyter, 2020.

Keller, Richard, *Colonial Madness: Psychiatry in French North Africa*, Chicago: University of Chicago Press, 2007.

Khanna, Ranjana, *Dark Continents: Psychoanalysis and Colonialism*, Durham: Duke University Press, 2003.

Kiev, Ari, ed., *Psychiatry in the Communist World*, New York: Science House, 1968.

———, *Transcultural Psychiatry*, New York: Free Press, 1972.

Kilroy-Marac, Katie, 'Nostalgic for Modernity: Reflecting on the Early Years of the Fann Psychiatric Clinic in Dakar, Senegal', *African Identities*, 2013, 11:4, 367–380.

———, *An Impossible Inheritance: Postcolonial Psychiatry and the Work of Memory in a West African Clinic*, University of California Press, 2019.

Kirmayer, 2013. Kirmayer, Laurence J., '50 Years of *Transcultural Psychiatry*', *Transcultural Psychiatry*, 2013, 50:1, 3–5.

Klain, Eduard, ed., *Ratna psihologija I psihijatrija*, Zagreb: Glavni Sanitetski Stozer, 1992.

———, *Kako sam prozivio domovinski rat*, Zagreb: Croatian Medical Journal, 1996.

Klajn, Hugo, *Ratna neuroza Jugoslovena*, Belgrade: Tersit, 1995 (Reprinted—Originally published in 1955).

Klajn, Petar, *Razvoj psihoanalize u Srbiji*, MA thesis, Unviersity of Belgrade, 1980.

———, *Razvoj psihoanalize u Srbiji*. Subotica: Pedagoska akademija, 1989.

Klajn, Vladislav, 'Problem Rehabilitacije -- Rehabilitacija Neuroticara', *VSP*, 1958, 7:8, 529–531.

———, *Ljubav, seks, porodica*, Belgrade and Novi Sad, 1981.

Kleinman Arthur, 'Depression, Somatization and the "New Cross-Cultural Psychiatry"', *Social Science and Medicine*, 1977, 11.

———, 'Depression, Somatization and the New Cross-Cultural Psychiatry', *Social Science and Medicine*, 1977, 11:1, 3–10.

Klepal, Jaroslav, 'The Only Thing I "Earned" in the Damned War Was PTSD.' Reconsidering Veteran Sociality and Politics in Bosnia and Herzegovina', *Southeast European and Black Sea Studies*, 2018, 18:4, 489–507.

Kocovic, Bogoljub, *Zrtve Drugog svetskog rata u Jugoslaviji*, London: Nase Delo, 1985.

Kondić, Ksenija, *Kako sačuvati mentalno zdravlje porodice u izbeglištvu*, Belgrade, 2000.

———, *Priručnik za primenu intervjua s decom lišenom roditeljske pratnje*, Belgrade: Cigoja, 1996.

Kordic, Boris, 'Istorija psihoanalize u Srbiji u XX veku', *Engrami*, 2001, 33:1.

Kosier, B., *Bezboznici* 2, Sarajevo: Svjetlost, 1991.

Kostic, Aleksandar, *Seksualno u nasoj narodnoj poeziji*, Belgrade and Zagreb: Medicinska naucna knjiga, 1978.

Kostic, Petar, *Psiholoska anatomija Golog Otoka*, Belgrade: Nezavisna izdanja Slobodana Masica, 2012.

Kovacevic, Dusan, *Sta je to u ljudskom bicu sto ga vodi prema picu*, Belgrade: Laguna, 2018.

Kovacevic, Filip, 'Marcuse in Yugoslavia', *Radical Philosophy Review*, 2013, 16:1, 205–222.

Krsmanovic, Tomislav, *Kaznena psihijatrija, 1975–2004*, Belgrade: Vedes, 2004.

———, *Roman o Briselu*, Sabac: Glas crkve, 2013.

Kruks, Sonia, Rayna Rapp, and Marilyn B. Young, eds, *Promissory Notes: Women in the Transition to Socialism*, New York: Monthly Review Press, 1989.

Kulic, Vladimir, 'Building the Non-aligned Babel: Babylon Hotel in Baghdad and Mobile Design in the Global Cold War', *Architecture Beyond Europe*, 2014, 6.

Kullaa, Rina, *Non-alignment and Its Origins in Cold War Europe: Yugoslavia, Finland and the Soviet Challenge*, London: I.B. Tauris, 2012.

Kurtovic, Larisa, 'Who Sows Hunger, Reaps Rage': On Protest, Indignation and Redistributive Justice in Post-Dayton Bosnia-Herzegovina', *Southeast European and Black Sea Studies*, 2015, 15:4, 639–659.

Lampe, John and Mark Mazower, eds, *Ideologies and National Identities: The Case of Twentieth-Century Southeast Europe*, Budapest: CEU Press, 2004.

Lavretsky, Helen, 'The Russian Concept of Schizophrenia: A Review of the Literature', *Schizophrenia Bulletin*, 1998, 24:4.

Lazic, Milorad, 'Neki problemi stranih studenata na jugoslovenskim univerzitetima šezdesetih godina XX veka, s posebnim osvrtom na afričke studente [Some Problems of Foreign Students at Yugoslav Universities in the 1960s, with Special Focus on African Students]', *Godišnjak za društvenu istoriju* 2009, 2, 61–78.

Leuenberger, Christine 'The End of Socialism and the Reinvention of the Self: A Study of the East German Psychotherapeutic Community in Transition', *Theory and Society*, 2002, 31:2.

———, 'Socialist Psychotherapy and Its Dissidents', *Journal of the History of the Behavioural Sciences*, 2001, 37:3.

Levi, Pavle, *Disintegration in Frames: Aesthetics and Ideology in the Yugoslav and Post-Yugoslav Cinema*, Stanford: Stanford University Press, 2007.

Linstrum, Erik, *Ruling Minds: Psychology in the British Empire*, Cambridge: Harvard University Press, 2016.

Liskova, Katerina, *Sexual Liberation, Socialist Style*, Cambridge: Cambridge University Press, 2018.

Littlewood, Roland and Maurice Lipsedge, *Aliens and Alienists: Ethnic Minorities and Psychiatry*, Abingdon: Routledge, 1997.

Littlewood, Roland, 'From Categories to Contexts: A Decade of the "New Cross-Cultural Psychiatry"', *British Journal of Psychiatry*, 1990, 156, 308–327.

MacBean, James Roy, 'Sex and Politics: Wilchelm Reich, World Revolution, and Makavejev's WR', *Film Quarterly*, 1972, 25:3, 2–13.

Mandler, Peter, *The English National Character: The History of an Idea from Edmund Burke to Tony Blair*, New Haven: Yale University Press, 2006.

Marcuse, Herbert, *Eros i civilizacija*, Zagreb: Naprijed, 1965.

———, *Negations: Essays in Critical Theory*, Boston: Beacon Press, 1968.

Mark, James and Peter Apor, 'Socialism Goes Global: Decolonization and the Making of a New Culture of Internationalism in Socialist Hungary 1956–1989', *Journal of Modern History*, 2015, 87, 852–891.

Mark, James, Artemy Kalinovsky, and Steffanie Marung, eds, *Alternative Globalizations. Eastern Europe and the Postcolonial World*, Bloomington: Indiana University Press, 2020.

Markovic, Mihailo, 'Marxist Philosophy in Yugoslavia: The *Praxis* Group', in R.T. De George and J.P. Scanlan, eds, *Marxism and Religion in Eastern Europe*, Fribourg and Munich: Sovietica, 1976, vol. 36, 63–89.
Markovic, Vladimir, *Za ljudska prava: Moje disidentske uspomene*, Belgrade: Slobodna Knjiga, 1999.
Marks, Sarah and Matthew Savelli, eds, *Psychiatry in Communist Europe*, London: Palgrave Macmillan, 2015.
Massino, Jill, 'Something Old, Something New: Marital Roles and Relations in State Socialist Romania,' *Journal of Women's History*, 2010, 22:1.
Matic, Vojin, *Kada pocinje vaspitanje deteta*, Belgrade, 1955.
Matthys Moore, Bradley, 'For the People's Health: Ideology, Medical Authority and Hygienic Science in Communist Czechoslovakia,' *Social History of Medicine*, 2014, 27:1, 122–143.
Matusevich, Maxim, 'Revisiting the Soviet Moment in Sub-Saharan Africa', *History Compass*, 2009, 10, 1–10.
———, *No Easy Row for a Russian Hoe: Ideology and Pragmatism in Nigerian-Soviet Relations*, 1960–1991, Trenton, NJ: Africa World Press, 2003.
———, 'Probing the Limits of Internationalism: African Students Confront Soviet Ritual', *Anthropology of East Europe Review*, 2009, 27:2 19–39.
McCulloch, Jock, *Colonial Psychiatry and the 'African Mind'*, Cambridge: Cambridge University Press, 1995.
McGovern, Mike, *Unmasking the State: Making Guinea Modern*, Chicago: University of Chicago Press, 2012.
Medvedev, R. and Z. Medvedev, *A Question of Madness*, London: Macmillan Ltd, 1971.
Mihailovic, Dragoslav, *Goli Otok*. Belgrade: NIP Politika, 1990.
———, *Goli Otok 5*, Belgrade: Sluzbeni Glasnik, 2012.
Milacic, Bozo, *Suncana putovanja i bijele noci*, Zagreb: Stvarnost, 1963.
Miller, Martin A., *Freud and the Bolsheviks: Psychoanalysis in Imperial Russia and the Soviet Union*, New Haven: Yale University Press, 1998.
Milosavljevic, Olivera, *Savremenici Fasizma 2: Jugoslavija u Okruzenju, 1933–1941*, Belgrade: Helsinski Odbor za Ljudska Prava u Srbiji, 2010.
Mishkova, Diana, Symbolic Geographies and Visions of Identity: A Balkan Perspective, *European Journal of Social Theory*, 2008, 11:2.
Mišković, Nataša, Harald Fischer-Tiné, and Nada Boškovska Leimgruber, eds, *The Non-Aligned Movement and the Cold War: Delhi, Bandung, Belgrade*, Routledge, 2014.
Mortimer, Lorraine, *Terror and Joy: The Films of Dusan Makavejev*, Minneapolis: University of Minnesota Press, 2009.
Murphy, H.B.M., 'A Crosscultural Survey of Schizophrenic Symptomatology', *International Journal of Social Psychiatry*, 1963, 9:4, 237–249.

Murphy, H.B.M., et al., 'Crosscultural Inquiry into the Symptomatology of Depression: A Preliminary Report', *Transcultural Psychiatry*, 1964, 1, 5–18.

Nandy, Ashis, *Savage Freud and Other Essays*, Princeton: Princeton University Press, 1995.

Nettelfield, Lara and Sarah Wagner, *Srebrenica in the Aftermath of Genocide*, Cambridge: Cambridge University Press, 2014.

Nikolic, Nikola, *Jasenovacki logor smrti*, Zagreb: Nakladni Zavod Hrvatske, 1948.

Panic, Rade, *Titovi Havaji*, Belgrade: Nezavisna izdanja Slobodana Masica, 1997.

Papadogiannis, Nikolaos, 'Political Travel Across the 'Iron Curtain' and Communist Youth Identities in West Germany and Greece in the 1970s and 1980s', *European Review of History*, 2016, 26:3, 526–553.

Paul, David W., *Politics, Art and the Commitment in the East European Cinema*, New York: St. Martin's Press, 1983.

Penn, Shana and Jill Massino, eds, *Gender Politics and Everyday Life in State Socialist Eastern and Central Europe*, Basingstoke: Palgrave Macmillan, 2009.

Perucica, Kosta, *Kako su nas prevaspitavali*. Belgrade: Dereta, 1990.

Petrovic, Gajo, 'Cemu Praxis?', *Praxis: Filozofski casopis,* September 1964, I:1.

Pick, Daniel, *The Pursuit of the Nazi Mind: Hitler, Hess and the Analysts*, Oxford: OUP, 2012.

Pollock, Ethan, *Stalin and the Soviet Science Wars*, Princeton, NJ and Oxford: Princeton University Press, 2006.

Pols, Hans, *Nurturing Indonesia: Medicine and Decolonisation in the Dutch East Indies*, Cambridge: Cambridge University Press, 2018.

Popovic, Miroslav, *Udri bandu*, Belgrade: Filip Visnjic, 1989.

Pringle, Yolana, *Psychiatry and Decolonisation in Uganda*, Basingstoke: Palgrave Macmillan, 2019.

Proctor, Hannah, *Psychologies in Revolution: Alexander Luria's 'Romantic Science' and Soviet Social History*, Basingstoke: Palgrave Macmillan, 2021.

Pupavac, Mladen and Vanessa Pupavac, 'Trauma Advocacy, Veteran Politics and the Croatian Therapeutic State', *Alternatives: Global, Local, Political*, 2012, 37:3, 199–213.

Radonjic, B., *Poruseni ideali,* Belgrade: Interpress, 1995.

Radonjic, Radovan, *Sukob KPJ s Kominternom i drustveni razvoj Jugoslavije, 1948–1950*, Zagreb: Narodno sveučilište grada Zagreba, Centar za aktualni politički studij, 1979.

Rajak, Svetozar, 'No Bargaining Chips, No Spheres of Interest: The Yugoslav Origins of Cold War Non-Alignment', *Journal of Cold War Studies,* 2014, 16:1.

Reich, Rebecca, 'Over the Cuckoo's Nest: Russian Variations on a Psychiatric Theme', in Marks and Savelli, eds, *Psychiatry in Communist Europe*, 196–215.

Reich, Rebecca, *State of Madness: Psychiatry, Literature, and Dissent After Stalin*, De Kalb, IL: Northern Illinois University Press, 2018.

Richmond, Yale, *Cultural Exchange and the Cold War: Raising the Iron Curtain*, Philadelphia: Pennsylvania State University Press, 2003.

Rieff, David, 'In Defense of Afro-Pessimism', *World Policy Journal*, 1998–1999, 15:4, 10–22.

Riviere, Claude, *Guinea: The Mobilization of a People*, New York: Ithaca, 1977; .

Robin, R.T., *The Making of the Cold War Enemy: Culture and Politics in the Military-Intellectual Complex*, Princeton, NJ: Princeton University Press, 2009.

Roelcke, Volker, Paul Weindling, and Louise Westwood, eds, *International Relations in Psychiatry: Britain, Germany and the United States to World War II*, University of Rochester Press, 2010.

Roll-Hansen, Nils, *The Lysenko Effect: The Politics of Science*, Amherst, NY: Humanity Books, 2005.

Romani, R., *National Character and Public Spirit in Britain and France, 1750–1914*, Cambridge: Cambridge University Press, 2002.

Sadowsky, Jonathan, *Imperial Bedlam: Institutions of Madness in Colonial South West Nigeria*, University of California Press, 1999.

Savelli, Matthew, '"Peace and Happiness Await Us:" Psychotherapy in Yugoslavia, 1945–1985,' *History of the Human Sciences*, 2018, 31:4, 38–57.

———, 'Diseased, Depraved or Just Drunk? The Psychiatric Panic Over Alcoholism in Communist Yugoslavia', *Social History of Medicine*, 2012, 25:2, 462–480.

———, 'The Peculiar Prosperity of Psychoanalysis in Socialist Yugoslavia', *Slavonic and East European Review*, 2013, 91:2, 262–288.

———, 'Beyond Ideological Platitudes: Socialism and Psychiatry in Eastern Europe', *Palgrave Communications*, 2018, 4:45. https://doi.org/https://doi.org/10.1057/s41599-018-0100-1.

Schmidt, Elizabeth, *Cold War and Decolonization in Guinea, 1946–1958*, Athens: Ohio University Press, 2007.

———, 'Cold War in Guinea: The RDA and the Struggle Over Communism, 1950–1958', *Journal of African History*, 2007, 48:1, 95–121.

———, 'Anticolonial Nationalism in French West Africa: What Made Guinea Unique?', *African Studies Review*, 2009, 52:2, 1–34.

———, *Mobilizing the Masses: Gender, Ethnicity and Class in the Nationalist Movement in Guinea, 1939–1958*, New Hampshire: Heinemann, 2005.

Schumann, Dirk, ed., *Raising Citizens in the 'Century of the Child:' Child-Rearing in the United States and German Central Europe in the Twentieth Century*, Studies in German History 12, New York: Berghahn Books, 2010.

Scott, Hilda, *Does Socialism Liberate Women? Experiences from Eastern Europe*, London: Beacon Press, 1974.

Segel, H.B., *The Walls Behind the Curtain: East European Prison Literature, 1945–1990,* Pittsburgh: University of Pittsburgh Press, 2012.

Sher, Gerson, *Praxis: Marxist Criticism and Dissent in Socialist Yugoslavia*, Bloomington: Indiana University Press, 1977, 129.

Simic, D. and B. Trifunovic, *Zenski logor na Golom Otoku: Ispovesti kaznenica i islednice*, Belgrade: ABC Produkt, 1990.

Sladojevic, Ana, 'Beyond the Photographic Frame: Interpretation of Photographs from the Museum of Yugoslavia's Collection in a Contemporary Context', in Radina Vučetić and Paul Betts, eds, *Tito in Africa: Picturing Solidarity*, Belgrade: Museum of Yugoslavia, 2017.

Sloan Mahone and Megan Vaughan, *Psychiatry and Empire*, Basingstoke: Palgrave Macmillan, 2007.

Slobodian, Quinn, ed., *Comrades of Color: East Germany in the Cold War World*, New York: Berghahn Books, 2015.

Spaskovska, Ljubica, 'Constructing the "City of International Solidarity": Non-aligned Internationalism, the United Nations and Visions of Development, Modernism and Solidarity, 1955–1975', *Journal of World History*, 2020, 31:3, 137–163.

Spiric, Zeljko, ed., *Ratna psihotrauma srpskih veterana*, Belgrade: Udruženje boraca rata Republike Srbije od 1990. godine, 2008.

Stajner-Popovic, Tamara, 'Childhood in a Time Tunnel', in Judit Szekacs-Weisz and Ivan Ward, eds, *Lost Childhood and the Language of Exile*, London: The Freud Museum, 2004.

Stanek, Lukasz, 'Architects from Socialist Countries in Ghana (1957–1967): Modern Architecture and Mondialisation', *Society of Architectural Historians' Journal*, 2015, 74:4, 416–442.

———, 'Architects from Socialist Countries in Ghana (1957–1967): Modern Architecture and Mondialisation', *Society of Architectural Historians' Journal*, 2015, 74:4, 416–442.

———, 'Mobilities of Architecture in the Late Cold War: From Socialist Poland to Kuwait, and Back', *International Journal of Islamic Architecture*, 2015, 4:2, 365–398.

Stanescu, M., *The Re-education Trials in Communist Romania, 1952–1960*, Boulder, CO: East European Monographs, 2010.

Stiglmayer, Alexandra, *Mass Rape: The War Against Women in Bosnia-Herzegovina*, University of Nebraska Press, 1994.

Stojanovic, Milinko, *Goli Otok: Anatomija zlocina*, Belgrade: Strucna knjiga, 1991.

Straker, Jay, *Youth, Nationalism and the Guinean Revolution*, Bloomington and Indianapolis: Indiana University Press, 2009.

Stubbs, Paul, 'Transforming Local and Global Discourses: Reassessing the PTSD Movement in Bosnia and Croatia', in David Ingleby, ed., *Forced Migration and Mental Health: Rethinking the Care of Refugees and Displaced Persons*, New York: Springer, 2006.

Subotic, Jelena and Srdjan Vucetic, 'Performing Solidarity: Whiteness and Status-Seeking in the Non-aligned World', *Journal of International Relations and Development*, 2019, 22, 722–743.

Sucic, Nikola, *Psihologija i Psihopatologija covjecanstva: Psihologija i Psihopatologija Nagona i Ljubavi*, Zagreb, 1939.

Supek, Rudi, 'Some Contradictions and Insufficiencies of Yugoslav Self-Managing Socialism', in Markovic and Petrovic, eds, *Praxis*, 249–272.

Tadic, Ljubomir, 'Bureaucracy—Reified Organization', in Mihailo Markovic and Gajo Petrovic, eds, *Praxis: Yugoslav Essays in the Philosophy and Methodology of the Social Sciences*, Dordrecht: D. Reidel, 1979.

Tadic, Ljubomir, *Poredak i sloboda*, Belgrade: Kult, 1976.

Tadic, Nevenka, *Psihijatrija detinjstva i mladosti*, Belgrade, 1989.

———, *Psihoterpija dece i omladine*, Belgrade: Naucna knjiga, 1984.

———, *Psihoanaliticka psihoterapija dece i omladine*, Belgrade, 1984.

Tirnanic, Bogdan, *Crni talas*, Belgrade: Filmski Centar Srbije, 2011.

Tolokontseva, D., 'Use of Correctional and Labour Measures on the Inmates of the Solovetsky Camp in the 1920s and 1930s', *Arctic Review on Law and Politics*, 2012, 2, 186–199.

Tomasevich, Jozo, *War and Revolution in Yugoslavia, 1941–1945: Occupation and Collaboration*, Stanford: Stanford University Press, 2001.

Trencsenyi, Balazs, *The Politics of 'National Character': A Study in Interwar East European Thought*, New York: Routledge Studies in Comparative Political Thought, 2012.

Tromly, Benjamin, 'Brother or Other? East European Students in Soviet Higher Education Establishments, 1948–1956', *European History Quarterly*, 2014, 44:1, 80–102.

Van Rahden, Till, 'Families Beyond Patriarchy: Visions of Gender Equality and Child Rearing among German Catholics in an Age of Revolution', in Nancy Christie, Michael Gauvreau, and Stephen Heathron, eds, *The Sixties and Beyond: Dechristianization as History in North America and Western Europe*, Toronto: University of Toronto Press, 2013, 270–293.

Van Voren, R., 'Comparing Soviet and Chinese Political Psychiatry', *Journal of the American Academy of Psychiatry and the Law*, 2002, 30:1.

Vaughan, Megan, *Curing Their Ills: Colonial Power and African Illness*, Stanford: Stanford University Press, 1991.

Verdery, Katherine, *What Was Socialism, and What Comes Next?* Princeton: Princeton University Press, 1996.

Vitorovic, Nikola, *Crne Suze Konga*, Belgrade: Biblioteka Marko Polo, 1961.

Vodovnik, Ziga, 'Democracy as a Verb: New Meditations on the Yugoslav Praxis Philosophy', *Journal of Balkan and Near Eastern Studies*, 2012, 14:4, 433–452.

Vucetic, Radina, 'We Shall Win: Yugoslav Film Cooperation with FRELIMO', *Revista de Ciencias Sociais*, 2019, 118, 130–151.

———, *Coca-Cola Socialism: Americanization of the Yugoslav Culture in the Sixties*, Budapest: CEU Press, 2018.

———, *Koka-kola socijalizam*, Belgrade: Sluzbeni Glasnik, 2016.

———, *Monopol na istinu: Partija, kultura i cenzura u Srbiji sezdesetih i sedamdesetih godina XX veka*, Belgrade: Clio, 2016.

Wachtel, Andrew, *Making a Nation, Breaking a Nation: Literature and Cultural Politics in Yugoslavia*, Stanford: Stanford University Press, 1998.

Watson, Peter, *War on the Mind: The Military Uses and Abuses of Psychology*, New York: Basic Books, 1978.

Windholz, George, 'Soviet Psychiatrists under Stalinist Duress: The Design for a 'New Soviet Psychiatry' and Its Demise,' *History of Psychiatry*, 1999, 10:39, 329–347.

Wing, John, *Reasoning About Madness*, New York: Transaction Publishers, 1978.

Wolfl, Dusko, ed., *Vladimir Hudolin and His Work*, Rijeka: Regional Centre for Alcoholism, 2007.

Yeomans, Rory, "Of 'Yugoslav Barbarians' and Croatian Gentlemen Scholars: Nationalist Ideology and Racial Anthropology in Interwar Yugoslavia," in Marius Turda and Paul Weindling, eds, *'Blood and Homeland:' Eugenics and Racial Nationalism in Central and Southeast Europe*, Budapest: CEU Press, 2007, 83–122.

Zajicek, Ben, 'Soviet Psychiatry and the Origins of the Sluggish Schizophrenia Concept, 1912–1936', *History of the Human Sciences*, 2018, 31:2, 88–105.

———, 'A Soviet System of Professions: Psychiatry, Professional Jurisdiction, and the Soviet Academy of Medical Sciences, 1932–1951', in Susan Grant, ed., *Russian and Soviet Health Care from an International Perspective: Comparing Professions, Practice and Gender, 1880–1960*, Basingstoke: Palgrave Macmillan, 2017, 97–117.

———, *Scientific psychiatry in Stalin's Soviet Union: The Politics of Modern Medicine and the Struggle to Define 'Pavlovian' Psychiatry, 1939–1953*, PhD dissertation, University of Chicago, 2009.

Index

A. Antić, *Non-Aligned Psychiatry in the Cold War*, Mental Health in Historical Perspective,
https://doi.org/10.1007/978-3-030-89449-8

The manufacturer's authorised representative in the EU is Springer Nature Customer Service Centre GmbH, Europaplatz 3, 69115 Heidelberg, Germany. If you have any concerns regarding our products, please contact ProductSafety@springernature.com

Printed and bound by CPI Group (UK) Ltd, Croydon, CR0 4YY
30/09/2026
02225499-0015